The
Smoothies
Bible

The
Smoothies
Bible

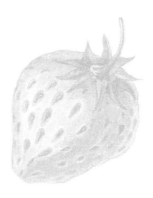

Pat Crocker

Robert
ROSE

The Smoothies Bible
Text copyright © 2003 Pat Crocker
Photographs copyright © 2003 Robert Rose Inc.

For complete cataloguing information, see page 309.

Disclaimer
The Smoothies Bible is intended to provide information about the preparation and use of smoothies containing whole foods and medicinal herbs. It is not intended as a substitute for professional medical care. The publisher and authors do not represent or warrant that the use of recipes or other information contained in this book will necessarily aid in the prevention or treatment of any disease, and specifically disclaim any liability, loss or risk, personal or otherwise, incurred as a consequence, directly or indirectly, of the use and application of any of the contents of this book. Readers must assume sole responsibility for any diet, lifestyle and/or treatment program that they choose to follow. If you have questions regarding the impact of diet on health, you should speak to a health-care professional.

Design & Production: PageWave Graphics Inc.
Editor: Judith Finlayson
Copy Editor: Christina Anson Mine
Recipe Editor: Jennifer MacKenzie
Illustrations: Kveta
Photography: Mark T. Shapiro
Food Stylist: Kate Bush
Prop Stylist: Charlene Ericson
Color Scans: Colour Technologies

The publisher and author wish to express their appreciation to the following supplier of props used in the food photography:

Homefront
371 Eglinton Ave. W.
Toronto, Ontario M5N 1A3
Tel: (416) 488-3189
www.homefrontshop.com

We acknowledge the financial support of the Government of Canada through the Book Publishing Industry Development Program (BPIDP) for our publishing activities.

Published by Robert Rose Inc.
120 Eglinton Ave. E., Suite 800, Toronto, Ontario, Canada M4P 1E2
Tel: (416) 322-6552 Fax: (416) 322-6936

Printed and bound in Canada by Canadian Printco Limited

7 8 9 10 CPL 11 10 09 08 07 06

Contents

I've been blessed with good friends.
This book is dedicated to the women
with whom I have raised a glass or two.
Claudia Wisdom-Good, Ruth MacDonald,
Joanna Esch, Pam Story, Susan Belsinger,
Myrna Ingleton, Gail Johnston, Helen Grant,
Joan McVean, Pie Aitkinson,
this one's for you.

Acknowledgments

DEVELOPING AND TESTING RECIPES IS CREATIVE, CHALLENGING AND, MOST often, fun. Still, it's always a daunting task. My work on this book took me further than I would have thought possible within the category of smoothies. When I began, my concept of smoothies revolved around the typical fruit juice combo that originated on the beaches of California. Developing the recipes for *The Smoothies Bible* forced me to expand that definition. I came to understand that there are a myriad of great combinations of vegetables, herbs and a wide variety of liquids that can also claim the moniker smoothie.

The challenges of writing this book were made easier with the support of the small-appliance industry. I thank the following blender manufacturers for providing the machines that tested the recipes in this book.

- Braun *(www.braun.com)*
- Cuisinart *(www.cuisinart.com)*
- Hamilton Beach/Proctor-Silex *(www.hamiltonbeach.com)*
- KitchenAid *(www.kitchenaid.com)*
- Krups *(www.krups.com)*
- Vitamix *(www.vitamix.com)*
- Waring *(www.waringproducts.com)*

In our family, depending on the season, we drink at least one smoothie a day. Our daughter, Shannon, helped design and name many of the recipes in this book. Thank you, Shannon and Gary, for your love and support in all my endeavors.

Once again, a personal thank-you goes to Susan Eagles, a member of the National Institute of Medical Herbalists, who provided the section on Health Conditions. Susan's work encompasses a positive framework for health and she teaches by example in living and eating to be well.

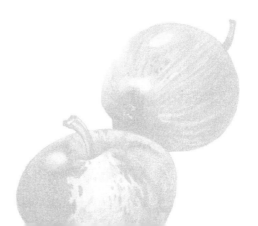

Introduction

WE KNOW WE NEED THEM. WE KNOW THEY PREVENT A HOST OF MODERN degenerative diseases, including cancer and heart disease. Although the United States Cancer Institute recommends that you eat five servings of fresh vegetables and three servings of fresh fruit each day, and Canada's Food Guide to Healthy Eating suggests five to 10 daily servings of fresh fruit and vegetables, research shows that significant numbers of people are not meeting these dietary objectives. One of the easiest ways to eat your fruits and vegetables is to drink them. And every year, more and more people are doing just that: according to the California-based Juice and Smoothie Association, by July 2002 the juice and smoothie business topped $1 billion in sales. Fast and easy to make, smoothies are also becoming the beverage of choice at home, where you can choose the ingredients you use, ensuring their freshness and quality.

Children are probably the biggest fans — and beneficiaries — of smoothies, which deliver the phytonutrients, vitamins and minerals that are so essential for growing bodies. By nine or 10 years of age, children are capable of learning the basics of operating a blender safely and cleaning it when they are finished. Teaching them how to make their own satisfying and nutritious drinks will build a healthy habit that will last a lifetime.

People at every point in the life cycle, from singles to empty nesters to the elderly, are discovering the simplicity and nutritional benefits of smoothies. Because they are so quick and easy to make and require minimal cleanup, smoothies are ideal to make in the small quantities that suit one or two people. They are also a delicious medium in which to take herbal or pharmaceutical medicine and nutritional supplements. Whisking in other healthful ingredients, such as soy protein, ginseng or wheat germ, boosts their already high nutritional value.

If your immune system is compromised, or if you are recovering from surgery or a major illness, vegetable smoothies will be of tremendous help. Make them with fresh vegetables and the healing herbs recommended for your health condition (see page 19). All of the vegetable smoothies may be served hot. They are especially beneficial to people who may not be able to take whole meals.

It has been said that you don't need a recipe book to make a smoothie. Although that's basically true — liquid and fresh fruits or vegetables are all it takes to make a basic blended drink — there is so much more to smoothies. In addition to a cornucopia of tangy fruit concoctions, this book offers hot smoothies, healing smoothies, vegetable smoothies, cheese smoothies and smoothies made with milk substitutes — all new and delicious ways to drink to your health.

Skoal, Pat Crocker
www.riversongherbals.com

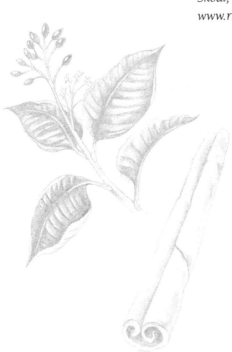

Guidelines to Good Health

What	Why	How
1. Make **complex carbohydrates** the main part of your meals; 60% of calories should come from complex carbohydrates.	• Complex carbohydrates (found in fruits, vegetables and whole grains) also supply vitamins, minerals, enzymes, phytochemicals and fiber. • Simple, refined carbohydrates (found in white sugar and flour) are stripped of nutrients and deliver only "empty" calories. White sugar can decrease immune function.	• Eat five different vegetables per day, one of which should be red or orange. • Eat two fruits per day, one of which should be citrus. • Drink at least one glass of raw, fresh fruit or vegetable juice or pulped drink per day. • Eat five servings of whole grains or cereals every day: whole-grain muesli or oatmeal for breakfast; whole wheat bread with meals; add rice, barley, amaranth or spelt to soups and stews; cook with whole wheat pastas and make whole-grain salads.
2. Protein should comprise 20% of total daily calories. Half (or more) of the protein should come from plant sources — preferably raw.[1]	• The body needs protein to maintain growth and health of cells. For more information, see entry for Protein in Glossary, page 300. • Meats contain saturated fat, which clogs blood vessels and, if not organic, can add toxins to the diet.	• Eat more plant proteins and reduce animal protein. • Eat foods in combinations that provide complete protein: whole grains with legumes, dairy products with nuts and seeds, legumes with nuts and seeds, dairy products with legumes. • Substitute tofu, soy milk or soy-based foods for meat products; use powdered soy protein in smoothies. • Use lean chicken and fish as "accents" to meals of grains, legumes and vegetables.
3. Fat should comprise 20% (or less) of total daily calories. • Eat polyunsaturated fat, restricting the saturated fat in the diet. • Ensure that essential fatty acids (such as omega-3) are part of the diet.	• Protein, carbohydrates and fat all supply food energy (calories), but fat contains twice as many calories as an equal amount of either of the other two. • Mono- and polyunsaturated fats contain less hydrogen and are higher in high-density lipoprotein (HDL), which protects arteries because it carries cholesterol away. Olive oil is a stable monounsaturated fat and the best choice for cooking. • See Glossary, page 298, for information on essential fatty acids.	• Eliminate or restrict use of whole milk, butter, cream, cream cheese, sour cream and fried foods. • Eliminate or restrict intake of saturated fats — particularly animal fats (butter, lard, fats in meats) and palm and coconut oils. • Use olive oil for cooking and unrefined cold-pressed extra-virgin olive, hemp, sunflower, safflower, soybean or corn oil for salad dressings. • Good sources of essential fatty acids include salmon and other cold-water fish, avocados, flax seeds, nuts and seeds.

[1] Rohé, Fred, *The Complete Book of Natural Foods* (Chicago: Shambhala Publications, 1983), p 31.

10

What	Why	How
4. Drink plenty of pure **water**, fruit juice and herbal tea daily.	• Water is necessary for the functioning of the body and its systems.	• Drink 8 glasses of water each day. • Fresh juices contain 80 to 90% water and may be substituted for water.

5. *Avoid the following:*

What	Why	How
• white sugar and flour...	• rob the body of nutrients and deplete the immune system	• Eat whole-grain foods and substitute stevia where possible or small amounts of maple syrup, honey or molasses for sugar.
• red meat...	• has a high fat content and leaves deposits on blood vessel walls	• Eat soy products and vegetable protein in combinations (see #2 or entry for Protein in Glossary, page 300).
• meat products (beef burgers, ham, bacon, sausages, processed meats, offal)...	• cause fat deposits and are high in salt and other additives	• Eat only organic chicken and fish.
• shellfish...	• often contain concentrated toxins from contaminants	• Eat shellfish only rarely.
• excess salt...	• causes fluid retention and hypertension	• Eat celery and other high-potassium vegetables; use herbs as salt substitutes.
• coffee and strong tea...	• contain caffeine, which has undesirable side effects	• Use coffee substitutes, fresh juices and herbal teas.
• excess* alcohol...	• acts as a depressant and robs the body of nutrients	• Substitute fresh juices; eat macrobiotically to reduce cravings.

* Moderate alcohol consumption means having one glass of beer or wine with a meal once or twice per week.

The A to Z of Smoothies

What Is a Smoothie?

SMOOTHIES CAME TO US VIA THE BEACHES OF CALIFORNIA, WHERE warm weather and cool, healthy drinks are part of the culture. With the introduction of blenders, Californians could buy blended thirst-quenching drinks made with orange juice, bananas and strawberries (with or without ice) right on the beach. Soon these coolers were known simply as "smoothies." It wasn't long before other combinations were created and a whole new category of beverages was invented. In 1961, Ann Seranne and Eileen Gaden included recipes for what they called "smoothees" in their *Blender Cookbook* (Doubleday & Co., Inc.). Even then, experimentation was spawning drinks such as their "Mocha Smoothee," "Orange-Pineapple Smoothee" and "Pineapple-Banana Smoothee" — all made with fruit juices and fresh bananas and enhanced with ice cream.

Types of Smoothies

Smoothies can be made from fruits, vegetables, herbs and/or a variety of other healthy ingredients. Smoothies require a liquid base — from juice to milk to broth to herbal tea. They can be served hot, cold, at room temperature — even frozen. During the heat of summer or after an intense workout, there is no better way to lower your body temperature than with a refreshingly cold smoothie.

Smoothies as Part of a Healthy Diet

A NUTRITIOUS DIET INCLUDES PROTEIN, CARBOHYDRATES, FAT, vitamins, minerals, enzymes, phytochemicals, fiber and water in proportions that promote growth and maintain healthy cells. It also includes ample quantities of vegetables and fruits. In fact, the phytochemicals in fruits and vegetables hold the key to preventing many diseases, such as cancer and heart disease, and debilitating conditions, such as asthma, arthritis and allergies. The problem is, even the most disciplined person can find it difficult to consume the quantities of fruits and vegetables that health professionals recommend. Adding a daily smoothie — or two — to your diet is one of the easiest ways to ensure that you eat enough fruits and vegetables to promote good health.

Our bodies thrive on food that is close to its natural state, which means that we should eat as much whole, fresh — and preferably organically produced — food as possible, while avoiding processed or refined foods, which contain artificial preservatives and additives (see Guidelines to Good Health, page 10). Two daily smoothies, brimming with fresh fruits or vegetables and juice, will help improve your immune system, boost your energy, strengthen your bones, clear your skin and lower your risk of disease. Consuming different kinds of smoothies made from a wide variety of herbs, fruits and vegetables will ensure that you receive a broad range of nutrients, which will help you achieve the best health possible.

How Big Is One Serving?

One whole orange, apple or carrot represents one serving of fruits or vegetables. For larger fruits, such as melons or pineapples, about one slice or wedge (about 1/2 cup/125 mL chopped) equals one serving, as does the same amount of a chopped vegetable. Calculate the total number of servings of fruits and vegetables you're getting in a smoothie by adding the amounts of fruits and vegetables in the recipe and dividing by the number of people who are sharing it.

Added Nutrition

Because smoothies are made in a powerful grinding machine and are thickly textured, it is easy to include nuts, grains, herbs and other supplements that you likely wouldn't add to milk or plain juice. This means that smoothies are a perfect base to which you can add nutrient-rich ingredients such as flax seeds, wheat and barley grass, organic soy protein powder, psyllium seeds and wheat germ. See Other Ingredient Profiles, page 145, for information on the dietary value of these and other nutritious additions.

Integrating Smoothies into Your Diet

It's easy to add smoothies to your diet, whether at the start of the day or the end. They are a natural choice for breakfast or as a quick pick-me-up after exercise or sports activities. They also make great after-school and nighttime snacks. Teenagers love making frozen smoothies and milk shakes for their friends. And fresh, tangy fruit-and-vegetable combinations make satisfying nonalcoholic cocktails for adults.

Tips for Making Smoothies Part of Your Daily Routine

- Position the blender in a convenient place on the counter.
- Always keep fresh bananas and seasonal fruit on hand.
- Stock the cupboards and freezer with favorite ingredients.
- Teach school-age children how to use the blender safely and clean it afterward.
- Write favorite recipes and ingredient combinations on cards and keep them in a place that is easily accessible.
- Introduce elders in your family and circle of friends to smoothies and show them how to add medicines or herbal remedies.
- Take a blender to work.

Healthful Benefits of Smoothies

FRUIT OR VEGETABLE SMOOTHIES ARE AN EXCELLENT WAY TO ENHANCE your health, because they provide vitamins, minerals and phytochemicals. Smoothies made with milk, cheese, yogurt or tofu deliver the goodness of protein and calcium. Depending upon the smoothie, here are some of the healthful nutrients that may be added to your diet in addition to vitamins (see page 16).

- **Antioxidants** are phytochemicals that counteract aging and reduce your susceptibility to cancers caused by cell-damaging free radicals that form in the body and initiate disease processes. Herbs, fruits and vegetables are high in antioxidants.
- **Calcium** is necessary to keep your heart, skin, teeth, bones and muscles healthy, and for proper blood clotting. Dairy-based smoothies and those rich in parsley, leafy greens, broccoli, prunes, almonds and pumpkin seeds are good sources of calcium.
- **Chlorophyll** has a unique structure that allows it to enhance the body's ability to produce hemoglobin and, therefore, increase the delivery of oxygen to cells. It is found only in plants.
- **Enzymes** are elements in fruits and vegetables that act as catalysts for chemical reactions in the body. They allow efficient digestion and absorption of food and support the metabolic processes involved in tissue growth. Enzymes give you a high energy level and promote good health. They are destroyed by heat, but smoothies made from fresh, raw fruits and vegetables leave them intact and readily absorbable.
- **Fiber** in the forms of cellulose, pectin, lignin and hemicellulose is found in fruits and vegetables and is essential to a healthy body. Fiber slows the absorption of food (increasing the absorption of nutrients), helps lower cholesterol and reduces the risk of heart disease. It also helps you eliminate toxins and carcinogens and prevents hemorrhoids, varicose veins, constipation, colitis and gallstones. Fibre adds bulk to fecal matter, facilitating its rapid elimination through the colon. Since toxins and bacteria are not given the chance to multiply when adequate fiber is present in the diet, the growth of diseases such as cancer is prevented. Along with all the vitamins, minerals, enzymes and phytochemicals, fiber in whole fruits and vegetables is retained when they are blended or pulped. Pulped fruit has a better cleansing effect on the body than juices because of its higher fiber content.
- **Iron** is a mineral that is present in the body, mostly in the blood. It carries oxygen in the blood to organs and muscles, which is necessary for life itself. The best plant sources of iron are parsley, dates, some nuts (including Brazil nuts and almonds), sesame seeds and pumpkin seeds.
- **Long-lasting satisfaction** is a benefit of including smoothies in your diet. Pulping different fruit-and-vegetable combinations and mixing them with herbs, nuts, seeds and whole grains nourishes the body and leaves you feeling fuller longer than fast foods, soft drinks or coffee.

- **Magnesium** is essential for strong bones and teeth, healthy muscles and abundant energy. The best plant sources are raisins, spinach and other dark green vegetables, garlic, nuts and wheat germ.

- **Manganese** benefits bones, nerves and cell tissue. Animals that are deficient in manganese develop severe osteoporosis, and some doctors think the same may apply to humans. The best plant sources of manganese are grapes, pineapples, raspberries, strawberries, blackberries, watercress, beets, celery and oats.

- **Phosphorous** assists in energy production and helps build bones, teeth and muscle tissue. All fresh fruits and vegetables deliver phosphorous.

- **Phytonutrients**, or **phytochemicals**, come in hundreds of forms and are found in fresh, whole foods. They are important to the growth and maintenance of healthy bodies. New nutrients or chemicals in food are constantly being discovered and researched. Adding smoothies to your diet is one way of ensuring that you consume the variety of fruits, herbs and vegetables necessary to guarantee that you're getting the full range of nutrients.

- **Potassium** keeps nerves and muscles healthy, and regulates bodily fluids, insulin secretion and metabolism. It also helps the body make use of nutrients. Diets high in potassium have been found to lower blood pressure. The best plant sources of potassium are cantaloupes, avocados, dried peaches, apricots, bananas, celery, parsley and watercress.

- **Sodium** is vital in our bodies because it assists in nerve activity and heart function. Processed foods contain large amounts of sodium — more than is needed by, or even safe for, the body. However, small amounts of sodium are found naturally in celery, beets and watercress and are enough to do the job in the body and lend a light, pleasant, salty taste.

- **The spark of life**, or the living "green power" that is present in all living plants, is available to the body when you consume fresh, raw fruits and vegetables. This "life force" is a natural, vital component that is lost in processing.

- **Sugar** in fruits and vegetables comes bundled with vitamins, minerals, enzymes and other phytochemicals that refined sugar lacks. Fruit and vegetable sugars are carbohydrates and, as such, deliver the same energy as pastries, candies and soft drinks, but without the chemicals and fat. *Caution:* People with diabetes and those who are prone to yeast infections and hypoglycemia must watch how and when they use fruits because they cause a rapid rise in blood sugar.

- **Water** is essential because human cells are made of at least 65% water and the body requires water to perform many functions. Drinking a minimum of eight large glasses of water a day is essential. Unlike coffee, soft drinks and alcohol, which remove water from the body as they are metabolized, smoothies are high in water, which replenishes lost fluids while supplying all the vitamins, minerals, enzymes and phytochemicals we need for life. In addition, fresh fruit-and-vegetable smoothies maintain the alkalinity of body fluids, which is vital for proper immune-system and metabolic function.

- **Zinc** is necessary for hormone control, growth, healing, and heart and nerve activity. The best plant sources of it are ginger, nuts and oats.

Drink Your Vitamins

By drinking a variety of smoothies often you can enhance your diet with the following vitamins:

- Vitamin A, which is found in bright orange fruits and vegetables, such as apricots, mangoes, melons, papayas, tangerines, carrots and tomatoes. It is important for healthy skin and tissue, improves night vision and acts as an antioxidant.
- B Vitamins, which are essential for brain function; conversion of protein, fat and carbohydrates to energy; glowing skin and hair; and nerve function. Watercress, peppers, tomatoes, strawberries, avocados, bananas, nuts and seeds all contain large doses of B vitamins.
- Vitamin C, which is present in citrus fruits, papayas, mangoes, pineapples, melons, kiwis, tomatoes and peppers and is a powerful antioxidant that fights infection and builds strong bones and joints.
- Vitamin E, which is a powerful antioxidant that promotes healing. It is found in large amounts in seeds, nuts and wheat germ.
- Vitamin K, which is important for blood clotting. Broccoli, lettuce and watercress are high in vitamin K.

Smoothie Equipment

Blenders

The recipes in this book are best made in a traditional blender that has a jar or jug with rotating blades set on a motor. Today, all blenders come with tight-fitting lids and openings that allow you to add ingredients while the motor is running. A food processor may be used for drinks that do not require ice. Today, many makes and models of blenders are available, in a wide range of prices.

Cleaning Your Blender

Disconnect the power cord before cleaning. Never immerse the motorized base in water; wipe it clean with a damp cloth. Drop $1/2$ tsp (2 mL) liquid dishwashing soap into the jug and fill to the halfway mark with hot water. Replace the lid securely and turn the switch to Pulse-Clean, Mix or Low. Run for several seconds. Pour soapy water out and rinse the jug and lid with hot water. From time to time, the jug can be disassembled and thoroughly cleaned in hot soapy water or in the dishwasher, according to the manufacturer's instructions.

Tip
- Before you buy, check how and where to order extra jugs, in case you want to have more than one or in the event that it breaks or cracks.

Buying a Blender?

Consider the following when determining which blender to purchase.

- **Base:** A heavy base stabilizes the machine and keeps it from vibrating or moving around on the counter. Washable heavy-duty stainless steel or heavy-gauge plastic are practical. Flat touch-pad buttons do not collect food debris and are easy to keep clean.

- **Motor:** Heavy-duty motors (120 volts, 60 hertz or more) are strong enough to chop ice cubes and the hard ingredients that some of the recipes call for. Less-powerful motors tend to burn out faster and may cause the machine to vibrate or jump around on the counter when ice, frozen fruit or hard vegetables are being processed.

- **Jug size, shape and capacity:** From tall to squat, fat to thin, the shape of blender jugs varies. Today, in response to consumer needs, many brands are moving to a wider jug that can process ice with less liquid. Jugs are usually made to hold between 5 and 6 cups (1.25 and 1.5 L), although some hold as much as 8 cups (2 L). When making your purchasing decision, consider the number of servings you will be making at one time to determine what size suits you best.

- **Jug materials:** Jugs are available in plastic, glass or stainless steel. Plastic is usually the least expensive. It is durable (a must if children are using the machine) and lightweight, but it scratches over time and is not recommended for processing ice. Glass is easier to clean, dishwasher-safe and fine for ice, and it doesn't wear out. Glass is more expensive than plastic, however. Stainless steel is top of the line: it is easy to clean and keeps frozen mixtures cold but is the most costly of the three.

- **Settings and speeds:** Some blenders only have two speeds (Low and High); others have several (from Mix to Puree to Liquefy and everything in between) Two speeds are essential, but if you plan to use ice in drinks (see Frozen Smoothies, page 272), look for a blender that has a Pulse or Ice Crush setting, which is designed to crush ice evenly without liquefying it.

- **Appearance:** Blenders have become sleeker, with rounded corners, and are available in a variety of colors (including stainless-steel or metallic finishes). While design does not affect performance, it is a consideration if the machine will be kept out on the counter where it is likely to be seen more often.

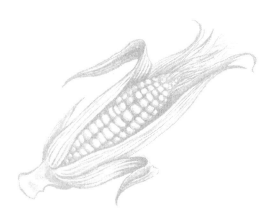

Health Conditions

Smoothies and Specific Health Conditions

ALTHOUGH THEY OFTEN DIFFER IN THEIR OPINIONS, SCIENTISTS, doctors and nutritionists agree that the foods we eat on a regular basis profoundly affect our health and well-being. Diet plays a significant role not only in keeping us healthy but also in preventing and controlling disease. The following are concise descriptions of many ailments that may be helped by consistently following specific dietary guidelines. For each condition, we have recommended the fruits, vegetables, herbs and other foods that provide the greatest benefits. Maximizing foods that have positive effects while minimizing or eliminating those that have negative effects will bring about a slow, steady improvement in health.

These recommendations are not intended to take the place of consultation with a health-care practitioner. For best results — especially if you are faced with a serious condition — contact a doctor, as well as a medical herbalist or natural-health specialist. Trained health-care professionals can provide you with sound medical advice, as well as a diet-and-lifestyle program that is tailored to your needs.

Consult the Glossary

As you read through this section on specific health conditions, you will come across a number of medical terms, some of which you may not understand. Consult the glossary, which begins on page 296, for definitions and explanations.

Fruits and vegetables
citrus fruits, peaches, pears, strawberries, asparagus, avocados, broccoli, carrots, cauliflower, leafy greens, onions, squash

AIDS & HIV
Acquired Immunodeficiency Syndrome & Human Immunodeficiency Virus

THERE IS NO KNOWN CURE FOR AIDS, AND ANYONE WITH HIV should be under a doctor's care. However, dietary therapy can improve immune function, promote resistance to infections associated with AIDS and reduce symptoms associated with HIV and AIDS.

Maximize

- Organic fruits and vegetables, which are free of chemicals
- Shiitake mushrooms, which studies have shown to strongly support the immune system
- Garlic — an antibacterial, antiviral and antifungal — which guards against opportunistic infections

Minimize

- Sweet foods, including honey and fruit juices, which encourage the growth of molds and yeast

Eliminate

- Refined flour
- Animal fats in meat and dairy products, as they decrease immunity
- Alcohol, which increases susceptibility to infection
- Food allergies and intolerances (see Appendix A: Food Allergies, page 304)
- Sugar

Other Recommendations

- Exercise daily, according to your fitness level. This helps improve circulation and eliminates toxins through sweating.
- Practice stress-reduction techniques, such as yoga, tai chi and meditation to strengthen the immune system by decreasing stress.

Healing Smoothies

- Allium Antioxidant, page 232
- C-Green, page 214
- Cauliflower Cocktail, page 206
- Green Energy (use ginseng instead of ginkgo), page 232
- Minestrone, page 203

Herbs

aloe vera, astragalus, burdock (leaf, root and seeds), evening primrose oil, garlic, ginseng, licorice*, turmeric

Other

cereal grasses, flax seeds, kelp, pumpkin seeds, sprouted seeds, soy yogurt, sunflower seeds, tofu, whole grains

---

★ Avoid licorice if you have high blood pressure. The prolonged use of licorice is not recommended under any circumstances.

Aging

SEVERAL SCIENTIFIC STUDIES SHOW THAT EATING A DIET high in nutrients but low in calories helps reduce signs of aging and increases life span. Recent studies also show that oxidation is one of the most important factors that contributes to aging. Oxidation occurs when cells are damaged by free radicals, by-products produced when the body converts oxygen to energy. The progression of Parkinson's disease and Alzheimer's disease have been linked to oxidative stress. Heart disease, cancer, arthritis and wrinkles are also signs of cell damage, often caused by free radicals. Antioxidants, which are found in many fruits and vegetables, protect the body from free-radical damage.

HEALING FOODS

Fruits and vegetables

apples, blueberries, grapefruit, oranges, pears, raspberries, strawberries, beets, broccoli, cabbage, carrots, celery, leafy greens, onions, pumpkin, sweet potatoes, tomatoes

Herbs

cayenne, German chamomile, garlic, ginger, ginkgo, green tea, lemon balm, milk thistle, oregano, parsley*, peppermint, rosemary, sage, spearmint, thyme, turmeric

Other

cereal grasses, flax seeds, nuts, extra-virgin olive oil, pumpkin seeds, sea herbs, sesame seeds, soy products, sunflower seeds, yogurt with active bacterial cultures

> * If you are pregnant, limit your intake of parsley to $1/2$ tsp (2 mL) dried or one sprig fresh per day. Do not take parsley if you are suffering from kidney inflammation.

HEALING FOODS

Fruits and vegetables

apples, blueberries, grapes, mangoes, oranges, raspberries, strawberries, asparagus, beets, carrots, onions, red and green bell peppers, spinach, watercress

Herbs

astragalus, burdock*** root, calendula***, cinnamon, dandelion*** leaf and root, elderflower, garlic, ginger, licorice**, parsley*, stinging nettle, thyme, turmeric, yarrow***

What to Do

Maximize

- Antioxidant-rich fruits and vegetables
- Antioxidant herbal teas (any combination of oregano, rosemary, lemon balm, sage, thyme and peppermint)
- Effective digestion. Remedying digestive problems (see Indigestion, page 57) will improve your body's ability to absorb nutrients

Minimize

- Animal fats in meat and dairy products. Replace some meat meals with fish and vegetable protein

Eliminate

- Unnecessary calories

Healing Smoothies

- Beta Blast, page 177
- Black Pineapple, page 161
- Blueberry, page 162
- Smart Smoothie, page 239
- Spa Special, page 236

Allergies
Hay Fever, Eczema & Asthma

THE SYMPTOMS OF ALLERGIC REACTIONS EVIDENCED IN HAY fever, eczema and asthma are caused by inflammation, which is the body's normal healing response to injury. Allergies are an example of chronic inflammation, in which factors such as food intolerance, stress and poor digestion allow a toxin to activate the immune system. This causes inappropriate inflammatory responses on the skin or in the eyes, nose or airways. Proper nutrition and the use of appropriate herbs can reduce the severity of the inflammation.

What to Do

Maximize

- Fruits and vegetables that provide flavonoids and antioxidants, which support appropriate immune response
- Essential fatty acids (found in oily fish, flax seeds and sunflower seeds, among other foods), which are anti-inflammatory and reduce the severity of allergies

Maximize

- Herbs that optimize digestion (dandelion root, as required), boost immunity (astragalus, garlic) and nourish the nervous system (oat straw, skullcap)

Eliminate

- Food allergies and intolerances (see Appendix A: Food Allergies, page 304)
- Sugar, including honey and fruit sugars. Studies have shown that sugars decrease immune function by impairing white-blood-cell activity. Excess sugar also promotes yeast infections, which increase allergic reactions
- Alcohol, which depresses immune function
- Mucus-forming foods (dairy products, bananas)

Other Recommendations

- Reduce stress. Stress and high emotion are factors in lowered immunity, which increases susceptibility to allergies. Sleep and relaxation help to produce immunity-enhancing compounds.
- Improve digestion. Poor digestion keeps the body from eliminating toxins and limits the absorption of nutrients. When food is completely digested, allergic reactions are often eliminated.
- Get adequate protein. Protein is essential for optimum immune function. The best sources of protein are fish, such as tuna, salmon, sardines, trout, cod and herring.

Other
flax seeds, nuts (except peanuts), pumpkin seeds, rice, soy products, yogurt with active bacterial cultures, whole grains

---

** Avoid licorice if you have high blood pressure. The prolonged use of licorice is not recommended under any circumstances.

*** People who are allergic to ragweed may also be allergic to herbs in the same botanical family (the *Compositae*, or daisy, family). The herbs in this family include burdock, calendula, chamomile, chicory, dandelion, echinacea, feverfew, milk thistle and yarrow (avoid yarrow if you are pregnant, see page 308).

Healing Smoothies

- Berry Fine Cocktail, page 189
- C-Green, page 214
- Green Energy (use a recommended herb instead of ginkgo), page 232
- Blueberry, page 162
- Citrus Cocktail, page 165
- Mango Madness (substitute $1/4$ cup/50 mL yogurt for banana), page 175

Alopecia

ALOPECIA IS A PARTIAL OR COMPLETE LOSS OF HAIR. IT CAN be caused by severe stress; skin diseases; excessive sunlight; thyroid imbalances; excessive sex hormones; or strong chemicals, such as those used for cancer treatment or on the hair, that interfere with the nutrition of the hair follicles.

Hair consists largely of protein, which is made from amino acids and minerals, and is greatly affected by nutrition. Rosemary is traditionally used to treat hair problems. A rosemary tea can be used both internally and externally to stimulate blood flow to the scalp.

Fruits and vegetables
broccoli, cabbage, garlic, onions, spinach

Herbs
ginger, rosemary, stinging nettle

Other

brown rice, eggs, flax seeds, nuts, soy products, sunflower seeds

Include in Your Diet

- High-protein foods (meat, fish, poultry, eggs, cheese, brown rice, nuts, seeds, soybeans)
- Foods that contain sulfur (egg yolks, cauliflower, cabbage, turnips, onions, garlic)
- Calcium-rich foods (dairy products, leafy greens, sea herbs)

Maximize

- Antioxidant-rich fruits and vegetables, especially broccoli, cabbage, garlic, onions and spinach

Minimize

- Stress. Relaxation techniques, such as meditation and yoga, can help alleviate the stresses and tensions of life

Healing Smoothies

- Allium Antioxidant, page 232
- Cabbage Cocktail, page 203
- Green Energy (use a recommended herb instead of ginkgo), page 232

HEALING FOODS

Fruits and vegetables

blueberries, citrus fruits, grapes, asparagus, broccoli, beets and beet greens, carrots, green bell peppers, kale, okra, onions, spinach, sweet potatoes, watercress, yams

Herbs

basil, garlic, German chamomile, ginger, ginkgo, ginseng, dandelion leaves and flowers, lemon balm, licorice*, stinging nettle, parsley**, red clover flowers, rosemary, sage, skullcap, turmeric

Alzheimer's Disease & Dementia

DEMENTIA IS CHARACTERIZED BY IMPAIRMENT OF MEMORY, judgment and abstract thinking. It may be caused by stress, by impaired circulation caused by a buildup of fatty deposits in the blood vessels of the brain or by a degenerative disease, such as Alzheimer's disease. Recognized risk factors for Alzheimer's disease include acetylcholine deficiency, free-radical damage and inflammation of brain tissue. Diet can play a role in the prevention of Alzheimer's by nourishing the brain; by lowering cholesterol, which causes fatty deposits to form in the blood vessels of the brain; and by providing antioxidants to protect against free radicals that cause brain-cell damage. Foods that contain choline, a building block of acetylcholine (a chemical that plays a key role in cognition and reasoning) may help prevent Alzheimer's disease.

What to Do

Minimize

- Meat and dairy products
- Environmental toxins

Maximize

- Fresh fruits and vegetables, which provide vitamins and minerals to feed brain tissue and antioxidants to eliminate free radicals

- Foods that contain choline, a building block of acetylcholine (Brazil nuts, lecithin, dandelion flowers, mung beans, lentils, fava beans)

- Nuts and seeds, which provide essential fatty acids to nourish the brain

Eliminate

- Refined and processed foods
- Alcohol
- Fatty foods, fried foods and oils (except extra-virgin olive oil)
- Aluminum in cookware, foil, deodorants and antacids. There is a suspected relationship between aluminum and Alzheimer's disease. Avoid preparing foods in aluminum cooking utensils. Although no direct link has been established between Alzheimer's and aluminum, high concentrations of aluminum have been found when autopsies were performed on Alzheimer's patients. It is probably wise to err on the side of caution. Don't prepare foods in aluminum cooking utensils, and avoid products that contain aluminum, such as most deodorants and some processed foods.

Other Recommendations

- Eat oily fish (salmon, sardines, mackerel, herring), which provide essential fatty acids to nourish brain and nerve tissue.

- Rosemary and sage traditionally have been used to improve memory. Both herbs are rich in antioxidants. Studies also show that they contain substances that conserve acetylcholine.

- Ginkgo biloba improves blood flow to the brain, which is helpful in cases in which a doctor has diagnosed that insufficient blood flow to the brain is causing dementia. If dementia is not caused by insufficient cerebral blood flow, do not use ginkgo biloba, as it may cause other problems.

- Take anti-inflammatory herbs (German chamomile, ginseng, licorice, turmeric) to reduce the inflammation of brain tissue associated with Alzheimer's disease.

Other

Brazil nuts, brown rice, cider vinegar, egg yolks, flax seeds, lecithin, legumes, lentils, nuts, oats, extra-virgin olive oil, pumpkin seeds, sea herbs, soy products, wheat germ

---

★ Avoid licorice if you have high blood pressure. The prolonged use of licorice is not recommended under any circumstances.

★★ If you are pregnant, limit your intake of parsley to 1/2 tsp (2 mL) dried or one sprig fresh per day. Do not take parsley if you are suffering from kidney inflammation.

Healing Smoothies

- Beet, page 201
- Black Pineapple, page 161
- Blueberry, page 162
- Brocco-Carrot, page 202
- C-Blend, page 166
- Smart Smoothie, page 239

Fruits and vegetables
apples, citrus fruits, grapes, peaches, strawberries, beets and beet greens, broccoli, carrots, fennel, green peas, Jerusalem artichokes, leafy greens, watercress

Herbs
burdock root, dandelion leaf and root, stinging nettle, parsley*

Other
almonds, dried apricots, figs, prunes, raisins, blackstrap molasses, kelp

* If you are pregnant, limit your intake of parsley to $1/2$ tsp (2 mL) dried or one sprig fresh per day. Do not take parsley if you are suffering from kidney inflammation.

Fruits and vegetables
apricots, bananas, broccoli, carrots, celery, fennel, leafy greens, onions, watercress

Herbs
alfalfa, borage, dandelion leaf, garlic, German chamomile, kava kava, lavender, lemon balm, parsley*, St. John's wort, skullcap, valerian**

Anemia

ANEMIA IS A DEFICIENCY OF HEMOGLOBIN IN THE BLOOD, which results in fatigue and facial pallor. Other symptoms depend on the type of anemia, which can be determined by a blood test. Iron-deficiency anemia is the most common type and may be precipitated by heavy menstrual flow, internal bleeding, dietary deficiency of iron, pregnancy or rheumatoid arthritis. To treat anemia, you must determine the type, then work to alleviate the underlying cause. For all types of anemia, increasing the body's ability to absorb nutrients is helpful.

What to Do

Maximize
- Iron-rich foods and herbs (sea herbs, beets, dried fruits, almonds, spinach, stinging nettle, parsley, watercress)
- Foods rich in vitamin C
- Herbal bitters, such as dandelion root, to improve iron absorption

Minimize
- Whole wheat bread, which limits iron absorption

Eliminate
- Foods that limit iron absorption (coffee, tea, chocolate, wheat bran)

Healing Smoothies
- Apricot Peach, page 159
- Beet, page 201
- Popeye's Power, page 229
- Sea-Straw, page 191

Anxiety States
Anxiety, Stress & Panic Attacks

ANXIETY IS CHARACTERIZED BY A MOOD OF FEAR AND IS often associated with insomnia. Panic disorders are recurrent attacks of severe anxiety. Causes may include fatigue, stress, nervous disorders, depression or hormone imbalance.

What to Do

Maximize
- Fresh fruits and vegetable fiber to boost general health, which allows you to cope better with stress
- Foods rich in B vitamins (whole grains, leafy greens) to support the nervous system

Maximize

- Foods that are high in calcium and magnesium (kelp, dulse, soy products, almonds, kale, parsley*), which help to ease nervous tension
- Herbs that help you relax and that improve sleep (German chamomile, lavender, skullcap)
- Meditation and relaxation exercises to help release nervous energy, allowing a more balanced emotional state

Eliminate

- Caffeine (found in coffee, black and green tea, chocolate and soft drinks)
- Alcohol
- Refined flour and sugar
- Artificial food additives
- Food allergies and intolerances (see Appendix A: Food Allergies, page 304)

Other

almond milk, dulse, honey, kelp, nuts (especially almonds), tofu, whole grains (especially oats)

> ** Valerian has an adverse effect on some people.
>
> *** Avoid licorice if you have high blood pressure. The prolonged use of licorice is not recommended under any circumstances.

Healing Smoothies

- Almond Banana, page 159
- Banana Frappé, page 265
- Calming Chamomile, page 232
- Lavender Smoothie, page 234
- Popeye's Power, page 229

Arthritis
Rheumatoid Arthritis & Osteoarthritis

RHEUMATOID ARTHRITIS IS THE MOST COMMON CHRONIC inflammatory joint disease. It can usually be diagnosed by the presence of antibodies (called rheumatoid factor) in the blood. Since it is blood-related rather than the result of wear and tear, rheumatoid arthritis is a disease that affects the whole body, often resulting in symptoms such as fever, weight loss, fatigue and a general decline in health. The joints (commonly the wrists, elbows, ankles, knees, hips, and hand and foot joints) become swollen and inflamed and are usually affected symmetrically. Neck pain and stiffness result from spinal inflammation. Joints can eventually become deformed due to a buildup of fluid that impairs the healing process in the joint tissue. Pain and stiffness is usually worst in the morning and may wear off during the day.

Osteoarthritis is a wear-and-tear disorder that usually starts after age 50. It is characterized by cartilage degeneration in weight-bearing joints, such as the hips, knees and spine, as well as joints in the hand. As the cartilage degenerates, new bone, cartilage and connective tissues are formed, which remodel the joint, leading to wasted muscle around the joint and limited movement. Inflammation is secondary to the degeneration of cartilage. Pain is usually provoked by movement and

Fruits and vegetables
apples, cherries, grapes, mangoes, papayas, asparagus, beets, broccoli, cauliflower, cabbage, carrots, celery, Jerusalem artichokes, turnips, onions, watercress

Herbs
alfalfa, celery seeds, dandelion root and leaf, fennel seeds, garlic, German chamomile, ginger, lemon balm, licorice***, meadowsweet, parsley*, rosemary, stinging nettle, turmeric

Other

cereal grasses, dulse, fish oils, kelp, legumes, blackstrap molasses, nuts (especially almonds), extra-virgin olive oil, soy products, seeds (flax, pumpkin, sesame, sunflower), wheat germ, whole grains (watch for allergies to wheat and corn), yogurt with active bacterial cultures

disappears with rest, so it typically gets worse as the day progresses. Because osteoarthritis pain is caused by placing weight on the joints, in overweight people it improves with weight loss. It is often related to a mineral imbalance in the diet and/or a defect that limits the body's ability to absorb minerals. As a result, it may improve with dietary changes and/or support for the digestive system.

Arthritis sufferers often have poor circulation (signified by constantly cold hands and feet), don't perspire, get constipated easily and are overweight. These factors contribute to the retention of waste products and must be addressed first by using some of the herbs listed below (see also Constipation, page 36, and Overweight, page 74). Visit a medical herbalist or other natural-health practitioner for additional advice for your individual situation.

What to Do

Maximize

- Fresh fruits and vegetables
- Fluid intake (drink at least eight large glasses of water, juice and/or herbal tea daily) to dilute and wash out toxins
- Oily fish (salmon, tuna, herring, sardines, trout, cod, mackerel), which are anti-inflammatory
- Herbs that support the digestive system (lemon balm, peppermint, chamomile) to improve nutrient absorption
- Herbal analgesics (German chamomile, meadowsweet) for pain relief

- Anti-inflammatory herbs (German chamomile, ginger, licorice, meadowsweet) to reduce pain and joint deterioration
- Herbal diuretics (dandelion leaf) and lymphatics (red clover flower) to encourage the elimination of waste products
- Herbs that support the liver (dandelion root, licorice) to help eliminate toxins
- Herbal circulatory stimulants (ginger, stinging nettle) to improve blood supply to the affected joints

Minimize

- Refined foods
- Tea, coffee and soft drinks
- Salt and salty foods
- Acidic fruits and vegetables (rhubarb, cranberries, plums, spinach, Swiss chard, beet greens)

Eliminate

- Junk food
- Food allergies and intolerances (see Appendix A: Food Allergies, page 304). Problem foods are often corn, dairy products, wheat, eggs, chocolate, peanuts and varieties of the nightshade family, which includes peppers, tomatoes, potatoes and eggplant

Eliminate

- Meat, especially red meat (beef, pork, lamb) and processed meat products (ham, hamburgers, sausages, cold cuts), which can stimulate inflammation
- Margarine, shortening and heat-processed oils (replace with extra-virgin olive oil)
- Shellfish. When protein from shellfish is digested, toxins (urea, uric acid, purines) in it are deposited in the fat and at the ends of the long bones (joints), where they lead to slow, chronic inflammation. Toxins created when shellfish are digested seem to cause more problems than other proteins
- Processed and refined foods
- Sugar and artificial sweeteners (replace with honey, maple syrup or stevia, page 120)
- Citrus fruits, which often cause allergic reactions in people with rheumatoid arthritis
- Vinegar and vinegared foods (pickles), which leach minerals from the body (except apple cider vinegar and brown rice vinegar)
- Alcohol
- Artificial food additives
- Food contaminants from pesticides (eat as much organically produced food as possible)

★ If you are pregnant, limit your intake of parsley to ¹/₂ tsp (2 mL) dried or one sprig fresh per day. Do not take parsley if you are suffering from kidney inflammation.

Healing Smoothies

- Allium Antioxidant, page 232
- Almond Banana, page 159
- Apple Spice Cocktail, page 158
- Aspirin in a Glass, page 235
- Breakfast Cocktail, page 175
- Calming Chamomile, page 232

ADD & ADHD
Attention Deficit Disorder & Attention Deficit Hyperactivity Disorder

A CHILD MAY BE DIAGNOSED WITH ADD IF HE OR SHE IS EASILY distracted, has a short attention span, has difficulty concentrating and impulsively moves from one activity to another. In ADHD, there are also signs of hyperactivity. Studies have shown that increasing a child's intake of whole, nutrient-rich foods increases the supply of nutrients to the brain and improves mental performance. Other studies show that iron deficiency can cause attention deficits.

Introducing fresh juice and smoothies into a child's diet is an easy way to help him or her eat more raw fruits and vegetables. Certain herbs can also help calm a child's nerves while the process of diet detoxification takes place.

HEALING FOODS

Fruits and vegetables
apples, pears, carrots, beets, broccoli, spinach

Herbs
catnip, cinnamon, German chamomile, lemon balm, parsley*, St. John's wort, stinging nettle

Other

almonds, kelp, sunflower seeds, pumpkin seeds, oats

★ If you are pregnant, limit your intake of parsley to $\frac{1}{2}$ tsp (2 mL) dried or one sprig fresh per day. Do not take parsley if you are suffering from kidney inflammation.

What to Do

Maximize

- Whole foods
- Antioxidant-rich fruits and vegetables
- Iron-rich foods (beets; leafy greens; almonds; sea herbs; watercress; and dried fruits, such as figs, raisins and apricots)
- Nuts and seeds to provide zinc, which is necessary for brain function

Minimize

- Foods that limit iron absorption (coffee, tea, chocolate, egg yolks, wheat bran)

Eliminate

- Artificial food additives, colorings, preservatives and sweeteners, which can be toxic to a child
- Sugar and sweet foods and drinks, which deplete the B vitamins necessary for nerve-cell function
- Refined foods, including white flour and white sugar products, which deplete the body's zinc supply
- Food allergies (see Appendix A: Food Allergies, page 304). They are often implicated in ADD, and some of the most common allergens are dairy products (see pages 245 and 246 for information on milk substitutes), eggs, wheat and oranges

Healing Smoothies

- Almond Banana, page 159
- Autumn Refresher, page 184
- Banana Frappé, page 265
- Date and Nut, page 268
- Green Energy (omit ginkgo), page 232
- Pear Pineapple, page 185

Fruits and vegetables

bananas, avocados, carrots, green beans, leafy greens, sweet potatoes, watercress

Herbs

alfalfa, borage leaves and flowers, dandelion leaf and root, fennel seeds, German chamomile, parsley*, red raspberry leaves, stinging nettle

Breastfeeding

A NOURISHING DIET THAT'S RICH IN MINERALS IS ESSENTIAL for the health of a nursing mother and her baby. Adding fennel, dill or anise to the mother's food or tea helps prevent infant colic. While weaning, drink sage tea to reduce breast milk production.

What to Do

Minimize

- Garlic, onions and hot peppers, which can create gas in the baby
- Refined foods (white flour, white sugar)

Eliminate

- Artificial food additives, colorings and sweeteners, which can be toxic to a child

Maximize

- Whole foods
- Foods that contain B vitamins (whole grains, leafy greens, sea herbs), which encourage a rich supply of breast milk
- Foods that contain calcium (leafy greens, sea herbs) to support Baby's bone development
- Mineral-rich herbal teas (stinging nettle, red raspberry leaf, alfalfa, red clover flower, dandelion)

Healing Smoothies

- Anise Anise, page 235
- Avocado Pineapple, page 197
- C-Green, page 214
- Green Gold, page 214
- Leafy Luxury, page 210
- Raspberry Raspberry, page 237

Bronchitis

BRONCHITIS IS AN INFLAMMATION OF THE BRONCHIAL TUBES that is usually characterized by chest congestion and a persistent cough. Typical causes include bacteria, virus, or exposure to smoke or chemicals. Without treatment, the condition can become chronic.

What to Do

Maximize

- Fruits and vegetables, especially those high in vitamin C and beta-carotene
- Raw garlic for its antibiotic effect on the lungs

Minimize

- Meat
- Salt and salty foods

Eliminate

- Dairy products
- Sugar
- Refined flour
- Alcohol
- Food allergies and intolerances (see Appendix A: Food Allergies, page 304)

Healing Smoothies

- Allium Antioxidant, page 232
- Autumn Refresher, page 184
- C-Blend, page 166
- C-Blitz, page 166
- Citrus Toddy, page 276
- Nectar of the Gods, page 179
- Orange Zinger, page 204

Other

almonds, blackstrap molasses, legumes, sunflower seeds, pumpkin seeds, sea herbs, wheat germ, whole grains, yogurt with active bacterial cultures

HEALING FOODS

Fruits and vegetables
apricots, citrus fruits, cranberries, pears, broccoli, cabbage, carrots, leafy greens, onions, red and green bell peppers, turnips, watercress

Herbs
cayenne, cinnamon, elderberries, fenugreek seeds, garlic, ginger, hyssop, licorice**, marshmallow, stinging nettle, parsley*, plantain, thyme

Other
legumes, sesame seeds, sunflower seeds, pumpkin seeds, soy products, soy yogurt

** Avoid licorice if you have high blood pressure. The prolonged use of licorice is not recommended under any circumstances.

Fruits and vegetables

apples, apricots, blueberries, cherries, citrus fruits, cranberries, figs, grapes, kiwis, mangoes, papayas, peaches, raspberries, strawberries, watermelon, asparagus, beets, broccoli, cabbage, carrots, leafy greens, onions, parsnips, squash, sweet potatoes, tomatoes, watercress

Herbs

astragalus, burdock root, calendula, cayenne, echinacea, garlic, green tea, licorice*, parsley**, red clover flower, rosemary, sage, turmeric

Other

extra-virgin olive oil, fish oil, flax seeds, legumes, nuts (except peanuts), pumpkin seeds, shiitake mushrooms, soy products, spirulina, sunflower seeds, yogurt with active bacterial cultures, wheat grass, whole grains

> ★ Avoid licorice if you have high blood pressure. The prolonged use of licorice is not recommended under any circumstances.

Cancer Prevention

RISK FACTORS FOR CANCER INCLUDE THE USE OF TOBACCO and alcohol, exposure to toxins in food and the environment, and family history of cancer. Factors that protect against cancer include eating a diet that consists primarily of fresh fruits, vegetables and other whole foods; a healthy, active lifestyle; and avoiding foods and toxins that have been linked to cancer (see Eliminate, below).

What to Do

Maximize

- Organic foods
- Soy products
- Antioxidant-rich fruits and vegetables
- Nuts and seeds

Minimize

- Animal protein in meat and dairy products

Other Recommendations

- Exercise daily, according to your fitness level.

Eliminate

- Margarine, shortening and cooking oils (except extra-virgin olive oil)
- Alcohol
- Sugar
- Coffee
- Salt; pickled and salt-cured foods
- Fried foods
- Fried, grilled or barbecued meat, fish and poultry
- Smoked or cured meats (ham, bacon, hot dogs, cold cuts)
- Artificial food additives
- Refined food

Healing Smoothies

- Allium Antioxidant, page 232
- Breakfast Cocktail, page 175
- C-Blitz, page 166
- Citrus Cocktail, page 165
- Eye Opener, page 165
- Minestrone, page 203
- Orange Zinger, page 204
- Tomato Juice Cocktail, page 217

Candida

CANDIDA IS A YEAST INFECTION THAT TYPICALLY OCCURS ON the external genitalia. It appears as a discharge in women and a rash in men. It may occur in the mouth, causing a burning sensation, or in the digestive system, causing bloating. General symptoms include fatigue, mood changes, depression, poor memory, headaches, cravings for sweets, bowel irregularities, muscle and joint problems, and skin problems.

Low thyroid function, diabetes, pregnancy, antibiotics, steroids, poor diet and sexual transmission can cause candida. Vaginal deodorants and scented soaps aggravate the condition by irritating the protective mucosa of the vagina. Stress, oral contraceptives, hormones and preservatives in food can encourage chronic candida. Reduce stress by using nerve-nourishing herbs, such as skullcap and oats.

What to Do

Maximize

- Antioxidant-rich vegetables
- Vegetable protein (soy products, legumes with rice)
- Raw garlic (several cloves a day) to kill the yeast fungus
- Yogurt with active bacterial cultures to control yeast growth

Minimize

- Fruits and fruit juices to reduce excess fruit sugars that encourage yeast growth
- High-carbohydrate vegetables (potatoes, corn, parsnips)

Eliminate

- Food allergies and intolerances (see Appendix A: Food Allergies, page 304)
- Bananas, citrus fruits, dried fruits and mushrooms
- Alcohol, coffee, chocolate and tea
- Dairy products, which contain sugars that encourage candida growth (except unsweetened yogurt with active bacterial cultures)

- Honey, molasses, soy sauce, sugar and sweeteners
- Meat
- Refined foods
- Vinegared foods (pickles, mustard, ketchup, salad dressings)
- Yeast (including bakery products made with yeast)

Healing Smoothies

- Allium Antioxidant, page 232
- Minestrone, page 203

Fruits and vegetables
cranberries, broccoli, cabbage, carrots, cauliflower, celery, leafy greens, onions, squash, sweet potatoes, red bell peppers

Herbs
calendula, cloves, dandelion leaf and root, echinacea, garlic, ginger, lemon balm, stinging nettle, parsley**, peppermint, rosemary, thyme

Other
caprylic acid, dulse, kelp, legumes, nuts, extra-virgin olive oil, seeds, soy products, whole grains, unsweetened yogurt with active bacterial cultures

---

** If you are pregnant, limit your intake of parsley to 1/2 tsp (2 mL) dried or one sprig fresh per day. Do not take parsley if you are suffering from kidney inflammation.

Fruits and vegetables
apples, bananas, citrus fruits, broccoli, carrots, green beans, green and red bell peppers, leafy greens, squash, sweet potatoes, tomatoes, watercress

Herbs
alfalfa, cayenne, dandelion leaf and root, echinacea, evening primrose oil, garlic, ginger, ginseng*, lemon balm, licorice**, milk thistle, parsley***, St. John's wort, stinging nettle

Other
brown rice, cereal grasses, dulse, fish oils, flax seeds, kelp, legumes, maitake mushrooms, oats, extra-virgin olive oil, pumpkin seeds, sesame seeds, shiitake mushrooms, sunflower seeds, whole grains, yogurt with active bacterial cultures

* Do not take ginseng if you have high blood pressure or if you drink coffee. Never take ginseng daily for longer than four weeks.

Chronic Fatigue Syndrome

CHRONIC FATIGUE SYNDROME IS NOT WELL UNDERSTOOD. It is characterized by overwhelming fatigue, lack of energy, sleep disturbances and depression, and often features headaches, sore throats or swollen glands. It often follows a viral infection that has weakened the immune system. Other possible causes are food allergies, poor digestion or nutrient absorption, antibiotic use and long-term stress.

What to Do

Maximize

- Immunity and proper digestion (see Immune Deficiency, page 54, and Indigestion, page 57)
- Antioxidant-rich fruits and vegetables
- Nuts and seeds

Minimize

- Animal protein in meat and dairy products

Other Recommendations

- Get regular daily exercise, according to your fitness level.

Eliminate

- Processed and refined foods
- Caffeine (found in coffee, black and green tea, chocolate and soft drinks)
- Sugar, alcohol, yeast (or foods made with yeast), which can encourage candida infection (see Candida, page 33), often a factor in the illness
- Foods allergies and intolerances (see Appendix A: Food Allergies, page 304). Common triggers are dairy products, wheat and corn
- Artificial food additives

Healing Smoothies

- Allium Antioxidant, page 232
- C-Blitz, page 166
- Green Gold, page 214
- Minestrone, page 203
- Popeye's Power, page 229
- Rustproofer #1, page 205
- Rustproofer #2 (substitute a recommended herb for peppermint), page 214

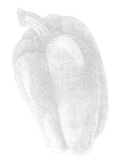

Common Cold

THE COMMON COLD IS A VIRAL INFECTION OF THE AIRWAYS.
During cold season, consuming a diet high in fresh fruits, vegetables
and garlic is an excellent preventive measure. The severity and duration
of any cold can be diminished by promoting elimination through the
skin (by sweating) and the bowel (by consuming an abundance of
fresh fruit and avoiding slow-digesting meat and dairy products).

Help for Common Cold

- Nausea: tea made from peppermint, chamomile, ginger
  or cinnamon
- Sore throat: gargle or tea made from sage****
- Cough: tea made from thyme, licorice**, hyssop, plantain
  or marshmallow root

What to Do

Maximize

- Fresh fruits and vegetables
  and their juices
- Hot herbs (cayenne, ginger)
  to promote body heat and
  discourage the virus
- Fluid intake (drink at least eight
  large glasses of water, juice
  and/or herbal tea daily)

Eliminate

- Animal protein. The large
  amount of energy required to
  digest meat and dairy products
  is better used as healing energy

Healing Smoothies

- Allium Antioxidant, page 232
- C-Blitz, page 166
- Citrus Toddy, page 276
- Flaming Antibiotic, page 208
- Green Gold, page 214
- Popeye's Power, page 229
- Rose Smoothie, page 238
- Rustproofer #1, page 205
- Sage Relief, page 238
- Tomato Juice Cocktail, page 217

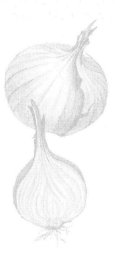

**Fruits and
vegetables**
lemons, onions, citrus
fruits, carrots

Herbs
astragalus, cayenne,
echinacea, elderflowers
and elderberries,
garlic, ginger,
licorice**, peppermint

Other
honey*****

** Avoid licorice if
you have high blood
pressure. The
prolonged use
of licorice is not
recommended under
any circumstances.

*** If you are pregnant,
limit your intake of
parsley to $1/2$ tsp
(2 mL) dried or one
sprig fresh per day.
Do not take parsley if
you are suffering from
kidney inflammation.

**** Do not take
sage if you have
high blood pressure
or are pregnant or
breastfeeding.

***** Do not feed
honey to children
under one year of age.

Fruits and vegetables

apples, pears, prunes, rhubarb, beets, leafy greens, leeks, onions

Herbs

burdock root, German chamomile, cinnamon, dandelion root, fennel seeds, garlic, ginger, lavender, lemon balm, licorice*, peppermint, yellow dock

Other

dried fruit, flax seeds, legumes, molasses, nuts, psyllium seeds, pumpkin seeds, sesame seeds, yogurt with active bacterial cultures

---

* Avoid licorice if you have high blood pressure. The prolonged use of licorice is not recommended under any circumstances.

Constipation

CONSTIPATION MAY BE CAUSED BY DISEASES, SUCH AS diverticulitis (see Diverticular Disease, page 40) or anemia (see Anemia, page 26), both of which require treatment. Less-serious causes include stress, lack of exercise, insufficient dietary fiber or the overuse of laxatives, which make the bowel lazy.

Constipation can often be relieved by increasing the amount of fiber in the diet, getting regular exercise and drinking an adequate amount of water (eight or more large glasses a day).

Constipation may be a result of either excessive relaxation or tension of the bowel muscles. Stimulation with cayenne or ginger can benefit a person who is too relaxed. A calming tea of German chamomile, lavender or lemon balm can relax a tense, overstimulated person. Dairy products cause constipation, especially in children. Replacing dairy products with soy or rice-based dairy substitutes often relieves constipation in a child.

What to Do

Maximize

- Whole foods
- Fiber (found in fresh, raw fruits and vegetables; legumes; nuts; seeds; and whole grains)
- Fluid intake (drink at least eight large glasses of water, juice and/or herbal tea daily)
- Bitter herbs (dandelion root; German chamomile; burdock leaf, root or seeds; ginger; fennel; yellow dock) to stimulate the bowel

Eliminate

- Refined foods

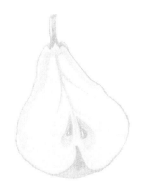

Healing Smoothies

- Anise Anise, page 235
- Apple Beet Pear, page 200
- Apple Pear, page 184
- Autumn Refresher, page 184
- Beet, page 201
- Blazing Beets, page 201
- Brocco-Carrot, page 202

- Green Gold, page 214
- Loosey-Goosey, page 172
- Prune, page 188
- Pump It Up, page 163
- Rhubarb Apple, page 190
- Spring Celebration, page 197

Depression

DEPRESSION, A PERSISTENTLY LOW MOOD, IS OFTEN accompanied by headaches, insomnia or constant drowsiness, inability to concentrate and low immunity. Although a long-term cure may require counseling, good nutrition promotes healing by helping to restore nervous-system function.

What to Do

Maximize

- A healthy diet
- Foods rich in B vitamins (whole grains, leafy greens) to improve nerve function
- Herbs that encourage relaxation and sleep and that counter stress and anxiety (borage, skullcap, St. John's wort, German chamomile, lemon balm)
- Herbs that support liver function (dandelion root, burdock root, rosemary)
- Nuts and seeds

Eliminate

- Artificial food additives, which can contribute to depression

Healing Smoothies

- Anti-Depression Tonic, page 223
- Brocco-Carrot, page 202
- C-Green, page 214
- Green Energy, page 232
- Smart Smoothie, page 239

Fruits and vegetables
black beans, broccoli, carrots, mangoes, soybeans, spinach, watercress

Herbs
borage, burdock root, cardamom, cayenne, cinnamon, cloves, dandelion root, garlic, German chamomile, ginger, ginkgo, lemon balm, oat seeds, parsley**, rosemary, skullcap, St. John's wort

Other
cereal grasses, evening primrose oil, flax seeds, kelp, nuts, oats (including bran), pumpkin seeds, sunflower seeds, whole grains

** If you are pregnant, limit your intake of parsley to 1/2 tsp (2 mL) dried or one sprig fresh per day. Do not take parsley if you are suffering from kidney inflammation.

Fruits and vegetables

apples, avocados, blueberries, grapefruit, lemons, limes, pears, broccoli, Jerusalem artichokes, leafy greens, onions

Herbs

cinnamon, cloves, coriander, dandelion root and leaf, evening primrose oil, fenugreek seeds, garlic, ginger, ginkgo, linden flower, stevia, turmeric, yarrow*

Other

fish oil, flax seeds, legumes, oats, extra-virgin olive oil, pumpkin seeds, spirulina, tofu, whole grains, unsweetened yogurt with active bacterial cultures

> * Avoid yarrow if you are pregnant.

Diabetes

DIABETES MELLITUS IS AN INSULIN DEFICIENCY THAT RESULTS in a high blood-sugar level. This deficiency affects the body's ability to metabolize carbohydrates, protein and fat, which often leads to an increase in the incidence of infections. It is important that a health-care practitioner monitor a patient with diabetes. If diabetes is not controlled, changes in the blood vessels can lead to high blood pressure and deterioration of circulation, causing kidney, nerve and eye problems.

Type I diabetes begins in childhood. The pancreas is unable to produce an adequate supply of insulin, so the disease is controlled with daily insulin injections.

Type II diabetes usually occurs in adulthood, and obesity is a major risk factor. The pancreas often produces sufficient insulin, but the body is unable to use it efficiently. High blood sugar can be reversed by diet and weight loss. In type II diabetes, diet and herbs can help regulate blood sugar, improve digestion and intestinal absorption of nutrients, support blood circulation and improve immunity.

What to Do

Maximize

- A mainly vegetarian diet of fresh organic fruits, vegetables, legumes and unrefined grains, which helps regulate blood sugar and boosts the immune system's ability to resist infection
- Omega-3 fatty acids (found in oily fish and fish oils, hemp oil, flax seeds, pumpkin seeds and soybean products), which are beneficial to blood circulation

Minimize

- Animal fats in meat and dairy products (replace some meat meals with fish and vegetable protein; replace dairy products with soy alternatives)

Eliminate

- Food allergies and intolerances (see Appendix A: Food Allergies, page 304)
- Dairy products
- Potatoes
- Dried fruits, sugar and sweeteners (except stevia and small amounts of raw honey)
- Fats and oils (except extra-virgin olive oil)
- Processed foods
- Refined foods
- Caffeine (found in coffee, black and green tea, and soft drinks)

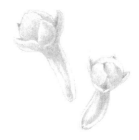

Other Recommendations

- Chronic stress affects sugar levels. Skullcap and oats can help calm nervous stress.

- Daily exercise makes an important contribution to regulating blood sugar levels.

Healing Smoothies

- Allium Antioxidant, page 232
- Apple Beet Pear, page 200
- Beta Blast, page 177
- Blue Cherry, page 163

- Green Energy, page 232
- Minestrone, page 203
- Spa Special, page 236

Diarrhea

DIARRHEA IS AN INFLAMMATION OF THE BOWEL CAUSED BY bacterial or viral infection, food allergies or intolerances, or malfunctions of the digestive system. Consult a health-care practitioner if diarrhea lasts longer than one week. Diarrhea causes dehydration, which can be life threatening for small children. In such cases, consult your health-care practitioner immediately.

What to Do

Maximize

- Water intake (to be safe, boil all water to eliminate any bacteria, then cool to drinking temperature)
- Herbal teas
- Starchy foods (potatoes, carrots, rice)

Minimize

- Raw fruits (except bananas), which can promote diarrhea
- Raw vegetables, as the fiber may irritate an inflamed bowel
- Dried fruits

Eliminate

- Alcohol, caffeine (found in coffee, black and green tea, chocolate and soft drinks), soft drinks
- Dairy products (except yogurt with active bacterial cultures)
- Sugar and sweeteners
- Food allergies and intolerances (see Appendix A: Food Allergies, page 304)

HEALING FOODS

Fruits and vegetables
cooked apples, bananas, lemons, limes, carrots, potatoes

Herbs
cardamom, German chamomile, fennel seeds, ginger, lemon balm, meadowsweet, nutmeg, red raspberry leaves, slippery elm bark powder

Other
evening primrose oil, flax seeds, pumpkin seeds, rice, sunflower seeds, whole grains, yogurt with active bacterial cultures

- Slippery Banana, page 240
- Vichyssoise (use yogurt with active bacterial cultures in place of milk, cream or tofu), page 211

HEALING FOODS

Fruits and vegetables
apples, bananas, grapes, mangoes, pears, prunes, broccoli, cabbage, carrots, celery, leafy greens, watercress

Herbs
cinnamon, fenugreek seeds, garlic, German chamomile, ginger, licorice*, marshmallow leaf and root, peppermint, psyllium seeds, slippery elm bark powder, valerian**

Other
flax seeds, legumes, oats, spirulina, wheat bran, whole grains, yogurt with active bacterial cultures

> ★ Avoid licorice if you have high blood pressure. The prolonged use of licorice is not recommended under any circumstances.

Diverticular Disease
Diverticulitis & Diverticulosis

DIVERTICULOSIS IS CHARACTERIZED BY THE PRESENCE OF multiple small pouches (diverticula) on the large intestine. Diverticulitis occurs when these pouches become inflamed. It is usually associated with constipation and caused by a low-fiber diet. Symptoms typically include continuous pain on the left side of the abdomen, flatulence and, sometimes, diarrhea.

What to Do

Maximize

- Fruits and vegetables
- Whole grains and legumes
- Water intake (drink at least eight large glasses daily)

Minimize

- Animal protein in meat and dairy products

Other Recommendations

- Gradually introduce a high-fiber diet to avoid digestive problems.
- During periods of inflammation, avoid high-fiber foods (raw vegetables, bran), which can irritate the bowel.
- Drink plenty of healing vegetable juices (spinach, cabbage, beet, garlic, carrot) with the addition of soothing slippery elm bark powder.

Eliminate

- Caffeine (found in coffee, black and green tea, chocolate and soft drinks)
- Alcohol
- Fried foods
- Pickled foods
- Ham, bacon and fatty meats
- Refined and processed foods
- Spicy foods
- Sugar
- Dairy products (except yogurt with active bacterial cultures)
- Constipation, if present (see Constipation, page 36)

Healing Smoothies

- Mango Madness, page 175
- Popeye's Power, page 229
- Prune, page 188
- Slippery Banana, page 240

Endometriosis

ENDOMETRIOSIS IS A CONDITION IN WHICH TISSUE THAT IS normally found in the uterus wall, or endometrium, is found in places outside the uterus, such as the bladder, bowel or fallopian tubes. This tissue responds to a woman's monthly hormonal cycle, shedding blood at these sites. Symptoms can include pain, irregular bleeding, depression and bowel problems.

What to Do

Maximize

- Antioxidants (preferably from vegetable sources) to support the immune system in eliminating imperfect or misplaced tissues
- Essential fatty acids (found in nuts, seeds and grains), which have a healing effect

Minimize

- Animal protein in meat and dairy products. Use organic meats, which are sure to be hormone-free, if possible
- Fruits, which may contribute to blood-sugar problems. Candida (see page 33) is often associated with endometriosis

Eliminate

- Sugar and sweeteners
- Yeast and foods made with yeast (bread)
- Coffee
- Alcohol
- Junk food
- Food allergies and intolerances (see Appendix A: Food Allergies, page 304). Dairy and wheat products are common culprits

Other Recommendations

- Balance hormones with chasteberry (*Vitex agnus-castus*).
- Take analgesic herbs (German chamomile, meadowsweet, passionflower, rosemary, valerian) for pain.
- Take nervous-system tonics (passionflower, valerian).
- Use turmeric for its antimicrobial/antiseptic/anti-inflammatory properties.
- Consume herbs that support the liver (calendula, dandelion root, rosemary).
- Evening primrose oil is antidepressant and helps to support the immune system in eliminating imperfect or misplaced tissues.

Fruits and vegetables
apples, apricots, cherries, grapefruit, strawberries, beets, broccoli, cabbage, leafy greens, peas, red and green bell peppers, squash, sweet potatoes

Herbs
calendula, chasteberry, dandelion leaf and root, evening primrose oil, German chamomile, meadowsweet, passionflower, rosemary, turmeric, valerian**

Other
barley, fish oils, legumes, nuts, oats, extra-virgin olive oil, seeds, tofu, whole grains, soy yogurt with active bacterial cultures

** Valerian has an adverse effect on some people.

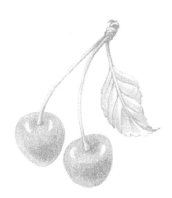

Healing Smoothies

- Beet, page 201
- Cherry Sunrise, page 164
- Peas Please, page 199

Eye Problems
Cataracts, Glaucoma & Macular Degeneration

RESEARCH SHOWS THAT YOUR RISK OF CATARACTS, GLAUCOMA and macular degeneration decreases if you eat a diet rich in antioxidants.

What to Do

Maximize

- Antioxidant-rich fruits and vegetables to protect the eyes from free-radical damage. Carrot juice, spinach and blueberries are especially effective
- Fresh garlic, which is strongly antioxidant

Minimize

- Fat in meat and dairy products

Eliminate

- Refined foods
- Fried foods
- Sugar and sweeteners

Healing Smoothies

- Black Pineapple, page 161
- Blue Water, page 163
- Blueberry, page 162
- C-Blend, page 166
- C-Blitz, page 166
- Citrus Cocktail, page 165
- Liquid Gold, page 185
- Mango Madness, page 175
- Squash Special, page 215
- Sunrise Supreme, page 173
- Tomato Juice Cocktail, page 217

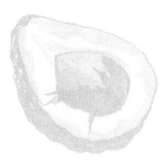

Fatigue

FATIGUE IS A SYMPTOM OF MANY DISEASES — INCLUDING anemia, diabetes, hepatitis, hypoglycemia and thyroid disease — and can be determined by blood tests and diagnosed by your doctor. Common nondisease factors often come from a lack of lifestyle balance, which includes diet, exercise, work and social life. A balanced diet provides the digestive enzymes the body requires for processing nutrients and converting food into energy.

What to Do

Maximize

- Fresh fruits and vegetables
- Whole grains
- Nuts and seeds
- Essential fatty acids

Minimize

- Fat in meat and dairy products
- Fried foods

Eliminate

- Caffeine and sugar, which can cause fatigue
- Refined flour products, which rob the body of nutrients
- Processed foods, which are often low in nutrients and high in chemical additives
- Margarine, shortening and salad oils (except extra-virgin olive oil)
- Alcohol

Other Recommendations

- Exercise daily, according to your fitness level.
- Eat smaller, more-frequent meals to maintain a constant blood-sugar level.
- Practice stress-reduction techniques, such as yoga, tai chi and meditation. Stress depletes vitality.
- Take herbs that support the liver (dandelion root, burdock root) to stimulate metabolism and remove toxins that can cause fatigue.

Healing Smoothies

- Apple Fresh, page 156
- B-Vitamin, page 187
- Brocco-Carrot, page 202
- Eye Opener, page 165
- Green Energy, page 232
- Mango Madness, page 175
- Pineapple-C, page 191
- Spiced Carrot, page 205
- Sunrise Supreme, page 173
- Taste of the Tropics, page 181

Fruits and vegetables
bananas, grapes, limes, mangoes, oranges, pineapple, strawberries, broccoli, carrots, leafy greens, onions, spinach, watercress

Herbs
alfalfa, burdock root, cardamom, cayenne, cinnamon, cloves, dandelion leaf and root, garlic, ginger, ginseng**, licorice***, parsley*, peppermint, red raspberry leaf, rose hips, stinging nettle, yellow dock

Other
almonds, cereal grasses, dates, fish oil, flax seeds, oats, pumpkin seeds, sea herbs, sunflower seeds, whole grains, tofu, wheat germ, yogurt with active bacterial cultures

** Do not take ginseng if you have high blood pressure or if you drink coffee. Never take ginseng daily for longer than four weeks.

*** Avoid licorice if you have high blood pressure. The prolonged use of licorice is not recommended under any circumstances.

Fruits and vegetables

apples, beets, broccoli, cabbage, cauliflower, celery, fennel, green beans, Jerusalem artichokes, onions, squash, sweet potatoes, watercress

Herbs

alfalfa, astragalus, burdock root and seeds, calendula, dandelion leaf and root, echinacea, evening primrose oil, garlic, licorice*, milk thistle, parsley**, passionflower, slippery elm bark powder, St. John's wort, turmeric

Other

barley grass, fish oils, flax seeds, legumes, pumpkin seeds, soy products, sunflower seeds, unsweetened yogurt with active bacterial cultures, whole grains (especially brown rice)

---

* Avoid licorice if you have high blood pressure. The prolonged use of licorice is not recommended under any circumstances.

** If you are pregnant, limit your intake of parsley to 1/2 tsp (2 mL) dried or one sprig fresh per day. Do not take parsley if you are suffering from kidney inflammation.

Fibromyalgia

FIBROMYALGIA IS CHARACTERIZED BY TENDER, ACHING muscles, joint pain similar to that of rheumatoid arthritis, fatigue and sleep disturbances. The areas typically affected are the neck, shoulders, lower back, chest and thighs. It is considered a form of chronic fatigue syndrome, with pain rather than fatigue as the dominant feature. Depression is often a feature, due to lack of sleep. The cause can be viral or a buildup of toxins. Food, drugs, allergies and nutritional deficiencies can also be involved. Neither the cause nor the cure is well understood, but good nutrition can help recovery.

What to Do

Maximize

- Antioxidant-rich vegetables
- Vegetable protein (see Guidelines to Good Health, page 10)
- Nuts and seeds
- Legumes

Minimize

- Fruits, which may contribute to low blood sugar (see Hypoglycemia, page 53)

Other Recommendations

- Eat oily fish (salmon, mackerel, sardines, tuna) two or three times a week.
- Practice stress-reduction techniques, such as tai chi, yoga and meditation.
- Exercise daily, according to your fitness level.

Eliminate

- Sugar; products that contain sugar; and high-sugar fruits, such as dried fruit, bananas and watermelon
- Refined flour
- Artificial food additives
- Alcohol
- Food allergies and intolerances (see Appendix A: Food Allergies, page 304). Gluten (in wheat products) and members of the nightshade family (potatoes, tomatoes, eggplant and all peppers) often cause problems
- Caffeine (found in coffee, black and green tea, chocolate and soft drinks), which decreases mineral absorption and contributes to the condition
- Dairy products (replace with soy- or rice-based alternatives)
- Salty and pickled foods
- Fried foods
- Pork, shellfish and fatty meats

Healing Smoothies

- Allium Antioxidant, page 232
- Apple Beet Pear, page 200
- Beet, page 201
- Blazing Beets, page 201
- Brocco-Carrot, page 202
- Minestrone, page 203
- Rustproofer #2, page 214

Flatulence

GAS IS A NORMAL RESULT WHEN FOOD IS DIGESTED. FOODS high in carbohydrates, such as beans, produce more gas because they are not entirely broken down by digestive enzymes. When bacteria ferment the undigested carbohydrates, gas is released. Other foods produce excess gas when the digestive enzyme they require is not available. The most common example is the enzyme needed to digest lactose in dairy products. Artificial sweeteners can also cause gas.

Changing your diet to include more high-fiber foods, such as beans and legumes, may also increase the incidence of gas. Consequently, dietary changes intended to increase the quantity of fiber should be made gradually, over a four- to six-week period.

Tip: To reduce the "gas effect" of legumes, soak them overnight in plenty of water. Discard the soaking water before cooking and rinse the cooked legumes well before adding them to recipes. Cook beans (and other foods) that give you gas with the recommended herbs, which expel gas from the digestive tract.

HEALING FOODS

Fruits and vegetables
apples, kiwis, papayas

Herbs
basil, cardamom, cayenne, German chamomile, cinnamon, cloves, coriander, cumin, dill, fennel seeds, garlic, ginger, mustard seeds, peppermint, thyme

Other
yogurt with active bacterial cultures

What to Do

Maximize

- Digestive herbal teas, such as chamomile and fennel, between meals
- Food-combining techniques (see Appendix B: Food Combining, page 306), taking care to eat fruits at least half an hour before or two hours after meals

Eliminate

- Artificial sweeteners and all foods that contain them
- Dairy products

Healing Smoothies

- Apple Mint, page 157
- Apple Pie, page 157
- Digestive Drink, page 227
- Gas Guzzler, page 228

Fruits and vegetables
apples, blackberries, blueberries, cherries, citrus fruits, lemons, pears, raspberries, red grapes, asparagus, beets, broccoli, carrots, celery, leafy greens, radishes, tomatoes, watercress

Herbs
dandelion leaf and root, garlic, ginger, milk thistle, parsley*, turmeric

Other
flax seeds, lecithin, oats, extra-virgin olive oil, whole grains

* If you are pregnant, limit your intake of parsley to ½ tsp (2 mL) dried or one sprig fresh per day. Do not take parsley if you are suffering from kidney inflammation.

Gallstones

CHOLESTEROL FROM ANIMAL FATS IS A MAJOR FACTOR IN THE formation of gallstones. Symptoms include indigestion, severe pain in the upper right abdomen, constipation, flatulence, nausea and vomiting. If a gallstone remains stuck in the bile duct, causing inflammation, it may need to be surgically removed.

Vegetarians are less likely to develop gallstones than people who eat meat, and dietary changes can reduce the risk of gallstone formation.

What to Do

Maximize

- Vegetable protein (see Guidelines to Good Health, page 10)
- Fruits, vegetables and whole grains

Minimize

- Fatty meats
- Dairy products

Eliminate

- Sugar
- Refined foods
- Coffee

Other Recommendations

- Eat oily fish (salmon, mackerel, sardines, tuna) to help lower cholesterol levels.
- Consume bitter foods (dandelion leaf, endive, radicchio, watercress) to increase bile flow, which helps prevent gallstone formation.
- Increase consumption of extra-virgin olive oil to discourage gallstone formation.
- Food allergies and intolerances (see Appendix A: Food Allergies, page 304). Often, eggs, pork, onions, coffee, milk, corn, beans and nuts affect gallstone sufferers

Healing Smoothies

- Apple Beet Pear, page 200
- Apple Mint, page 157
- Autumn Refresher, page 184
- Beet, page 201
- Berry Best, page 177
- Brocco-Carrot, page 202
- C-Blitz, page 166
- C-Green, page 214
- Cherry Berry, page 164
- Digestive Drink, page 227
- Raspberry, page 189
- Red, Black and Blue, page 162
- Tomato Juice Cocktail, page 217
- Zippy Tomato, page 217

Gout

GOUT IS AN INFLAMMATORY JOINT PROBLEM CHARACTERIZED by increased production of uric acid, which is deposited in the joints, especially those of the fingers and toes. It may be hereditary or may be caused by the consumption of excess alcohol, meat or starchy food, which increases the production of uric acid. Decreasing the production of uric acid and increasing its excretion in the urine helps control gout.

What to Do

Maximize

- Water intake (drink at least eight large glasses daily) to assist in the elimination of uric acid
- A vegetarian diet
- Herbal teas that dissolve uric acid (celery seed) and help eliminate uric acid (dandelion leaf, stinging nettle)

Minimize

- Protein (chicken, turkey and whitefish are fine in moderation)
- Fat in meat and dairy products
- Salt and salty foods
- Eggs (those from free-range chickens are preferable)
- Wheat, which is acid forming (use brown rice and buckwheat, which produce less acid)

Eliminate

- Foods and substances that form acid in the body, including:
- pork and beef;
- preserved meats, such as salami;
- tomatoes and spinach;
- vinegar (except apple cider vinegar);
- refined sugar and flour;
- coffee and tea;
- cheese;
- artificial food additives; and
- alcohol.
- Foods that are high in purines, including:
- organ meats (kidney, liver);
- shellfish, herring, sardines, anchovies and mackerel;
- peanuts;
- asparagus;
- mushrooms; and
- legumes (peas, beans, lentils).

Healing Smoothies

- Berry Best, page 177
- Cherry Berry, page 164
- Gout Gone, page 225

Fruits and vegetables
apples, bananas, lemons, limes

Herbs
cumin, evening primrose oil, ginger, German chamomile, lavender, meadowsweet, slippery elm bark powder

Other
foods that are rich in B vitamins (whole grains, leafy greens)

Hangover

DRINKING TOO MUCH ALCOHOL CAN RESULT IN HEADACHE, fatigue, nausea, dizziness and depression, which together are called hangover. Hangovers occur because alcohol dehydrates the body, increases acidity in the digestive system, causes the loss of potassium and vitamins, and affects the liver and nervous system. You may get faster relief from hangover symptoms if you follow these recommendations, preferably before retiring.

What to Do

Maximize

- Water to hydrate the body before, during and after drinking
- Juices that are high in vitamin C
- Herbal teas that settle the stomach (chamomile)
- Slippery elm bark powder to protect the stomach from excess acid

Healing Smoothies

- Calming Chamomile, page 232
- Hangover Remedy, page 240
- Morning After, page 237
- Slippery Banana, page 240

Fruits and vegetables
apples, bananas, broccoli, leafy greens, watercress

Herbs
cayenne, evening primrose oil, German chamomile, lavender, lemon balm, linden flower, passionflower, rosemary, skullcap, thyme, valerian*

Headaches
(Non-Migraine)

HEADACHES, OTHER THAN MIGRAINES, CAN BE CAUSED BY many factors, including muscular and nervous tension, digestive disorders, blood pressure changes, low blood sugar, caffeine, alcohol or drug withdrawal, eye strain, food allergies, a stuffy room, weather changes or poor posture. Avoiding foods that are common headache triggers (see Eliminate, right) may help reduce the incidence of headaches.

What to Do

Maximize

- Foods that are high in magnesium (whole grains, legumes, sea herbs, wheat germ, apples, bananas, nuts, seeds, fish), which relaxes muscles and helps reduce spasms

Minimize

- Salt and salty foods
- Fatty foods

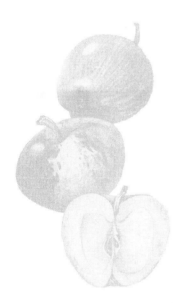

Eliminate

- Artificial food additives, especially monosodium glutamate (MSG)
- Food allergies and intolerances (see Appendix A: Food Allergies, page 304). Dairy products, wheat, corn, oranges and eggs commonly trigger headaches
- Meats preserved with nitrates (bacon, ham, hot dogs)
- Aspartame and foods that are sweetened with aspartame
- Caffeine (found in coffee, black and green tea, chocolate and soft drinks)
- Cheese and red wine

Other Recommendations

- Lemon balm and meadowsweet tea may help relieve headaches caused by digestive disorders.
- Skullcap and valerian* teas can be helpful for stress-related headaches.
- Antispasmodic herbs (cayenne, German chamomile, lemon balm, linden flower, passionflower, skullcap, thyme, valerian*) may help when a headache is caused by muscular tension.

Other
almonds, legumes, oats, sunflower seeds, tofu, walnuts, wheat germ, whole grains, yogurt with active bacterial cultures

> * Valerian has an adverse effect on some people.

Healing Smoothies

- Brocco-Carrot, page 202
- C-Green, page 214
- Green Energy (substitute skullcap for ginkgo), page 232

Fruits and vegetables
apples, apricots, blueberries, blackberries, cranberries, grapefruit*, grapes, kiwis, mangoes, melons, oranges, papayas, pineapple, strawberries, asparagus, avocados, broccoli, carrots, celery, leafy greens, lettuce, onions, parsnips, all peppers, peas, squash, watercress

Herbs
cayenne, dandelion leaf and root, fenugreek seeds, garlic, ginger, linden flowers, parsley**, rosemary, stinging nettle, turmeric

Other
almonds, barley, fish oil, kelp, lecithin, legumes, oats, extra-virgin olive oil, seeds (flax, pumpkin, sesame, sunflower), soy products, sprouted seeds and beans, walnuts, whole grains, yogurt with active bacterial cultures

Heart Problems
High Cholesterol, High Blood Pressure, Cardiovascular Disease, Heart Failure & Stroke

FAMILY HISTORY, CIGARETTE SMOKING, HIGH ALCOHOL consumption and high "bad" cholesterol are major risk factors for high blood pressure, circulation disorders and cardiovascular disease. In most cardiovascular diseases and circulation disorders, cholesterol deposits narrow the arteries, constricting the flow of blood.

Cholesterol is necessary to sustain life. There are two types in human blood: low-density lipoprotein (LDL, or "bad" cholesterol), which increases the risk of high blood pressure, heart disease and gallstones; and high-density lipoprotein (HDL, or "good" cholesterol), which reduces these risks. To improve health, eat a diet that lowers LDL and raises HDL.

What to Do

Maximize

- Fresh fruits and vegetables, whole grains, nuts and seeds, all of which help regulate blood pressure, reduce LDL and raise HDL
- Garlic and onions to reduce blood pressure and cholesterol
- Antioxidant-rich fruits and vegetables to help prevent cholesterol deposits from forming on artery walls
- Red grape juice to prevent blood clotting

Minimize

- Alcohol
- Coffee
- Eggs
- Salt and salty foods (processed foods)
- Sugar and products that contain sugar

Eliminate

- High-fat meats (such as bacon, pork, beef) and dairy products (except skim milk)
- Margarine and salad oils (except extra-virgin olive oil)
- Fried foods
- Pastries
- Milk chocolate
- Alcohol
- Refined sugar and flour
- Coconut

Other Recommendations

- Supportive therapy for heart problems includes daily exercise (such as walking for 30 minutes a day, depending on your level of fitness) and stress-reduction techniques, such as yoga, tai chi and meditation.

- Eat oily fish (salmon, mackerel, sardines, tuna) two to three times a week.
- Substitute vegetable protein for some meat meals (see Guidelines to Good Health, page 10).
- Use herbs (see left) to help lower cholesterol and improve circulation.

Healing Smoothies

- Allium Antioxidant, page 232
- Apple Fresh (use rosemary instead of ginseng), page 156
- Black Pineapple, page 161
- Brocco-Carrot, page 202
- C-Blend, page 166
- C-Blitz, page 166

- Citrus Cocktail, page 165
- Eye Opener, page 165
- Grape Heart, page 173
- Melon Morning Cocktail, page 178
- Spring Celebration, page 197

★ Avoid grapefruit if you are using calcium channel blocker medication.

★★ If you are pregnant, limit your intake of parsley to $\frac{1}{2}$ tsp (2 mL) dried or one sprig fresh per day. Do not take parsley if you are suffering from kidney inflammation.

★★★ Avoid licorice if you have high blood pressure. The prolonged use of licorice is not recommended under any circumstances.

Heartburn

HEARTBURN IS A BURNING SENSATION IN THE CHEST THAT is related to digestive problems. It may be caused by a hiatal hernia, indigestion or inflammation of the stomach. Check with your health-care practitioner to determine the cause. It is especially important to eliminate the possibility of heart disease. Frequent drinks of therapeutic fruit and vegetable juices, antacid herbs (dandelion root, meadowsweet) and soothing herbs (marshmallow root, slippery elm bark powder) can offer relief.

What to Do

Maximize

- Fresh fruits and vegetables
- Water intake (drink at least eight large glasses daily, between meals only)

- Slippery elm bark powder (especially at night) to protect the stomach from excess acid

HEALING FOODS

Fruits and vegetables
bananas, papayas, beets, cabbage, carrots, celery, cucumbers, parsnips

Herbs
calendula, cardamom, dandelion root, dill, fennel, ginger, German chamomile, licorice★★★, marshmallow root, meadowsweet, parsley★★, slippery elm bark powder

Other
flax seeds

Eliminate

- Coffee, soft drinks, alcohol and chocolate
- Fried, fatty and spicy foods
- Citrus fruits and tomatoes
- Pickled foods
- Refined flour and sugar
- Cigarette smoking
- Large meals
- Antacid and anti-inflammatory drugs, which can irritate the stomach lining

Minimize

- Acid-forming foods (meat, dairy products)

Healing Smoothies

- Beet, page 201
- Slippery Banana, page 240

- Beet, page 201
- Slippery Banana, page 240

Herpes Simplex
Cold Sores & Genital Herpes

HERPES SIMPLEX VIRUS TYPE 1 CAN CAUSE COLD SORES. Genital herpes is caused by herpes simplex virus type 2 and should always be treated by a doctor. Once contracted, the virus remains dormant in the nerve endings and may reactivate when triggered by factors such as lowered immune system function; high stress; alcohol; or certain foods, such as processed foods and foods that are high in arginine (see Eliminate, right). Diet can be used to complement therapy prescribed by a qualified health-care practitioner. The most effective therapy is to avoid outbreaks by keeping immunity high, managing stress and avoiding foods that trigger the virus. Herbs can help by supporting the immune system and nourishing the nerves, where the virus resides.

What to Do

Maximize

- Antioxidant-rich vegetables
- Fish (salmon, sardines, tuna, halibut), legumes and nutritional yeast. These foods are high in the amino acid lysine, which appears to inhibit the virus from replicating
- Antiviral herbs (astragalus, calendula, echinacea, garlic, lemon balm, St. John's wort)
- Immunity-boosting herbs (astragalus, echinacea, burdock (leaf, root or seeds)
- Antistress herbs (ginseng, St. John's wort, lemon balm)

HEALING FOODS

Fruits and vegetables
apples, apricots, berries, grapes, papayas, pears, asparagus, broccoli, cabbage, carrots, leafy greens, onions, squash, watercress

Herbs
astragalus, burdock (leaf, root and seeds), calendula, cayenne, cloves, dandelion root, echinacea, elderflowers, garlic, ginseng, lemon balm, parsley*, St. John's wort, yarrow**

Other
legumes (except chickpeas), nutritional yeast, sea herbs, sprouted beans, yogurt with active bacterial cultures

Health Conditions

Minimize

- Fruits
- Whole grains, seeds and brown rice. While these foods are high in arginine (see Eliminate, right), they can be balanced with vegetables that are high in lysine

Other Recommendations

- Practice stress-reduction techniques, such as meditation, yoga and breathing exercises.

Eliminate

- Foods that are high in arginine (nuts, wheat, caffeine, chocolate, carob, bacon, coffee, sugars, tomatoes, eggplants, all peppers, mushrooms). Arginine is an amino acid that encourages the herpes virus to replicate
- Alcohol, processed foods and refined foods, which depress the immune system

★ If you are pregnant, limit your intake of parsley to ¹/₂ tsp (2 mL) dried or one sprig fresh per day. Do not take parsley if you are suffering from kidney inflammation.

★★ Avoid yarrow if you are pregnant.

★★★ Avoid licorice if you have high blood pressure. The prolonged use of licorice is not recommended under any circumstances.

Healing Smoothies

- Allium Antioxidant, page 232
- Breakfast Cocktail, page 175
- Brocco-Carrot, page 202
- C-Green, page 214
- Herb-eze, page 223

Hypoglycemia

HYPOGLYCEMIA, OR LOW BLOOD SUGAR, IS A DISORDER characterized by an overproduction of insulin. Symptoms can include aches and pains, constant hunger, dizziness, headache, fatigue, insomnia, digestive disorders, palpitations, tremors, sweating, nausea and nervous tension. You may notice some of these symptoms if you miss a regular meal. Attention to diet can help control blood-sugar levels.

What to Do

Maximize

- Whole grains, vegetables and legumes
- Smaller meals, eaten more frequently
- Cruciferous vegetables (broccoli, cabbage, cauliflower) to help control blood sugar
- Protein with each meal

HEALING FOODS

Fruits and vegetables
apples, cherries, grapefruit, plums, raw beets, broccoli, cabbage, cauliflower, raw carrots, Jerusalem artichokes, leafy greens, tomatoes

Herbs
dandelion root, German chamomile, ginseng, licorice***

Other
cereal grasses, flax seeds, kelp, legumes, nuts, seeds, spirulina, whole grains, yogurt with active bacterial cultures

Minimize

- Sweet foods, including fruits (particularly bananas, watermelon and dried fruits)

Eliminate

- Refined flour and sugar
- Black tea, coffee, soft drinks and alcohol
- Cigarette smoking, which interferes with blood-sugar mechanisms

Healing Smoothies

- Cauliflower Cocktail, page 206
- Cherry Sunrise, page 164

Cauliflower Cocktail, page 206 · Cherry Sunrise, page 164

Fruits and vegetables
brightly colored fruits and vegetables, such as apricots, carrots, melons, broccoli, leafy greens

Herbs
astragalus, burdock (leaf, root and seeds), cayenne, cloves, echinacea, elderflower and elderberries, garlic, ginseng, green tea, licorice*, parsley**, red clover, rosemary, sage, St. John's wort, thyme, turmeric, yarrow***

Other
cereal grasses, legumes, nuts, seeds, shiitake mushrooms, whole grains, yogurt with active bacterial cultures

Immune Deficiency

A HEALTHY IMMUNE SYSTEM IS THE KEY TO RESISTING infections, allergies and chronic illnesses. The immune system protects and defends the body against viruses, bacteria, parasites and fungi. If it is not in top condition, it won't be able to resist these disease-causing agents. Balance in all areas of life — diet, exercise, mental perspective, social activity and spirituality — helps protect the immune system and keep it functioning well.

What to Do

Maximize

- Whole foods
- Fresh, raw, organic fruits and vegetables to provide the vitamins, minerals, digestive enzymes and antioxidants necessary for a healthy immune system
- Whole grains
- Essential fatty acids (found in legumes; nuts; seeds; and oily fish, such as salmon, mackerel, sardines and tuna), which is necessary for growth and maintenance of cells
- Fluid intake (drink at least eight large glasses of water, juice and/or herbal tea daily)

Minimize

- Non-organic meat, which is likely to contain antibiotics and steroid hormones, which depress immunity
- Excess animal fat, which suppresses immunity
- Antibiotics and corticosteroids. While these drugs can be lifesaving, overuse can deplete the immune system, causing more-complex health problems

Eliminate

- Sugar, which depletes vitamins and minerals, impairs the immune system and promotes yeast infections
- Refined, processed or preserved foods and soft drinks, which disrupt mineral levels in the body, leading to poor metabolism of essential fatty acids
- Artificial food additives and pesticides likely found in non-organic food
- Alcohol, which depresses immune function
- Margarine, salad dressings and cooking oils (except extra-virgin olive oil and some other cold-pressed oils)
- Nitrites in bacon and sausage, which are converted to toxic substances in the body
- Food allergies and intolerances (see Appendix A: Food Allergies, page 304). Dairy products, gluten, corn products, eggs, oranges, strawberries, pork, tomatoes, coffee, tea, peanuts and chocolate often affect the immune system

Other Recommendations

- Consume sufficient protein. Protein provides the amino acids necessary for building healthy tissue and organs and for antibody production.
- Optimize digestion to improve the absorption of nutrients (see Indigestion, page 57).
- Stress depletes the immune system. Practice stress-reduction techniques, such as yoga, meditation and tai chi.
- Use herbs that are immune-system regulators (astragalus, echinacea, garlic, licorice*, thyme).
- Use antibiotic herbs (burdock leaf, root and seeds; cayenne; cloves; echinacea; garlic; red clover flower; thyme).
- Use antiviral herbs (burdock leaf, root and seeds; elderflower and elderberries; garlic; ginger; lemon balm; licorice*; marjoram; St. John's wort; yarrow***).
- Use antioxidant herbs (astragalus, ginkgo, green tea, hawthorn, milk thistle, rosemary, sage, turmeric).

★ Avoid licorice if you have high blood pressure. The prolonged use of licorice is not recommended under any circumstances.

★★ If you are pregnant, limit your intake of parsley to ½ tsp (2 mL) dried or one sprig fresh per day. Do not take parsley if you are suffering from kidney inflammation.

★★★ Do not take yarrow if you are pregnant.

Healing Smoothies

- Allium Antioxidant, page 232
- Apple Beet Pear, page 200
- Berry Best, page 177
- Black Pineapple, page 161
- Blazing Beets, page 201
- Breakfast Cocktail, page 175
- Brocco-Carrot, page 202
- C-Green, page 214
- Cranberry Pineapple, page 168
- Grape Heart, page 173
- Ki-Lime, page 174
- Leafy Luxury (use apple juice), page 210
- Minestrone, page 203
- Rustproofer #2, page 214
- Spiced Carrot, page 205

Fruits and vegetables
all

Herbs
cinnamon, cayenne, dandelion leaf, evening primrose oil, garlic, ginger, ginkgo, ginseng, nutmeg, saw palmetto, stinging nettle

Other
legumes, fish oil, flax seeds, kelp, nuts, oats, sunflower seeds, pumpkin seeds, soy products, wheat germ

Impotence

IMPOTENCE, A MAN'S INABILITY TO ACHIEVE OR MAINTAIN AN erection, may be caused by stress, insufficient blood supply to the penis (from cholesterol deposits in the blood vessels), excess alcohol, drugs, tobacco, diabetes, prostate enlargement or low testosterone.

A whole-food diet helps provide the vitamins and minerals necessary for sexual health. Herbal circulatory stimulants, such as ginger and cayenne, are often helpful for impotence caused by deficient circulation. See Anxiety States, page 26, for suggestions on alleviating emotional stress.

What to Do

Maximize

- Fresh fruits and vegetables, whole grains, nuts and seeds
- Foods that contain vitamin E (whole-grain cereals, brown rice, nuts, seeds, wheat germ, soy products, kelp, dandelion leaf, extra-virgin olive oil) to protect the arteries that go to the penis from free-radical damage. Recent studies indicate better antioxidant effects occur when vitamin E comes from food rather than supplements

Minimize

- Animal protein (except for that in fish and chicken)

Eliminate

- Fried foods and junk foods
- Sugar
- Caffeine (found in coffee, black and green tea, chocolate and soft drinks)
- Refined flour
- Alcohol

Healing Smoothies

- B-Vitamin, page 187
- Blazing Beets, page 201
- Cajun Cocktail, page 207
- Flaming Antibiotic, page 208
- Green Energy, page 232

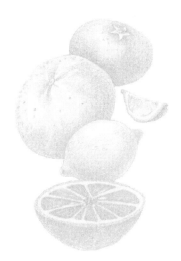

Indigestion

OVEREATING, IRREGULAR EATING, EXCESS ALCOHOL OR nervous tension may cause occasional indigestion. Symptoms can include abdominal discomfort, nausea or gastric reflux (flowing of stomach and small-intestine contents backward into the esophagus). Chronic indigestion can be caused by irritable bowel syndrome, food intolerances, ulcer or gallbladder disorder. Symptoms of chronic indigestion can include bloating, fatigue, diarrhea and constipation.

What to Do

Maximize

- Relaxed, unhurried meals
- Daily intake of yogurt with active bacterial cultures
- Antioxidant-rich fruits and vegetables
- Digestive herbal teas, such as chamomile, fennel, ginger, lemon balm or peppermint, taken regularly between meals

Minimize

- Alcohol
- Tea
- Eggs and meat

Eliminate

- Food allergies and intolerances (see Appendix A: Food Allergies, page 304)
- Sugar and artificial sweeteners
- Cold drinks, especially during or after meals
- Fruit juices
- High-fat and fried foods
- Dairy products (except yogurt with active bacterial cultures)
- Salty and spicy foods
- Refined foods
- Heavy meals
- Coffee

Natural Digestive Aids

- Acidophilus (see Yogurt, page 245). Lactobacillus acidophilus is "friendly" bacteria used to ferment milk into yogurt. This bacteria can replace intestinal bacteria necessary for digestion when it has been destroyed by antibiotics.

- Calendula (*Calendula officinalis*), page 93. Because it stimulates bile production, calendula aids digestion. Calendula may be included in smoothies (use 1 tbsp/15 mL fresh petals) and makes an attractive garnish for drinks.

HEALING FOODS

Fruits and vegetables
apricots, bananas, lemons, mangoes, melons, papayas, pineapple, Jerusalem artichokes, leafy greens, squash, sweet potatoes

Herbs
cardamom, cayenne, coriander seeds, dandelion root, dill, cinnamon, cumin, fennel, German chamomile, ginger, lemon balm, meadowsweet, peppermint, slippery elm bark powder, turmeric

Other
almonds, barley, apple cider vinegar, flax seeds, rice, yogurt with active bacterial cultures

To avoid indigestion, be sure to wait at least one hour after a meal before drinking fruit smoothies. If fruit is eaten immediately after a meal, digestive problems may result (see Appendix B: Food Combining, page 306).

- Cinnamon (*Cinnamomum zeylanicum*), page 97. A warming carminative used to promote digestion, cinnamon adds a pleasant taste to smoothies.
- Dandelion root (*Taraxacum officinale*), page 98. An easily obtained, fairly mild but bitter laxative. Dandelion stimulates the liver and gallbladder and increases the flow of bile to aid digestion. Dandelion leaf acts as a diuretic.
- Fennel (*Foeniculum vulgare*), page 101. Add a chopped fresh fennel bulb or an infusion of fennel seeds to smoothies to aid digestion and soothe discomfort from heartburn and indigestion.
- Fiber. Insoluble fiber in fruits, vegetables and whole grains helps prevent constipation and digestive diseases, such as diverticulosis and colon cancer.
- German chamomile (*Matricaria recutita*), page 103. As Peter Rabbit's mother knew, chamomile soothes upset tummies and inflammations and reduces flatulence and gas pains.
- Ginger (*Zingiber officinale*), page 103. Ginger is used to stimulate blood flow to the digestive system and to increase the absorption of nutrients. It increases the action of the gallbladder while protecting the liver against toxins.
- Kiwi (*Actinidia chinensis*), page 130. The enzymes in kiwis help digestion.
- Licorice (*Glycyrrhiza glabra*), page 109. Soothes gastric mucous membranes and eases spasms of the large intestine. Avoid licorice if you have high blood pressure.
- Papaya (*Carica papaya*), page 131. Papaya is a traditional remedy for indigestion. It contains an enzyme called papain, which is similar to pepsin, an enzyme that helps digest protein in the body.
- Peppermint (*Mentha piperita*), page 114. Because it contains flavonoids that stimulate the liver and gallbladder, peppermint increases the flow of bile. It has an antispasmodic effect on the smooth muscles of the digestive tract, making peppermint tea a good choice as an after-dinner drink.
- Pineapple (*Ananas comosus*), page 132. Pineapple is rich in the antibacterial enzyme bromelain. It is also anti-inflammatory and helps in the digestive process. Due to its digestive properties, raw pineapple prevents gelatin from setting and cannot be used in molded salads.
- Turmeric (*Curcuma longa*), page 122. Increases bile production and bile flow, which improves digestion.

Healing Smoothies

- Breakfast Cocktail, page 175
- Digestive Drink, page 227
- Peppermint Aperitif (replace ice cubes with $1/4$ cup/50 mL water), page 237
- Slippery Banana, page 240

Health Conditions

Infertility — Female

FACTORS THAT AFFECT FEMALE FERTILITY INCLUDE AGE, vaginal infections, artificial lubricants, surgical scarring, ovarian cysts, endometriosis, uterine fibroids, low thyroid function and diets deficient in the nutrients required for healthy pregnancy, stress relief and hormone balance.

The most important factor in ensuring a healthy pregnancy and birth is the mother's health before and during pregnancy. Whole, fresh, natural foods provide the vitamins and minerals necessary for good health. To help ensure the baby's good health, it is worth taking a few months to improve the mother's health before pregnancy.

An irregular menstrual cycle is a sign of hormonal imbalance. The herb chasteberry, also known as *Vitex agnus-castus* (see page 96), and herbs that support the liver, such as dandelion root (see page 99), may be used to regulate hormone production.

What to Do

Maximize

- Whole foods
- Antioxidant-rich fruits and vegetables
- Nuts and seeds
- Foods that contain folic acid (bulgur, orange juice, spinach, beans, sunflower seeds, wheat germ)

Minimize

- Acid-forming foods (meat, fish, grains, cheese, eggs, tea, coffee, alcohol, cranberries, plums, prunes, lentils, chickpeas, peanuts, walnuts), which can make cervical mucus acidic, which will destroy sperm

Eliminate

- Refined flour
- Cigarette smoking
- Sugar
- Artificial food additives

Other Recommendations

- Drink tea made from nerve-nourishing herbs (German chamomile, skullcap, oat straw) and regularly include relaxing activities, such as walking, meditation, yoga and tai chi, to reduce stress.
- Balance your intake of meat and fish protein (organic if possible) with vegetable protein, such as that in soybean products or beans with rice.

Healing Smoothies

- Apricot Peach, page 159
- B-Vitamin, page 187
- Beet, page 201
- Beta Blast, page 177
- Brocco-Carrot, page 202
- Raspberry, page 189
- Rustproofer #2, page 214

HEALING FOODS

Fruits and vegetables
apricots, oranges, peaches, raspberries, asparagus, avocados, beets, broccoli, carrots, leafy greens, sweet potatoes

Herbs
dandelion leaf and root, evening primrose oil, red clover flower, red raspberry leaf, rosemary, stinging nettle

Other
almonds, adzuki beans, Brazil nuts, bulgur, kidney beans, sea herbs, seeds (sunflower, pumpkin, flax, sesame), soy products, wheat germ, yogurt with active bacterial cultures

Fruits and vegetables
berries, cantaloupe, grapefruit, kiwis, oranges, strawberries, asparagus, avocados, broccoli, cabbage, cauliflower, leafy greens (especially spinach), red and green bell peppers

Herbs
astragalus, cayenne, ginger, ginkgo, ginseng, red raspberry leaf

Other
bran, fish oils, legumes, nuts, oats, seeds (especially sunflower and pumpkin), soybean products, whole grains

Infertility — Male

MALE INFERTILITY IS CHARACTERIZED BY LOW SPERM COUNT and low sperm motility (a situation in which the semen is too thick to allow proper sperm mobility). Causes can be related to a deficiency in dietary nutrients, hormone imbalance or stress. There is some evidence that suggests that the estrogens in pesticides and other chemical pollutants may be a cause of declining sperm counts over the past 50 years.

What to Do

Maximize

- Antioxidant-rich fruits and vegetables, especially those that contain vitamin C. Studies have shown that high sperm motility requires a sufficient intake of vitamin C
- Foods that contain zinc (seafood, legumes, whole grains, sunflower seeds, pumpkin seeds), which is required for sperm motility
- Herbs that improve circulation (cayenne, ginger) of all body fluids, including semen

Eliminate

- Alcohol, coffee, tea and soft drinks, which decrease sperm health

Minimize

- Iodized salt. Excess iodine lowers sperm count
- Refined foods (white rice, white flour, white sugar)
- Animal fats in meat and dairy products

Other Recommendations

- Drink tea made from nerve-nourishing herbs (German chamomile, skullcap, oat straw) and regularly include relaxing activities, such as walking, meditation, yoga and tai chi, to reduce stress.

Healing Smoothies

- Berry Fine Cocktail, page 189
- C-Blitz, page 166
- Citrus Cocktail, page 165

Health Conditions

Influenza

INFLUENZA (FLU) IS A VIRAL INFECTION OF THE RESPIRATORY tract. Symptoms include chills, fever, cough, headache, aches, fatigue and lack of appetite. Treating the flu early can shorten recovery time and help prevent more-serious disease. Top priorities are getting rest to allow the body's energies to focus on healing and drinking plenty of fluids to encourage the elimination of toxins.

Eating small meals, mainly of vegetable juices, reduces the energy required for digestion, allowing more energy to be focused on healing. "Hot" herbs, such as ginger and cayenne, increase body temperature, which discourages the influenza virus from multiplying.

What to Do

Maximize
- Fresh fruits and vegetables
- Fluid intake (drink at least eight large glasses of water, juice and/or herbal tea daily)

Eliminate
- Alcohol, sugar and sugar products, which decrease immunity

Healing Smoothies

- Brocco-Carrot, page 202
- Flaming Antibiotic, page 208
- Flu Fighter #2, page 229
- Hot Flu Toddy, page 230
- Pineapple Citrus, page 186
- Spring Celebration, page 197

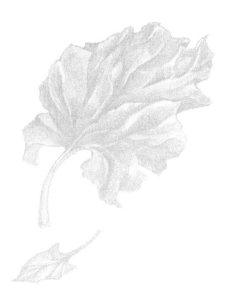

HEALING FOODS

Fruits and vegetables
lemons, oranges, pineapple, strawberries, broccoli, carrots, Jerusalem artichokes, spinach, watercress

Herbs
cayenne, cinnamon, echinacea, elderflower and elderberries, garlic, ginger, licorice*, parsley**, peppermint, thyme, yarrow***

Other
kelp, psyllium seed, well-cooked (mushy) rice

---

* Avoid licorice if you have high blood pressure. The prolonged use of licorice is not recommended under any circumstances.

** If you are pregnant, limit your intake of parsley to 1/2 tsp (2 mL) dried or one sprig fresh per day. Do not take parsley if you are suffering from kidney inflammation.

*** Do not take yarrow if you are pregnant.

Fruits and vegetables
apples, bananas, lettuce, leafy greens

Herbs
German chamomile, hops*, lavender, lemon balm, passionflower, skullcap, St. John's wort, valerian**, wild lettuce

Other
honey, nuts, oats, sunflower seeds, brown rice, yogurt with active bacterial cultures

---

★ Do not take hops if you are suffering from depression.

★★ Valerian has an adverse effect on some people.

Insomnia

INSOMNIA, OR THE INABILITY TO SLEEP, MAY BE CAUSED BY low blood-sugar levels (see Hypoglycemia, page 53), anxiety, depression, temperature (too hot or too cold) or caffeine ingestion. Foods high in B vitamins, calcium and magnesium supply nutrients that calm the nervous tension that can prevent sleep (see Anxiety States, page 26, and Depression, page 37).

What to Do

Maximize
- Calming, caffeine-free drinks
- Foods that are high in B vitamins (whole grains, leafy greens, broccoli, wheat germ), calcium (yogurt, tofu, broccoli) and magnesium (apples, avocados, dark grapes, nuts, brown rice)

Eliminate
- Alcohol
- Caffeine (found in coffee, black and green tea, chocolate and soft drinks)
- Artificial food additives

Healing Smoothies
- Almond Banana, page 159
- Sleepytime Smoothie, page 227

Fruits and vegetables
apples, apricots, kiwis, lemons, papayas, pineapple, broccoli, cabbage, carrots, spinach, tomatoes

Herbs
cinnamon, dandelion (root, leaves and flowers), fennel, German chamomile, ginger, lemon balm, licorice***, parsley****, peppermint, slippery elm bark powder

Irritable Bowel Syndrome

IRRITABLE BOWEL SYNDROME IS A LONG-STANDING BOWEL dysfunction for which no organic cause can be found. It is characterized by bloating, abdominal pain, and diarrhea or constipation. Healing factors include diet, stress management and elimination of allergens. Herbs can be used to soothe the intestines, reduce inflammation, improve digestion, calm the nerves and promote intestinal healing.

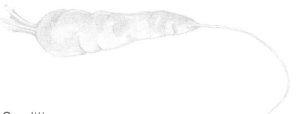

Maximize

- Fish and vegetable proteins (nuts, seeds, tofu, beans, legumes)
- Raw fruits and vegetables to provide immunity-boosting vitamins C and E, improve bowel function and eliminate toxins
- Flax seeds and flaxseed oil, which are soothing and anti-inflammatory and help heal the bowel and improve bowel function

Eliminate

- Alcohol
- Coffee
- Red meat
- Refined sugar and flour
- Artificial sweeteners
- Fats and oils (except extra-virgin olive oil)
- Foods allergies and intolerances (see Appendix A: Food Allergies, page 304). Common culprits are dairy products and citrus fruits
- Caffeine, wheat and corn

Healing Smoothies

- Beet, page 201
- Brocco-Carrot, page 202
- Calming Chamomile, page 232
- Cauliflower Cocktail, page 206
- Rustproofer #1, page 205
- Slippery Banana, page 240
- Spiced Carrot (omit cayenne), page 205

Other
flax seeds, nuts, oat bran, tofu, yogurt with active bacterial cultures

*** Avoid licorice if you have high blood pressure. The prolonged use of licorice is not recommended under any circumstances.

**** If you are pregnant, limit your intake of parsley to 1/2 tsp (2 mL) dried or one sprig fresh per day. Do not take parsley if you are suffering from kidney inflammation.

Kidney Stones

KIDNEY STONES ARE 60% LESS COMMON IN PEOPLE WHO follow vegetarian diets. A high-fiber, high-fluid, low-protein diet is the best preventive medicine. Diets high in animal protein encourage stone formation.

Kidney stones are usually made of calcium and oxalic acid. For this type of stone, limit foods that contain oxalic acid and large amounts of salt (sodium can stimulate calcium excretion). Stones that are made of uric acid and other minerals are less common. Eliminating shellfish can help prevent uric acid stones. Consult your health-care practitioner to determine which type of stone you have and what the possible causes are.

HEALING FOODS

Fruits and vegetables
apricots, mangoes, melons, peaches, asparagus, broccoli, celery, corn, fennel, leeks, onions

Herbs
goldenrod, marshmallow leaf and root, plantain, stinging nettle

Other
brown rice, seeds (flax, pumpkin, sesame, sunflower), whole grains

Maximize

- Water intake (drink at least two large glasses of water four times a day between meals) to flush out stones and prevent bacterial buildup
- Alkaline-forming foods (oranges, lemons, all vegetables) for uric acid stones

Minimize

- Animal protein in meat and dairy products

Eliminate

- Salt and high-sodium foods (bacon, processed foods)
- Sugar
- High-oxalate foods (leafy greens, rhubarb, coffee, tea, chocolate, grapefruit, parsley, peanuts, strawberries, tomatoes) for oxalic acid stones
- Seafood for uric acid stones
- Alcohol
- Refined flour

Other Recommendations

- Replace animal protein with soy and other vegetable proteins.
- Marshmallow leaf tea, which is soothing to the urinary system, may help break up stones.

Healing Smoothies

- Allium Antioxidant, page 232
- Apricot Peach, page 159
- Mango Madness, page 175
- Peachy Melon, page 183

Fruits and vegetables
all fruits, carrot juice

Herbs
garlic, ginger, sage*, thyme

Other
honey**

> * Avoid sage if you have high blood pressure or are pregnant or breastfeeding.
>
> ** Do not give honey to children under one year of age.

Laryngitis

LARYNGITIS IS AN INFLAMMATION OF THE VOCAL CORDS that may be associated with a cold or other infection, or caused by excessive use of the voice. It is important to rest the voice for a few days. If laryngitis is accompanied by fever and a cough or lasts longer than two days, consult your health-care practitioner.

What to Do

Maximize

- Fruits and fruit juices
- Herbal teas and gargles (thyme and sage)

- Apricot Peach, page 159
- C-Blend, page 166
- Beta Blast, page 177

Liver Problems

THE LIVER IS RESPONSIBLE FOR REMOVING TOXINS FROM the blood that can interfere with the functions of the heart, nervous system, digestive system and circulatory system. Excess fat, chemicals, intoxicants, and refined and processed foods disrupt liver function. Anger, nervous tension, mood swings, depression, skin problems, gallbladder problems, menstrual and menopausal difficulties and candida infections can result from poor liver function. It can be improved by diet, and the following dietary suggestions can complement traditional treatment of liver diseases, such as hepatitis, which must be treated by a physician.

What to Do

Maximize

- Fruits and vegetables
- Legumes and whole grains
- Bitter foods and herbs (asparagus; citrus peel; dandelion leaf, root and flowers; milk thistle seeds; German chamomile flowers) to stimulate liver function
- Water intake (drink at least eight large glasses of water daily)
- Dandelion root tea

Minimize

- Animal protein (replace with small amounts of fish and vegetable protein)

Eliminate

- Foods that interfere with liver function (animal fats, dairy products, eggs, refined foods, margarine, shortening, oils — except extra-virgin olive oil — alcohol, processed foods)
- Fried foods
- All tobacco products
- Sugar, sweets and junk foods
- Non-organic foods, which may contain pesticide residues or toxins

Healing Smoothies

- Apple Beet Pear, page 200
- Apple Fresh, page 156
- Beet, page 201
- Popeye's Power, page 229
- Sunrise Supreme (use blackberries instead of strawberries), page 173

HEALING FOODS

Fruits and vegetables
apples, blackberries, dark grapes, plums, raspberries, beets, carrots, celery, leafy greens, onions, tomatoes, watercress

Herbs
alfalfa, astragalus, burdock root, cayenne, dandelion leaf and root, fennel, fenugreek, German chamomile, ginger, lemon balm, licorice***, garlic, milk thistle, parsley****, rosemary, stinging nettle, turmeric, yellow dock

Other
cereal grasses, flax seeds, lecithin, legumes, extra-virgin olive oil, sea herbs, spirulina, whole grains

*** Avoid licorice if you have high blood pressure. The prolonged use of licorice is not recommended under any circumstances.

**** If you are pregnant, limit your intake of parsley to $1/2$ tsp (2 mL) dried or one sprig fresh per day. Do not take parsley if you are suffering from kidney inflammation.

Fruits and vegetables
apples, lemons, red grapes, beets, leafy greens, leeks, onions, watercress

Herbs
cayenne, cinnamon, cloves, fennel seeds, garlic, ginger, ginseng, mustard, parsley*, peppermint, rose petals, rosemary, stinging nettle

Other
almonds, Brazil nuts, fish oil, flax seeds, honey, legumes, oats, pumpkin seeds, soy products, cereal grasses, sunflower seeds, walnuts, wheat germ, whole grains

* If you are pregnant, limit your intake of parsley to 1/2 tsp (2 mL) dried or one sprig fresh per day. Do not take parsley if you are suffering from kidney inflammation.

Low Libido

YOU CAN REMEDY LOW LIBIDO, A LACK OF SEXUAL INTEREST or energy, by nourishing the reproductive organs and boosting your overall energy level. A diet that consists of whole foods, which provide basic vitamins and minerals, as well as valuable phytochemicals, will encourage sexual health. Antioxidant-rich fruits and vegetables improve circulation by preventing cholesterol deposits from forming on blood-vessel walls. The essential fatty acids in nuts and seeds are especially important in regulating sexual response. If stress is a factor, use nerve-nourishing oats, lemon balm or skullcap.

What to Do

Maximize

- Antioxidant-rich fruits and vegetables
- Nuts and seeds
- Whole grains
- Herbs that stimulate circulation and energy (cayenne, cinnamon, cloves, garlic, ginger, rosemary)
- Other herbs, such as ginseng, fennel, parsley*, nutmeg, lavender, mustard and rose, which have been traditionally used as aphrodisiacs

Minimize

- Meat

Eliminate

- Alcohol
- Coffee
- Dairy products
- Refined and processed foods
- Sugar

Healing Smoothies

- Allium Antioxidant, page 232
- Apple Fresh, page 156
- Beet, page 201
- Blazing Beets, page 201
- Green Energy, page 232

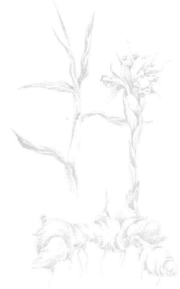

Lupus

THERE ARE TWO FORMS OF THIS AUTOIMMUNE DISEASE: discoid lupus erythematosus (DLE), which affects only the skin, and systemic lupus erythematosus (SLE), which affects the connective tissues throughout the body. In DLE, the skin lesions are red and scaly. Early symptoms of SLE are fatigue, weight loss and fever, which progress to arthritis-like joint pain. In the later stages, SLE may affect the kidneys and heart. Because this disease attacks the body's immune system, it is important to avoid viral infections, stress and fatigue. Nutrition and herbs can help by providing support and nourishment to the immune system and the organs through which detoxification takes place: skin, lungs, kidneys, liver and bowels. Relaxation exercises and plenty of sleep also support the immune system.

What to Do

Maximize

- Antioxidant-rich fruits and vegetables
- Water intake (drink at least eight large glasses of water daily) to eliminate toxins
- Essential fatty acids (found in nuts and seeds, especially freshly ground flax seeds) to strengthen the immune system and improve blood flow

Eliminate

- Animal protein in meat and dairy products, which contributes to the progression of lupus. Substitute vegetable proteins in soy products and legumes with rice
- Food allergies and intolerances (see Appendix A: Food Allergies, page 304). Keep a diet diary to note symptom changes in relation to food eaten
- Salad and cooking oils (except extra-virgin olive oil), which promote inflammation
- Sugar and alcohol, which inhibit immune function
- Alfalfa seeds and sprouts, which can cause inflammation

Other Recommendations

- Eat oily fish (salmon, mackerel, sardines and tuna), which provide healing omega-6 oils, three times a week.
- Use anti-inflammatory herbs (German chamomile, elderflower, fennel, ginger, meadowsweet, turmeric).
- Use herbs that help eliminate toxins (burdock leaf, root and seeds; dandelion root and leaf; parsley*).
- Consume herbs and foods that support the immune system (echinacea, garlic, shiitake mushrooms, cereal grasses).
- Exercise daily, according to your fitness level.

Fruits and vegetables
apples, apricots, blackberries, black currants, blueberries, cantaloupe, cherries, grapes, pineapple, avocados, broccoli, cabbage, carrots, cauliflower, fennel, leafy greens, onions, squash, watercress

Herbs
burdock root, dandelion root and leaf, echinacea, elderflower, evening primrose oil, fennel, garlic, ginger, lemon balm, licorice**, meadowsweet, parsley*, red clover flower, St. John's wort, stinging nettle, thyme, turmeric

Other
cereal grasses, fish oil, flax seeds, legumes, extra-virgin olive oil, seeds, shiitake mushrooms, soy products, whole grains, soy yogurt

> ** Avoid licorice if you have high blood pressure. The prolonged use of licorice is not recommended under any circumstances.

Healing Smoothies

- Apricot Peach, page 159
- Black Pineapple, page 161
- Brocco-Carrot, page 202
- C-Green, page 214
- Pine-Berry, page 186

HEALING FOODS

Fruits and vegetables
apples, avocados, bananas, berries, grapes, peaches, pears, asparagus, carrots, celery, fennel, green bell peppers, leafy greens, tomatoes, watercress

Herbs
dandelion root, fennel, garlic, ginseng, lemon balm, licorice*, motherwort, red clover flower, rosemary, sage

Other
dried fruits, flax seeds, lentils, sea herbs, soy products, sunflower seeds, extra-virgin olive oil, pumpkin seeds, wheat germ, whole grains, yogurt with active bacterial cultures

* Avoid licorice if you have high blood pressure. The prolonged use of licorice is not recommended under any circumstances.

Menopause

MENOPAUSE OCCURS WHEN MENSTRUATION CEASES. Hormonal changes around that transitional time can result in irregular menstruation and other symptoms, such as hot flashes, mood swings and vaginal dryness. Stress magnifies these symptoms.

After menopause, a woman's estrogen level decreases. Decreased estrogen is one of the many factors involved in the development of osteoporosis and heart disease. Daily exercise, relaxation and good diet will help you make a smooth transition and decrease your risk of heart disease and osteoporosis. Nutritional and herbal support help balance hormone levels, improve blood circulation, eliminate toxins and reduce nervous tension.

In addition to the transition-smoothing herbs listed on the left, use the following herbs for specific conditions and symptoms:

- chasteberry (also known as *Vitex agnus-castus*) to balance hormones;
- ginseng, skullcap or oats for stress and nervous tension;
- valerian for insomnia;
- black cohosh for joint pain, hot flashes or depression; and
- hawthorn berries for women with a family history of heart disease.

What to Do

Maximize
- Antioxidant-rich fruits and vegetables
- Nuts and seeds
- Whole grains

Minimize
- Animal fats in meat and dairy products

Eliminate
- Caffeine (found in coffee, black and green tea, chocolate and soft drinks)
- Sugar
- Cigarette smoking
- Alcohol

Healing Smoothies

- Apple Fresh, page 156
- Best Berries, page 191
- Green Energy (use ginseng instead of ginkgo), page 232
- Pear Fennel, page 184
- Peppery Tomato Cocktail, page 213
- Spring Celebration, page 197

Menstrual Disorders

AMENORRHEA (ABSENCE OF MENSTRUATION), DYSMENORRHEA (painful menstruation) and premenstrual syndrome (PMS) are often caused by a hormone imbalance, which is sometimes related to excess stress, exercise or animal products in the diet. Other factors can include poor circulation and insufficient blood or lymphatic circulation.

The natural approach is to:

- balance hormones;
- support blood (and lymphatic) circulation to the pelvic organs;
- promote relaxation, regular moderate exercise and good nutrition; and
- improve digestion and elimination to improve nutrient absorption and regulate hormones.

What to Do

Maximize

- Fruits and vegetables, especially those listed on the right

Minimize

- Salt and salty foods
- Alcohol

Other Recommendations

- Balance your intake of lean meat or fish protein with vegetable protein.
- Ensure that you get sufficient dietary calcium by eating foods such as yogurt, broccoli and tofu.
- Exercise daily, according to your fitness level.

Eliminate

- Refined foods, which lack minerals and vitamins and contain potentially harmful additives
- Caffeine (found in coffee, black and green tea, chocolate and soft drinks), which depletes calcium and other minerals
- Sugar and sweeteners
- Non-organic meat and dairy products, which can contain artificial hormones and toxins

HEALING FOODS

Fruits and vegetables
apricots, blueberries, blackberries, citrus fruits, grapes, strawberries, beets and beet greens, broccoli, carrots, leafy greens

Herbs
chasteberry, dandelion root and leaf, evening primrose oil, garlic, ginger, parsley**, skullcap, stinging nettle, yarrow***

Other
almonds, dulse, fish oil, flax seeds, kelp, lecithin, legumes, nuts, pumpkin seeds, sesame seeds, soy products, sunflower seeds, whole grains

** If you are pregnant, limit your intake of parsley to 1/2 tsp (2 mL) dried or one sprig fresh per day. Do not take parsley if you are suffering from kidney inflammation.

*** Do not take yarrow if you are pregnant.

HEALING FOODS

Fruits and vegetables
blackberries, cantaloupe, beets, broccoli, carrots, celery, leafy greens, onions

Herbs
cayenne, cinnamon, dandelion leaf and root, feverfew, garlic, German chamomile, ginger, lemon balm, parsley*

Other
brown rice and rice bran, flax seeds, legumes, pumpkin seeds, sunflower seeds, whole grains

> * If you are pregnant, limit your intake of parsley to 1/2 tsp (2 mL) dried or one sprig fresh per day. Do not take parsley if you are suffering from kidney inflammation.

Migraines

A MIGRAINE HEADACHE STARTS WITH THE CONSTRICTION OF blood vessels in the brain, which is then followed by an expansion, which causes pain. Warning symptoms (such as vision changes or mood swings) can come with the blood-vessel constriction. The pain usually starts on one side of the head, but may spread to both sides, and may be accompanied by nausea or dizziness. Migraine triggers can include strong emotions, hormonal changes, food allergies and some medications, including oral contraceptives.

What to Do

Maximize

- Vegetable protein
- Fresh fruits and vegetables

Minimize

- Animal fats in meat and dairy products
- Sugar

Eliminate

- Caffeine (found in coffee, black and green tea, chocolate and soft drinks)
- Foods that precipitate migraine attacks by causing constriction of the blood vessels (red wine, cheese, corn, smoked or pickled fish, sausages, hot dogs and all other preserved meats, pork, shellfish, walnuts)
- Artificial food additives
- Alcohol
- Food allergies and intolerances (see Appendix A: Food Allergies, page 304), which are usually the cause of migraine headaches. Migraine sufferers are commonly intolerant of dairy products, wheat, eggs, oranges and/or monosodium glutamate (MSG). When food allergies and intolerances are alleviated, the incidence of migraines is either eliminated or greatly reduced

Other Recommendations

- Eat oily fish (salmon, mackerel, sardines and tuna) two or three times a week to maintain steady blood flow to the brain.

- Eat a leaf or two of fresh feverfew daily.
- Practice food-combining techniques (see Appendix B: Food Combining, page 306).

Healing Smoothies

- Beet, page 201
- Brocco-Carrot, page 202

- C-Green, page 214
- Migraine Tonic, page 231

Multiple Sclerosis

MULTIPLE SCLEROSIS IS THE BREAKDOWN OF THE PROTECTIVE myelin sheaths around the brain and spinal cord. Symptoms may include muscular weakness, numbness, blurred vision, light-headedness and urinary incontinence. Although a cure is not known, dietary changes, such as those recommended below, have shown impressive results in slowing the disease's progress by preventing the breakdown of myelin sheaths and returning to health.

What to Do

Maximize

- Foods that are low in saturated fat
- Essential fatty acids (found in evening primrose oil, flax seeds, fish oils)
- Immunity (see Immune Deficiency, page 54)
- Foods that are high in B vitamins (fish, wheat germ, sea herbs) and magnesium (apples, avocados, bananas, leafy greens, fish, nuts, soy products, brown rice, wheat germ) to nourish nerve tissue
- Lifestyle quality. Evaluate and reduce stress in your life by practicing meditation, yoga, tai chi or taking daily long walks in natural surroundings

Minimize

- Animal fats

Eliminate

- Candida infections (see Candida, page 33)
- Food allergies and intolerances (see Appendix A: Food Allergies, page 304)
- Coffee
- Red meat and dark meat of chicken or turkey
- Dairy products and eggs
- Gluten
- Fats and oils (except cold-pressed oils, such as extra-virgin olive oil)

Healing Smoothies

- Almond Banana, page 159
- B-Vitamin, page 187
- Beet, page 201
- Minestrone, page 203
- Smart Smoothie, page 239

HEALING FOODS

Fruits and vegetables
all raw fruits, except those that are acid forming (cranberries, plums, prunes). Broccoli, cabbage, leafy greens and watercress are especially good sources of calcium

Herbs
alfalfa, dandelion leaf, German chamomile, oat straw, parsley*, plantain, stinging nettle

Other
blackstrap molasses, dried fruits, fish and fish oil, legumes, nuts, seeds, feta cheese, sardines, salmon, spirulina, tofu, whole grains, yogurt with active bacterial cultures

Sea herbs are especially good sources of calcium

* If you are pregnant, limit your intake of parsley to ¹/₂ tsp (2 mL) dried or one sprig fresh per day. Do not take parsley if you are suffering from kidney inflammation.

Osteoporosis

OSTEOPOROSIS IS A DISEASE CHARACTERIZED BY PROGRESSIVE bone loss and decreased bone density and strength. It is caused when bones lose calcium. Consumption of calcium- and nutrient-rich foods helps keep bones strong. In order for the body to absorb calcium, it requires adequate levels of certain vitamins and minerals, especially vitamin D and magnesium.

Factors in bone loss are:

- age;
- decreased estrogen level (estrogen enhances calcium absorption);
- not doing weight-bearing exercise, which decreases calcium absorption (doing weight-bearing exercise increases it);
- some prescription drugs, such as corticosteroids, anticonvulsants, diuretics and antacids, which contain aluminum, which interferes with calcium absorption;
- chronic stress, which depletes calcium;
- lack of minerals and vitamins in the diet, which inhibits calcium absorption; and
- disease of the thyroid or adrenal glands.

What to Do

Maximize

- Foods that promote calcium absorption:
- raw fruits;
- green vegetables;
- nuts and seeds; and
- legumes.

Minimize

- Foods high in oxalic acid (almonds, Swiss chard, rhubarb, spinach), which inhibits calcium uptake
- Foods that use up calcium while being metabolized by the body (citrus fruits, vinegar, wine)

- Sodium fluoride (found in drinking water, soft drinks, canned food, preserved meats, boxed cereals, and residues of insecticides and fertilizers on commercially grown produce). Although fluoride is needed in bone formation, an excess inhibits the process.
- Sugar, salt and caffeine, which cause calcium to be excreted through the urine;
- Alcohol;
- High-protein (meat and dairy) diets, which lead to bone loss through calcium excretion in the urine. (This is partly because calcium is used in the process of protein breakdown.) Moderate amounts of fish, poultry, eggs and dairy products can be included in the diet. Note that a lack of protein will also cause weakness in the whole system, including all of the bone-making organs and systems

- Phosphorus-rich foods, especially soft drinks, which contribute most to bone loss. Although phosphorous is necessary to bone health, an excess inhibits calcium metabolism
- Refined flour, which is nutrient-depleted, leading to a loss of minerals in the diet
- Vegetables in the nightshade family (tomatoes, potatoes, eggplants, all peppers), which contain the calcium inhibitor solanine
- Commercially prepared foods that contain chemicals, which add toxins and deplete minerals
- Food grown with non-organic fertilizers, which cause depletion of their minerals
- Grains and brans, particularly raw bran, which are high in phytic acid, which binds to calcium, making it unavailable to the body. Soak grains overnight to neutralize the phytic acid and make the vitamins and minerals available to the body

Healing Smoothies

- Apple Beet Pear, page 200
- Avocado Pineapple, page 197
- B-Vitamin, page 187
- Beet, page 201
- Black Pineapple, page 161
- Brocco-Carrot, page 202
- C-Green, page 214
- Cherry Berry, page 164
- Eye Opener, page 165
- Leafy Luxury, page 210
- Red, Black and Blue, page 162
- Rustproofer #2, page 214
- Watercress, page 219

Fruits and vegetables

apples, blackberries, cherries, citrus fruits, grapes, pineapple, strawberries, watermelon, asparagus, broccoli, cabbage, celery, cucumber, fennel, leafy greens, lettuce, Jerusalem artichokes, radishes, watercress

Herbs

cayenne, chickweed, dandelion leaf and root, evening primrose oil, fennel, garlic, ginger, parsley*, psyllium seeds

Other

cider vinegar, flax seeds, kelp, legumes, soy products, walnuts, whole grains

---

* If you are pregnant, limit your intake of parsley to 1/2 tsp (2 mL) dried or one sprig fresh per day. Do not take parsley if you are suffering from kidney inflammation.

Overweight

EXCESSIVE WEIGHT IS MOST OFTEN CAUSED BY INSUFFICIENT exercise relative to the amount eaten. In a few cases, weight gain can be attributed to hormonal imbalances and some drugs (including corticosteroids and birth control pills). Long-term weight loss is most effectively achieved by adopting a whole-food diet and increasing exercise.

What to Do

Maximize

- Fresh fruits and vegetables, which help speed up the metabolism and eliminate toxins
- Water intake (drink at least eight large glasses daily) to reduce appetite and eliminate toxins

Minimize

- Refined flour products, fast foods and junk foods
- Fats in meat, dairy products and salad oils (except extra-virgin olive oil)
- Starchy foods (breads, corn, parsnips, potatoes, squash, sweet potatoes)

Eliminate

- Sugar and artificial sweeteners
- Fried foods
- Artificial food additives
- Food allergies and intolerances (see Appendix A: Food Allergies, page 304). Milk products, eggs, oranges and gluten may affect digestion

Other Recommendations

- Eat oily fish (salmon, sardines, mackerel, tuna) two or three times a week to help the body burn excess fat.
- Eat fruit between meals for optimum digestion and to discourage snacking on inappropriate foods.
- Exercise daily, according to your fitness level.
- Replace empty-calorie drinks and snacks with nutrient-rich smoothies.

Healing Smoothies

- B-Vitamin, page 187
- Black Pineapple, page 161
- C-Green, page 214
- Popeye's Power, page 229
- Sea-Straw, page 191

Parkinson's Disease

SYMPTOMS OF PARKINSON'S DISEASE INCLUDE MUSCLE RIGIDITY, loss of reflexes, slowness of movement, trembling and shaking. It is caused by the degeneration of nerve cells within the brain, which leads to a deficiency of the neurotransmitter dopamine. While there is no cure for Parkinson's disease, dietary therapy can help prevent further degeneration of neurons by neurotoxins. Choose foods that are high in antioxidants and avoid pollutants by choosing fresh, organic foods.

What to Do

Maximize

- Raw antioxidant-rich organic fruits and vegetables to optimize vitamin and mineral intake and provide digestive enzymes
- Legumes, nuts and seeds (especially sunflower seeds) to provide vitamin E, which can slow progression of the disease

Minimize

- Animal protein in meat and dairy products, which aggravates symptoms

Eliminate

- Refined and processed foods
- Sugar and artificial sweeteners
- Alcohol
- Wheat and liver, which contain manganese, which may aggravate the disease
- Fatty foods, fried foods, margarine and oils (except extra-virgin olive oil)

Other Recommendations

- Eat fava beans (broad beans), which contain levodopa, a precursor to dopamine. Eating $1/2$ cup (125 mL) a day can decrease the amount of medication required. Discuss this with your doctor to avoid overdosing.
- Passionflower can help reduce tremors.
- Ginkgo improves blood circulation to the brain, bringing it more nutrients, which helps prevent cell damage.
- Avoid antacids, cookware, deodorants and water that contain aluminum, which may have adverse effects on Parkinson's sufferers.
- Ground flax seeds help cure and prevent constipation and provide essential fatty acids to nourish brain and nerve tissue.
- Oily fish (salmon, sardines, mackerel, tuna) provides essential fatty acids that nourish brain and nerve tissue.

HEALING FOODS

Fruits and vegetables
bananas, blueberries, strawberries, beets, carrots, leafy greens, lettuce, potatoes

Herbs
alfalfa, evening primrose oil, ginger, ginkgo, milk thistle seed, passionflower, St. John's wort

Other
legumes, nuts, oats, extra-virgin olive oil, peanuts, seeds (flax, sesame, sunflower, pumpkin), soy lecithin, spelt flour, whole grains (except wheat)

Healing Smoothies

- Beet, page 201
- C-Green, page 214
- Eye Opener, page 165
- Smart Smoothie, page 239
- Spa Special, page 236
- Pump It Up (use flax seeds instead of protein powder), page 163

HEALING FOODS

Fruits and vegetables
apples, apricots, bananas, blueberries, cantaloupe, cherries, red grapes (with seeds), mangoes, papayas, pears, avocados, cabbage, carrots, cucumbers, broccoli, leafy greens, onions, watercress

Herbs
calendula, cinnamon, cloves, dandelion root, echinacea, garlic, German chamomile, ginger, green tea, licorice*, marshmallow root, meadowsweet, parsley**, slippery elm bark powder, turmeric

Other
barley, cereal grasses, extra-virgin olive oil, honey, legumes, seeds, oats

Peptic Ulcers
Gastric & Duodenal Ulcers

STOMACH AND INTESTINAL ULCERS, CALLED PEPTIC ULCERS, occur when the protective mucous lining of the stomach or intestine breaks down. Ulcers can be caused by infection from *Heliobacter pylori* bacteria; a breakdown of the protective mucous lining of the intestine caused by steroid medications, such as Aspirin, or nonsteroidal anti-inflammatory medications, which increase acid secretions that break down the lining; stress; and food allergies. Healing involves minimizing the consumption of acids that erode the stomach and intestinal lining, protecting and soothing the intestinal lining, stimulating the immune system and inhibiting the growth of harmful bacteria. Anti-inflammatory, antibacterial, calming and mucous-protective herbs are also helpful in healing ulcers.

What to Do

Maximize

- Fruits and vegetables, which provide healing vitamins and protection from infection. Fully ripe, sweet fruits are more soothing than sour fruits
- Slippery elm bark powder (especially at bedtime) to form a coating in the intestinal tract that protects against acid
- Fluid intake (drink at least eight large glasses of water, juice and/or herbal tea daily, between meals only, to ensure that your digestive juices are not diluted)

Minimize

- Salt

Eliminate

- Caffeine (found in black and green tea, coffee, chocolate, soft drinks and decaffeinated coffee), which stimulates secretion of stomach acid
- Dairy products, which lead to increased stomach acidity
- Alcohol, soft drinks and refined grains, which promote ulceration
- Refined flour and sugar
- Ulcer-causing drugs (steroids, such as Aspirin, and nonsteroidal anti-inflammatories)
- Cigarette smoking

Eliminate

- Very hot liquids, which irritate ulcers
- Fried foods and oils (except extra-virgin olive oil)

Other Recommendations

- Eat smaller, more-frequent meals and avoid eating late at night.
- Try stress-reducing techniques, such as meditation, yoga and tai chi.
- Drink raw cabbage juice (1 cup/250 mL taken four times a day on an empty stomach immediately after juicing is effective in healing ulcers).
- Practice food-combining techniques (see Appendix B: Food Combining, page 306).

Healing Smoothies

- Berry Best, page 177
- Blue Cherry, page 163
- Mango Madness (use apple juice instead of orange juice), page 175
- Pear Fennel, page 184
- Peptic Tonic, page 226
- Pump It Up, page 163

★ Avoid licorice if you have high blood pressure. The prolonged use of licorice is not recommended under any circumstances.

★★ If you are pregnant, limit your intake of parsley to 1/2 tsp (2 mL) dried or one sprig fresh per day. Do not take parsley if you are suffering from kidney inflammation.

Pregnancy

NUTRITION IS VITAL TO A BABY'S HEALTH, FROM PRECONCEPTION to birth. Ideally, a mother should get enough nutrients from food rather than supplements. Whole foods provide high-quality, easily digestible nutrients in forms and proportions that your body can use more easily than supplements. Make natural, unprocessed whole grains, beans, fruits, vegetables, nuts and seeds the basis of your diet. Add sufficient protein in the form of lean meat, fish or soy products.

What to Do

Maximize

- Fruits and vegetables
- Nuts and seeds
- Folic acid (found in egg yolks, wheat germ, leafy greens, soybeans, asparagus, oranges), which is necessary for normal fetal development
- Foods that are rich in omega-3 fatty acids (found in flax seeds; walnuts; and oily fish, such as salmon, tuna, mackerel and sardines), which are needed to maintain a mother's hormone balance and for proper fetal development

HEALING FOODS

Fruits and vegetables
bananas, cantaloupe, citrus fruits, strawberries, avocados, carrots, leafy greens, peas, sweet potatoes, watercress

Herbs
alfalfa, dandelion root and leaf, lemon balm, oat straw, red raspberry leaf, rose hips, stinging nettle

Other

dulse, flax seeds, kelp, legumes, blackstrap molasses, nuts (especially almonds), extra-virgin olive oil, soy products, seeds (especially sunflower), wheat germ, whole grains, yogurt with active bacterial cultures

Note: See Appendix C: Herbs to Avoid During Pregnancy, page 308

Minimize

- Foods that increase calcium loss (common in pregnancy), such as:
- sugar and sweeteners;
- tea, coffee and soft drinks;
- fats;
- refined flour; and
- bran, tomatoes, potatoes, eggplant and all peppers.

Eliminate

- Alcohol
- Artificial food additives
- Non-organic foods, which can contain pesticide residues
- Junk foods

Healing Smoothies

- Avocado Pineapple, page 197
- Best Berries, page 191
- Beta Blast, page 177
- C-Green, page 214
- Citrus Cocktail, page 165
- Green Gold, page 214
- Peas Please, page 199
- Pineapple Citrus, page 186
- Raspberry Raspberry, page 237
- Rustproofer #2 (replace peppermint with red raspberry leaf), page 214
- Sea-Straw, page 191
- Spring Celebration, page 197
- Watercress, page 219

HEALING FOODS

Fruits and vegetables
apples, bananas, berries, citrus fruits, pears, asparagus, beets, broccoli, cabbage, cauliflower, leafy greens, onions, red and green bell peppers, tomatoes, watercress

Herbs
garlic, ginger, goldenrod, green tea, fresh stinging nettle root, parsley*, plantain, saw palmetto berries, turmeric

Prostate Enlargement, Benign

PROSTATE ENLARGEMENT OCCURS IN 50% OF MEN AGED 50, 60% of men aged 60 and so on to 100% of men aged 100. The enlarged prostate blocks the urinary tract, obstructing the flow of urine.

What to Do

Maximize

- Antioxidant-rich fruits and vegetables
- Tomatoes, which reduce the risk of prostate cancer
- Soy products, which protect the prostate from disease
- Foods that are rich in zinc (shellfish, brown rice, legumes, leafy greens, dried fruits, onions, sunflower seeds, pumpkin seeds, egg yolks) to reduce prostate size

- Foods that contain vitamin C (citrus fruits, berries, leafy greens, parsley, all peppers) to aid zinc absorption

- Foods that are rich in vitamin B6 (bananas, cabbage, egg yolks, leafy greens, legumes, prunes, raisins, soybeans, sunflower seeds) to improve the effectiveness of zinc

Other
almonds, Brazil nuts, cashews, flax seeds, kelp, legumes, pecans, pumpkin seeds, sesame seeds, soy products, sunflower seeds

Eliminate

- Caffeine (found in coffee, black and green tea, chocolate and soft drinks), which limits calcium absorption
- Alcohol, which flushes zinc out of the system
- Foods that contain artificial additives, pesticides or hormones
- Margarine and cooking oils (except extra-virgin olive oil)
- Fried foods
- Sugar and sugar products

Minimize

- Animal fat in meat and dairy products

Other Recommendations

- Eat oily fish (salmon, mackerel, sardines, tuna) two or three times a week.
- Ensure that you get sufficient dietary protein to help absorb zinc.

> ★ If you are pregnant, limit your intake of parsley to $^1/_2$ tsp (2 mL) dried or one sprig fresh per day. Do not take parsley if you are suffering from kidney inflammation.

Healing Smoothies

- Allium Antioxidant, page 232
- Apple Pear, page 184
- Autumn Refresher, page 184
- B-Vitamin, page 187
- Beet, page 201
- Berry Best, page 177
- Berry Fine Cocktail, page 189
- C-Blend, page 166
- C-Blitz, page 166
- C-Green, page 214
- Cabbage Cocktail, page 203
- Cauliflower Cocktail, page 206
- Citrus Cocktail, page 165
- Leafy Luxury, page 210
- Pear Pineapple, page 185
- Prostate Power, page 239
- Pure Tomato, page 216
- Spring Celebration, page 197
- Tomato Juice Cocktail, page 217
- Watercress, page 219

Sinusitis

SINUSITIS IS AN INFLAMMATION OF THE SINUSES, WHICH is caused by colds, influenza, allergies or dental infections. The most-effective prevention and treatment strategies are to avoid mucus-producing foods and to identify, then avoid, food allergies (see Appendix A: Food Allergies, page 304).

Herbs
cayenne, dandelion leaf and root, elderflowers, ginger, echinacea, garlic, parsley*

apricots, cantaloupe,
citrus fruits, mangoes,
pumpkin, strawberries,
watermelon,
asparagus, broccoli,
cabbage, carrots, green
beans, leafy greens,
papayas, red and green
bell peppers

Other

legumes, lentils,
pumpkin seeds, sea
herbs, sunflower seeds,
wheat germ

* If you are pregnant,
limit your intake of
parsley to 1/2 tsp
(2 mL) dried or one
sprig fresh per day.
Do not take parsley if
you are suffering from
kidney inflammation.

What to Do

Maximize

- Foods that are rich in vitamin C (citrus fruits, strawberries, parsley*)
- Foods that are rich in vitamin E (wheat germ, nuts, seeds, cabbage, soy lecithin, spinach, asparagus)
- Foods that are rich in beta-carotene (carrots, mangoes, cantaloupes, apricots, watermelon, red bell peppers, pumpkin, leafy greens, parsley*, papayas)
- Foods that are rich in zinc (pumpkin seeds, fish, sea herbs)
- Liquid intake (drink at least eight large glasses of water a day)
- Raw garlic to reduce and prevent sinus congestion (take daily)

Minimize

- Starchy foods

Eliminate

- Alcohol
- Bananas
- Dairy products (except yogurt with active bacterial cultures)
- Eggs
- Food allergies and intolerances (see Appendix A: Food Allergies, page 304)
- Refined sugar and flour

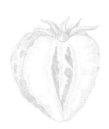

Healing Smoothies

- Allium Antioxidant, page 232
- Beta Blast, page 177
- Brocco-Carrot, page 202
- C-Blitz, page 166

Fruits and
vegetables
apples, apricots,
berries, cantaloupe,
grapes, mangoes,
papayas, pears, carrots,
cucumbers, leafy
greens, beets and beet
greens, pumpkin,
squash, watercress

Skin Conditions
Acne, Dry Skin, Psoriasis & Rosacea

ACNE: THIS CONDITION, CHARACTERIZED BY RAISED RED
pimples, usually responds to the dietary changes and cleansing herbs
listed on the right. When acne is related to the menstrual cycle,
include the hormone-balancing herb chasteberry (*Vitex agnus-castus*).

Dry Skin: Adding essential fatty acids to your diet helps nourish
dry skin. Food sources include extra-virgin olive oil, freshly ground
flax seeds, fresh walnuts and hazelnuts, and oily fish (mackerel,
sardines, salmon, tuna).

Psoriasis: This condition is caused by an increase in the production of skin cells, causing red, scaly plaques. It usually affects the elbows and knees. The cause is unknown, but it is often related to stress and emotional state; herbs such as German chamomile, skullcap and lemon balm can help calm and relax you. Exposing the plaques to sunlight and bathing in the sea are also helpful. Relaxation techniques, such as meditation, yoga and tai chi, can help bring balance to your life. Avoid nuts, citrus fruits and tomatoes, all of which can aggravate psoriasis.

Rosacea: Acne rosacea is a chronic inflammatory skin disease in which too much oil is produced by the glands in the skin. It is often associated with digestive disorders, and the dietary suggestions and cleansing herbs (right) are usually effective in clearing rosacea up.

What to Do

Maximize

- Fresh fruits and vegetables
- Foods that are rich in beta-carotene (carrots, broccoli, leafy greens, apricots, papayas)
- Blood-cleansing herbs (dandelion root, burdock root, yellow dock)
- Herbal nerve relaxants (German chamomile, skullcap, lemon balm, oat seeds)
- Seeds (flax, pumpkin, sunflower)

Minimize

- Salt and salty foods
- Animal protein (replace with vegetable protein)

Eliminate

- Red meat
- Shellfish
- Sugar
- Fried foods
- Oranges
- Chocolate
- Refined flour
- Coffee and black tea
- Dairy products
- Soft drinks
- Artificial food additives, including sweeteners
- Alcohol

Other Recommendations

- Drink at least eight glasses of water, juice and/or herbal tea daily to flush out toxins.
- Eat oily fish (salmon, sardines, mackerel, tuna) two or three times a week.

Herbs

burdock root, leaf and seeds; calendula; dandelion root and leaf; echinacea; evening primrose oil; licorice**; fennel seeds; red clover flower; stinging nettle; yellow dock

Other

extra-virgin olive oil, soy products, pumpkin seeds, sesame seeds, sunflower seeds, flax seeds, lentils, oats, sea herbs, spirulina, whole grains, yogurt with active bacterial cultures

** Avoid licorice if you have high blood pressure. The prolonged use of licorice is not recommended under any circumstances.

Healing Smoothies

- Beet, page 201
- Breakfast Cocktail, page 175
- Pear Fennel, page 184
- Popeye's Power, page 229
- Psoria-Smoothie, page 230
- Teenage Tonic, page 226

Fruits and vegetables
cantaloupe, citrus fruits, broccoli, carrots, leafy greens

Herbs
German chamomile, red clover (flowering tops), skullcap

Other
oats, oat bran, pumpkin seeds, sunflower seeds, tofu

Smoking — Quitting

IN ADDITION TO BEING A MAJOR CAUSE OF HEART AND LUNG disease and cancer, smoking encourages the loss of calcium (leading to osteoporosis) and is a risk factor for high blood pressure and ulcers. Smoking constricts the blood vessels, decreasing circulation to peripheral parts of the body, and increases the risk of stroke for both men and women, as well as impotence in men. It also causes wrinkles.

Reduce Cravings

- Maintain constant blood sugar by eating six meals a day that consist mainly of fresh fruits and vegetables, with a little protein and whole grains.
- Ease withdrawal symptoms with a mainly vegetarian diet, which slows down the removal of nicotine from the body.

- Exercise regularly. Walking and breathing exercises are excellent.
- Snack on sunflower and pumpkin seeds — the zinc content may reduce cravings by blocking taste enzymes.
- Eat plenty of oats. Studies show that oats diminish cravings.
- Drink calming herbal teas to soothe your nerves.

Healing Smoothies

- Beta Blast, page 177
- Brocco-Carrot, page 202
- C-Blitz, page 166

- Green Energy, page 232
- Orange Zinger, page 204

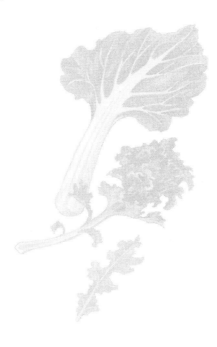

Urinary Tract Infections

URINARY TRACT INFECTIONS CAN BE CAUSED BY YEAST OR bacteria. The infection can then pass into the bladder. Cystitis, an inflammation of the bladder, is caused when yeast or bacteria settle into the irritated tissue of the bladder. It is characterized by frequent, painful urination.

What to Do

Maximize

- Liquid intake (drink 8 to 10 cups/2 to 2.5 L water, vegetable juice and/or herbal tea daily) to dilute and wash out bacteria
- Unsweetened cranberry and blueberry juices to prevent bacteria from adhering to the bladder wall
- Onions and garlic, which are antibacterial. Raw garlic is best. Add it to main dishes, sauces, dips and smoothies; add freshly crushed to salads and vegetables; or chop into pieces small enough to swallow
- Antibacterial herbs (buchu, yarrow) to soothe the bladder and herbs that promote urination (marshmallow root, buchu, dandelion leaf)

Minimize

- Meat (replace with vegetable protein, such as that found in tofu, or legumes and rice)
- Alcohol, sugar and artificial food additives, which irritate an inflamed bladder
- Refined sugar and flour
- Dairy products

Eliminate

- Caffeine (found in coffee, black and green tea, chocolate and soft drinks)

Healing Smoothies

- Blue Water, page 163
- Cran-Orange, page 168
- Healthy Bladder Blitz, page 225
- Watermelon, page 193

HEALING FOODS

Fruits and vegetables
blueberries, cranberries, lemons, watermelon, carrots, celery, fennel, onions, parsnips, turnips

Herbs
buchu, cinnamon, coriander, cumin, dandelion leaf, echinacea, fennel seeds, garlic, marshmallow root, slippery elm bark powder, stinging nettle, yarrow*

Other
pumpkin seeds, yogurt with active bacterial cultures, barley

> * Do not take yarrow if you are pregnant.

Fruits and vegetables
apples, beets, carrots, celery, leafy greens, watercress

Herbs
burdock root, chasteberry, cinnamon, dandelion leaf and root, garlic, ginger, red clover, red raspberry leaf, stinging nettle, yarrow*, yellow dock

Other
kelp, tofu, whole grains

> ★ Do not take yarrow if you are pregnant.

Uterine Fibroids

UTERINE FIBROIDS ARE BENIGN GROWTHS THAT ARE STIMULATED by estrogen. They can cause pain, heavy menstrual bleeding, anemia and bladder problems. With the drop in estrogen that occurs at menopause, fibroids usually shrink. Plenty of exercise to improve pelvic circulation is helpful.

What to Do

Maximize

- Sea herbs to reduce fibroid growth
- Fiber from fresh fruits and vegetables and whole grains to improve the elimination of toxins
- Hormone-balancing herbs (chasteberry), liver-supporting herbs (dandelion root, burdock root, milk thistle seed) and vegetables (beets, carrots)
- Organic foods

Eliminate

- Caffeine (found in coffee, black and green tea, chocolate and soft drinks), which increases estrogen levels
- Fried foods, margarine and oils (except extra-virgin olive oil)
- Alcohol
- Artificial food additives, preservatives and colorings, which contribute to the accumulation of toxins and hormone imbalance

Other Recommendations

- Correct anemia if present (see Anemia, page 26).
- Correct constipation if present (see Constipation, page 36).

Healing Smoothies

- Apple Pie, page 157
- Beet (add one 1/2-inch/1 cm long piece of peeled ginger), page 201
- Spiced Carrot, page 205

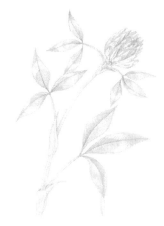

Varicose Veins & Hemorrhoids

VARICOSE VEINS DEVELOP IN THE LEGS WHEN THERE IS A restriction in blood flow to the heart, causing blood to pool and stretch the veins. Age and genetic predisposition are factors. Possible causes include heart-valve damage, which alters the flow of blood; high blood pressure, which causes blockage; blood-flow restriction (from tight clothing); excess weight; and lack of exercise. The risk increases during pregnancy and with age. Keep veins in good shape with a diet full of natural foods.

Hemorrhoids are varicose veins around the anus. They may be caused by constipation, pregnancy, obesity, lack of exercise or standing for long periods of time, all of which put extra pressure on the perineal area.

What to Do

Maximize

- Foods that are high in vitamin E (whole grains, wheat germ, legumes, nuts, seeds, leafy greens, sea herbs, soy products) to improve circulation

- Foods that are high in vitamin C (citrus fruits, red and green bell peppers, berries, leafy greens) to strengthen blood vessels

Other Recommendations

- Remedy constipation (see Constipation, page 36), which worsens hemorrhoids.
- Eat oily fish (salmon, sardines, mackerel, tuna) two or three times a week to provide essential fatty acids, which maintain elasticity of veins and help circulation.
- Exercise daily, according to your fitness level.

- Avoid hot baths, which relax the veins, or tone the veins immediately afterward by rinsing your legs with cold water and wiping gently with witch hazel.
- Do not massage varicose veins.
- Avoid standing for long periods of time.
- Raise feet whenever possible.

Healing Smoothies

- Berry Best, page 177
- Berry Fine Cocktail, page 189
- C-Blend, page 166

- C-Blitz, page 166
- C-Green, page 214
- Cherry Sunrise, page 164

HEALING FOODS

Fruits and vegetables
berries (blueberries, strawberries, raspberries, blackberries), cherries, citrus fruits, pears, red grapes, broccoli, cabbage, leafy greens, onions, watercress

Herbs
alfalfa, burdock seed and root, cayenne, dandelion leaf and root, garlic, ginger, horse chestnut, parsley**, witch hazel, yarrow*

Other
buckwheat, dulse, kelp, legumes, nuts, oats, extra-virgin olive oil, soy products, seeds (flax, sunflower, pumpkin, sesame), wheat germ, whole grains

** If you are pregnant, limit your intake of parsley to $1/2$ tsp (2 mL) dried or one sprig fresh per day. Do not take parsley if you are suffering from kidney inflammation.

- Orange Zinger, page 204
- Real Raspberry, page 189
- Sea-Straw, page 191

- Spa Special (use a recommended herb instead of milk thistle), page 236
- Sunrise Supreme, page 173

Water Retention
Edema

WATER RETENTION CAN BE A SYMPTOM OF A SERIOUS condition, such as high blood pressure, heart disease, kidney disease or liver disease. Or it may simply be the result of medications, poor circulation, allergies, anemia or protein deficiency. Consult with your health-care practitioner to determine the cause.

Cases of water retention in the late stages of pregnancy must always be referred to a doctor. Strong diuretics and water-loss diets can reduce water retention in the short term but may result in kidney damage over the long term. Water retention can result from too much (or too little) dietary protein, insufficient water intake or as a side effect of premenstrual syndrome (PMS) or menopause. Consult with your health-care practitioner in all cases of water retention.

What to Do

Maximize
- Water intake (drink at least eight large glasses daily)
- Raw fruits and vegetables

Minimize
- Table salt, sea salt, soy sauce and salted snacks, which can cause water retention
- Tea and coffee, which are strong diuretics that can cause kidney strain if used excessively

Eliminate
- Food allergies and intolerances (see Appendix A: Food Allergies, page 304). Dairy products and wheat can cause water retention
- Sugar
- Refined flour

HEALING FOODS

Fruits and vegetables
blueberries, cantaloupe, grapes, strawberries, watermelon, asparagus, beets, broccoli, cabbage, carrots, celery, corn, cucumbers, leafy greens, squash, watercress

Herbs
burdock leaf, root and seeds; dandelion leaf and root; garlic; parsley*; stinging nettle

Other
adzuki beans and other legumes, fish oils, whole grains

* If you are pregnant, limit your intake of parsley to ½ tsp (2 mL) dried or one sprig fresh per day. Do not take parsley if you are suffering from kidney inflammation.

Other Recommendations

- Exercise daily, according to your fitness level, to improve circulation and reduce water retention.

- Use stronger diuretics (parsley*, celery) only occasionally.

- Include tonic diuretics (dandelion root, stinging nettle, asparagus, corn, grapes, cantaloupe, cucumbers, watermelon) regularly in your diet. The herbs can be made into teas, which can be used as liquid bases of smoothies.

Healing Smoothies

- Berry Best, page 177
- Blue Water, page 163
- Brocco-Carrot, page 202

- C-Green, page 214
- Diuretic Tonic, page 225
- Popeye's Power, page 229

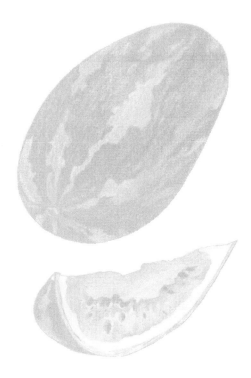

Ingredient Profiles

Use the Glossary

• If you come across terms in this section that you don't understand,
consult the Glossary, pages 296 to 301.

Alfalfa

Medicago sativa
A hardy perennial easily grown in most parts of North America.

Parts Used
Leaves, flowers and sprouted seeds.

Healing Properties
Actions: Tonic, nutritive, lowers blood cholesterol, antianemia.
Uses: Alfalfa is a cell nutritive and overall tonic for the body. It promotes strong teeth, bones and connective tissues. Alfalfa is one of the best sources of chlorophyll, which stimulates new skin growth; heals wounds and burns; diminishes the symptoms of arthritis, gout and rheumatism; lowers blood cholesterol level; reduces inflammation; and improves the body's resistance to cancer.

Caution
Alfalfa seeds and sprouts are rich in the amino acid canavanine, which can contribute to inflammation in rheumatoid arthritis, systemic lupus erythematosus and other rheumatoid and inflammatory conditions. Alfalfa leaves are not a source of canavanine and can be used for inflammatory and rheumatic conditions.

Availability
Whole or cut dried leaves are available in alternative/health stores. Sprouted seeds are readily available in supermarkets.

How to Use in Smoothies
Fresh sprigs: Wash, pat dry and remove leaves and flowers from stem. Use leaves and flower petals; discard stem and green flower center. Use 1 tbsp (15 mL) for each smoothie recipe.

Dried leaves and flowers: Crush dried leaves and flowers to a fine powder. Use up to 1 tbsp (15 mL) per smoothie.

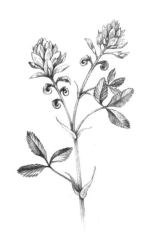

Infusion: In a teapot, pour $1/4$ cup (50 mL) boiling water over 2 tbsp (25 mL) chopped fresh leaves (or 2 tsp/10 mL powdered dried leaves). Cover and steep for 10 minutes. Cool (no need to strain) and use to replace $1/4$ cup (50 mL) liquid in smoothie recipes.
Tincture: Add 1 tsp (5 mL) tincture to each smoothie recipe.

Healing Smoothies
- Aspirin in a Glass, page 235
- Good Health Elixir, page 223

Astragalus

Astragalus membranaceus
A hardy shrub-like perennial native to eastern Asia but grown in temperate regions.

Parts Used
Root.

Healing Properties
Actions: Immunostimulant, antimicrobial, cardiotonic, diuretic, promotes tissue regeneration.

Uses: Used throughout Asia as a tonic, astragalus is a powerful immune-system stimulator for virtually every kind of immune-system activity. It has also been shown to alleviate the adverse effects of steroids and chemotherapy on the immune system, and can be used during traditional cancer treatment.

Availability
While more and more North American herb farms are growing this exceptional medicinal herb, the most-reliable sources for the dried root are Asian herb stores in large urban areas. However, alternative/health stores carry cut or ground dried astragalus, as well as the tincture form.

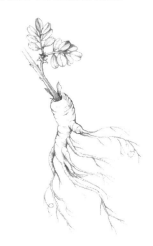

How to Use in Smoothies
Ground dried root: Add 1 tsp (5 mL) to each 1 cup (250 mL) of smoothie.
Decoction: In a small saucepan, combine $1/4$ cup (50 mL) boiling water with one 1-inch (2.5 cm) slice dried root (or 1 tsp/5 mL chopped dried root). Cover and simmer for 10 minutes. Remove from heat; steep for 10 minutes. Strain, discard root and let cool. Use to replace $1/4$ cup (50 mL) liquid in smoothie recipes.

Tincture: Add 10 to 20 drops tincture to each 1 cup (250 mL) of smoothie.

Healing Smoothies
• Herb-eze, page 223

Basil

Oscimum basilicum
A bushy annual with large, waxy, deep green leaves and small tubular flowers on long spikes.

Parts Used
Leaves and flowering tops.

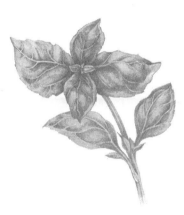

Healing Properties
Actions: Antispasmodic, soothing digestive, antibacterial, antidepressant, adrenal gland stimulant.
Uses: Indigestion, nervous tension, stress, tension headaches.

Availability
Fresh sprigs are sold in season at farmer's markets and supermarkets. Sifted chopped dried leaves are available at natural-food stores.

How to Use in Smoothies
Fresh leaves: Use 1 to 3 leaves for each 1 cup (250 mL) of smoothie. Wash, pat dry and strip leaves off stem. Discard stem and roughly chop leaves before adding to the blender.

Healing Smoothies
• Anti-Depression Tonic, page 223
• Pear Basil Raspberry, page 224

Black Cohosh

Cimicifuga racemosa
A tall, wild woodland perennial native to North America with broad leaves and spikes of fragrant white flowers.

Parts Used
Root and rhizome.

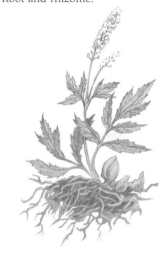

Healing Properties
Actions: Antirheumatic, antispasmodic, mild pain reliever, estrogenic, sedative, anti-inflammatory, uterine stimulant.
Uses: A bitter, tonic herb that soothes aches and pains, black cohosh is used to treat rheumatoid arthritis, sciatica, bronchial spasms, menstrual cramps, menopausal problems, and labor and postpartum pains.

Caution
Do not take black cohosh if you are pregnant or breastfeeding unless otherwise advised by your health-care practitioner. Excessive doses can cause headaches.

Availability
Seeds, rootlets and plants are available for growing. Dried roots and tinctures are available at alternative/health stores.

How to Use in Smoothies
Decoction: In a small saucepan, combine $1/4$ cup (50 mL) boiling water with $1/2$ tsp (2 mL) chopped or ground dried root. Cover and simmer for 10 minutes. Remove from heat; steep for 10 minutes. Strain, discard root and let cool. Use to replace $1/4$ cup (50 mL) liquid in smoothie recipes.
Tincture: Add 8 drops tincture to each 1 cup (250 mL) of smoothie.
Note: Do not add to smoothies more than once a day.

Healing Smoothies
• Cramp Crusher, page 224
• Pain Reliever, page 228

Borage

Borago officinalis
A self-seeding annual with a branching, hollow stem that supports alternating long oval leaves. Small blue star-shaped flowers hang in wide, drooping clusters. The whole plant is covered with prickly silver hairs.

Parts Used
Leaves and flowering tops.

Healing Properties
Actions: Adrenal gland restorative, expectorant, increases milk in breastfeeding.
Uses: Coughs, depression, stress, to strengthen adrenal glands after treatment with corticosteroid drugs.

Caution

Borage leaves contain very small amounts of pyrrolizidine alkaloids, which can be toxic to the liver but are considered safe for occasional use under the supervision of a qualified health-care practitioner.

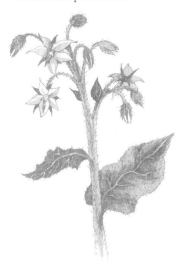

Availability

Easy to grow in containers or gardens, fresh borage is not readily available to purchase. Dried leaves are sometimes available in natural-food stores. Use fresh whenever possible, as dried leaves have lost most of their medicinal effectiveness.

How to Use in Smoothies

Fresh sprigs: Use half to 1 whole leaf and up to 4 fresh flowers. Wash, pat dry and strip leaves and flowers off stem. Discard stem and chop leaf and flowers before adding to the blender.
Infusion: In a teapot, pour $1/4$ cup (50 mL) boiling water over 1 tbsp (15 mL) chopped fresh leaves. Cover and steep for 10 minutes. Cool (no need to strain) and use to replace $1/4$ cup (50 mL) liquid in smoothie recipes.

Healing Smoothies

• Courage, page 224

Buchu
Barosma betulina

A small green shrub native to South Africa. Plants in this genus have attractive flowers and aromatic bright green ovate leaves that make them popular as ornamentals.

Parts Used

Leaves.

Healing Properties

Actions: Diuretic, urinary antiseptic.
Uses: Used to treat urinary disorders, such as painful urination, cystisis, prostatitis and urethritis. Research indicates that buchu contains properties that block ultraviolet light, which could be helpful in skin preparations.

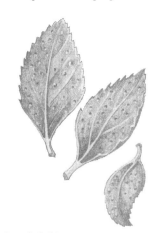

Availability

Dried leaves and tinctures are available in alternative/health stores.

How to Use in Smoothies

Ground dried leaves: Use 1 tsp (5 mL) ground dried leaves for each smoothie recipe. Add to other ingredients before blending.

Infusion: In a teapot, pour $1/4$ cup (50 mL) boiling water over 1 tsp (5 mL) chopped or ground dried leaves. Cover and steep for 10 minutes. Cool (no need to strain) and use to replace $1/4$ cup (50 mL) liquid in smoothie recipes.
Tincture: Add 20 to 40 drops tincture to each 1 cup (250 mL) of smoothie.

Healing Smoothies

• Healthy Bladder Blitz, page 225

Burdock
Arctium lappa

A hardy biennial that produces fruiting heads covered with hooked burrs that catch on clothing and animal fur. Grows wild extensively in North America. Due to its wide availability in rural and urban waste areas, burdock can be easily foraged. Avoid collecting it from roadsides, ditches, streams close to field runoff, or other areas likely to be polluted by car exhaust or chemical runoff.

Parts Used

Root, stalk, leaves and seeds.

Burdock Leaf
Healing Properties

Actions: Mild laxative, diuretic.
Uses: Leaves may be used in the same way that the root is (see Burdock Root, page 93), though they are less effective.

Availability

Dried leaves and tinctures are available in alternative/health stores.

How to Use in Smoothies

Fresh leaves: Use 1 tbsp (15 mL) chopped fresh leaves in any smoothie recipe. Add to other ingredients before blending.

Dried leaves: Crush to a fine powder. Use 1 to 2 tsp (5 to 10 mL) for each 1 cup (250 mL) of smoothie. Add to other ingredients before blending.
Infusion: In a teapot, pour 1/4 cup (50 mL) boiling water over 1 tbsp (15 mL) chopped fresh leaves (or 1 tsp/5 mL chopped or ground dried leaves). Cover and steep for 10 minutes. Cool (no need to strain) and use to replace 1/4 cup (50 mL) liquid in smoothie recipes.
Tincture: Add 10 to 40 drops tincture to each 1 cup (250 mL) of smoothie.

Healing Smoothies
• Diuretic Tonic, page 225

Burdock Root
Healing Properties
Actions: Mild laxative, antirheumatic, antibiotic, diaphoretic, diuretic, skin and blood cleanser, soothing demulcent, tonic, soothes kidneys, lymphatic cleanser.
Uses: Burdock root is used as a cleansing, eliminative remedy. It helps remove toxins that cause skin problems (including eczema, acne, rashes and boils), digestive sluggishness and arthritis pain. It supports the liver, lymphatic glands and digestive system.

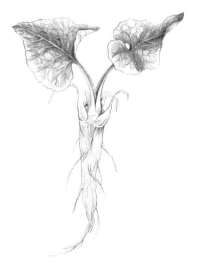

Availability
Dig roots in the wild in the fall. Scrub and chop, then dry for storage. Chopped dried root and tinctures are available in alternative/health stores.

How to Use in Smoothies
Fresh root: Scrub, coarsely chop and add to other ingredients before blending. Use 1 tbsp (15 mL) chopped fresh root for each 1 cup (250 mL) of smoothie.
Dried root: Crush to a fine powder. Use 1 tsp (5 mL) for each 1 cup (250 mL) of smoothie. Add to other ingredients before blending.
Decoction: In a small saucepan, gently simmer 1 tsp (5 mL) dried root in 1/4 cup (50 mL) water for 15 minutes. Strain, discard root and let cool. Use to replace 1/4 cup (50 mL) liquid in smoothie recipes.
Tincture: Add 10 to 20 drops tincture to each 1 cup (250 mL) of smoothie.

Healing Smoothies
• Gout Gone, page 225
• Psoria-Smoothie, page 230

Burdock Seeds
Healing Properties
Actions: Antipyretic, anti-inflammatory, antibacterial, reduce blood sugar level.
Uses: Lymphatic cleanser, soothing demulcent, tonic, soothe kidneys.

Availability
Seeds can be gathered easily in the wild in late summer and early fall (see Burdock, page 92). They are not always available in alternative/health stores, but burdock tinctures are.

How to Use in Smoothies
Infusion: In a teapot, pour 1/4 cup (50 mL) boiling water over 1 tsp (5 mL) bruised fresh or dried seeds. Cover and steep for 10 minutes. Strain, discard seeds and let cool. Use to replace 1/4 cup (50 mL) liquid in smoothie recipes.
Tincture: Add 10 to 40 drops tincture to each 1 cup (250 mL) of smoothie.

Healing Smoothies
• Teenage Tonic, page 226

Calendula
(Pot Marigold)
Calendula officinalis
A prolific annual easily grown from seed, with bright yellow to orange marigold-like flowers.

Parts Used
Petals.

Healing Properties
Actions: Astringent, antiseptic, antifungal, anti-inflammatory, heals wounds, menstrual regulator, stimulates bile production.
Uses: Calendula acts as a digestive aid and general tonic. It improves menopausal problems, menstrual pain, gastritis, peptic ulcers, gallbladder problems, indigestion and fungal infections.

Availability
Whole dried flower heads are available in alternative/health stores.

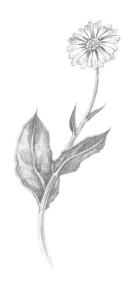

How to Use in Smoothies

Infusion: In a teapot, pour ¼ cup (50 mL) boiling water over 1 tbsp (15 mL) fresh petals (or 1 tsp/5 mL dried petals). Cover and steep for 10 minutes if using dried petals, or 15 minutes if using fresh. Cool (no need to strain) and use to replace ¼ cup (50 mL) liquid in smoothie recipes.
Tincture: Add 5 to 20 drops tincture to each 1 cup (250 mL) of smoothie.

Healing Smoothies

- Peptic Tonic, page 226
- Teenage Tonic, page 226

Cardamom

Elettaria cardamomum

A rhizomatous perennial with large lanceolate leaves originally from the Indian rain forests. For centuries it has been exported to Europe, mainly for its fragrance. When coaxed into bloom, the flowers are white with dark pink–striped lips.

Parts Used

Seeds.

Healing Properties

Actions: Antispasmodic, carminative, digestive stimulant, expectorant.
Uses: A pungent herb with stimulating, tonic effects that work best on the digestive system, cardamom relaxes spasms, stimulates appetite and relieves flatulence.

Availability

Whole or ground dried seeds are widely available in supermarkets and natural-food stores.

How to Use in Smoothies

Ground dried seeds: Add 1 tsp (5 mL) ground dried seeds to other ingredients before blending.
Infusion: In a teapot, pour ¼ cup (50 mL) boiling water over 1 tsp (5 mL) lightly crushed dried seeds. Cover and steep for 10 minutes. Strain, discard seeds and let cool. Use to replace ¼ cup (50 mL) liquid in smoothie recipes.

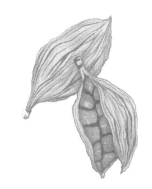

Healing Smoothies

- Digestive Drink, page 227

Catnip

Nepeta cataria

A hardy perennial — and a favorite of cats — with erect branched stems that bear gray-green toothed ovate leaves and whorls of white tubular flowers.

Parts Used

Leaves, stems and flowers.

Healing Properties

Actions: Antispasmodic, astringent, carminative, diaphoretic, cooling, sedative.
Uses: Catnip lowers fever, relaxes spasms, increases perspiration and is often taken at night to ensure sleep. It is also used for diarrhea, stomach upsets, colic, colds, flu, inflammation, pain and convulsions. It is especially useful for lowering children's fevers.

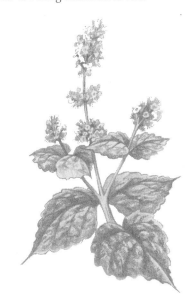

Availability

Catnip is easily grown in North America, but dried leaves, stems and flowers are available in natural-food stores.

How to Use in Smoothies

Fresh sprigs: Use 2 or 3 leaves for each 1 cup (250 mL) of smoothie. Wash, pat dry and strip leaves and flowers from stem. Discard stem and coarsely chop leaves and flowers.
Dried leaves and flowers: Crush to a fine powder. Use 1 tsp (5 mL) for each 1 cup (250 mL) of smoothie. Add to other ingredients before blending.

Infusion: In a teapot, pour $1/4$ cup (50 mL) boiling water over 1 tbsp (15 mL) chopped fresh catnip (or 1 tsp/5 mL chopped or ground dried). Cover and steep for 10 minutes. Cool (no need to strain) and use to replace $1/4$ cup (50 mL) liquid in smoothie recipes.

Healing Smoothies
- Sleepytime Smoothie, page 227

Cayenne

Capsicum annuum and
Capsicum frutescens
A tropical perennial grown as an annual in temperate zones (see also Chile Peppers, page 138). Although many varieties of chile peppers are used in cooking to add flavor and heat, the cayenne pepper is also used frequently as an herb because of its healing powers.

Parts Used
Red pepper fruit.

Healing Properties
Actions: Stimulant, tonic, carminative, diaphoretic, rubefacient, antiseptic, antibacterial.
Uses: Cayenne stimulates blood circulation, purifies the blood, promotes fluid elimination and sweating, and is most often used as a stimulating nerve tonic. Applied externally, over-the-counter creams and ointments that contain active capsaicin extract are often effective in relieving the pain of osteoarthritis, rheumatoid arthritis and shingles, as well as the burning pain in the toes, feet and legs caused by diabetic neuropathy and fibromyalgia.

Caution
Cayenne contains an irritating compound that, when applied externally, heals inflammations on unbroken skin by bringing blood to the surface. If used on broken skin, cayenne will irritate the wound and not be as effective. Natural-medicine practitioners often advise that capsicum not be taken internally in cases of chronic inflammation of the intestinal tract, such as in irritable bowel syndrome, ulcerative colitis and Crohn's disease. It should be used sparingly during pregnancy.

Availability
Fresh whole cayenne peppers are available in Latin American markets, supermarkets and natural-food stores. Dried whole cayenne peppers and ground cayenne pepper are widely available.

How to Use in Smoothies
Use fresh or reconstituted dried cayenne peppers, ground dried cayenne pepper or canned cayenne peppers in smoothies. If unavailable, whisk in a drop of hot pepper or jerk sauce. Taste and add more if desired.
Fresh pepper: Wash and handle carefully and wash hands thoroughly after handling, as capsaicin will irritate the skin and is very painful if it gets into the eyes or nasal passages or onto lips. Remove and discard stem, ribs and seeds. When first using cayenne peppers, add half of the recommended amount to the blender after all other ingredients have been pureed. Taste and add more if desired.
Ground dried pepper: Add $1/8$ to $1/4$ tsp (0.5 to 1 mL) ground dried cayenne pepper to other ingredients before blending. Gradually add more (up to 1 tsp/5 mL) if taste allows.

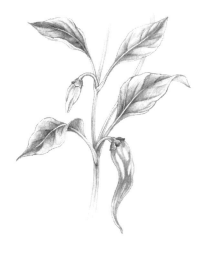

Healing Smoothies
- Hot Flu Toddy, page 230
- Migraine Tonic, page 231
- Pain Reliever, page 228

Celery Seeds

Apium graveolens
A biennial with a bulbous, fleshy root and thick, grooved stems. Although the stalk, leaves and, sometimes, the seeds are used in cooking (see Celery and Celeriac, page 137), it is the seeds collected from wild celery that are used for medicinal purposes.

Parts Used
Seeds.

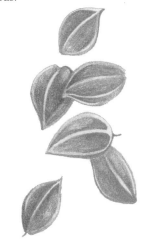

Healing Properties

Actions: Anti-inflammatory, antioxidant, carminative, sedative, urinary antiseptic.

Uses: Celery seeds are an aromatic, tonic herb that relieves muscle spasms and are used to treat gout, inflammation of the urinary tract, cystitis, osteoarthritis and rheumatoid arthritis.

Caution

Do not use celery seeds if you are pregnant.

Availability

Purchase celery seeds from herbalists or natural-food stores only.

How to Use in Smoothies

Dried seeds: Crush to a fine powder. Use ¼ tsp (1 mL) for each 1 cup (250 mL) of smoothie. Add to other ingredients before blending.

Infusion: In a teapot, pour ¼ cup (50 mL) boiling water over ¼ tsp (1 mL) lightly crushed dried seeds. Cover and steep for 10 minutes. Strain, discard seeds and let cool. Use to replace ¼ cup (50 mL) liquid in smoothie recipes.

Healing Smoothies
- Muscle Relief, page 228
- Turmeric Cocktail, page 241

Chamomile

See German Chamomile

Chasteberry

Chaste Tree

Vitex agnus-castus

A deciduous aromatic shrub or small tree native to southern Europe that grows in temperate climates (zones 7 to 10). Chaste trees bear palmate leaves, small lilac-scented tubular flowers and fleshy red-black fruits.

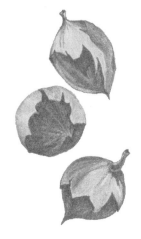

Parts Used

Berries.

Healing Properties

Actions: Balances female sex hormones by acting on the anterior pituitary gland.

Uses: Premenstrual syndrome (PMS), painful menstruation (dysmenorrhea), menopausal symptoms.

Caution

Do not take chasteberry with drugs that contain progesterone.

Availability

Dried berries and tinctures are available in alternative/health stores.

How to Use in Smoothies

Infusion: In a teapot, pour ¼ cup (50 mL) boiling water over 1 tbsp (15 mL) lightly crushed fresh chasteberries (or 1 tsp/5 mL lightly crushed dried). Cover and steep for 10 minutes. Strain, discard berries and let cool. Use to replace ¼ cup (50 mL) liquid in smoothie recipes.

Tincture: Add 10 to 20 drops tincture to each 1 cup (250 mL) of smoothie.

Healing Smoothies
- Woman's Smoothie (add 1 tsp/5 mL crushed dried chasteberries to the other herbs in Step 1), page 236

Chickweed

Stellaria media

A low, spreading annual with diffusely branched stems, ovate leaves and white star-shaped flowers found in most parts of North America.

Parts Used

Roots, leaves, flowers and stems.

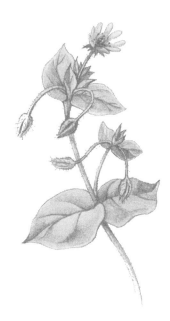

Healing Properties

Actions: Anticancer, anti-inflammatory, antirheumatic, astringent, heals wounds, demulcent.

Uses: Chickweed is used internally to treat rheumatism, constipation, mucus in the lungs, coughs, colds, tumors and blood disorders. It is used externally to treat eczema, psoriasis and other skin conditions.

Availability

A common weed, chickweed may be wildcrafted from summer through fall. Dried aerial parts (stem, leaves and flowers) and roots are available in natural-food stores.

How to Use in Smoothies

Fresh sprigs: Use 1 or 2 leaves and/or flowers in each smoothie recipe. Wash, pat dry and strip leaves and flowers off stem. Discard stem and coarsely chop leaves and flowers before blending.

Dried leaves and flowers: Crush to a fine powder. Use 2 tsp (10 mL) for each 1 cup (250 mL) of smoothie. Add to other ingredients before blending.

Infusion: In a teapot, pour $1/4$ cup (50 mL) boiling water over 2 tbsp (25 mL) chopped fresh leaves, flowers or stems (or 2 tsp/10 mL chopped or ground dried). Cover and steep for 10 minutes. Cool (no need to strain) and use to replace $1/4$ cup (50 mL) liquid in smoothie recipes.

Healing Smoothies

• Add 1 or 2 chopped fresh leaves and/or flowers to any smoothie recipe

Cinnamon

Cinnamomum zeylanicum

The dried smooth inner bark of a cultivated laurel-like tree that grows in the hot, wet tropical regions of India, Brazil, the East and West Indies, and islands in the Indian Ocean.

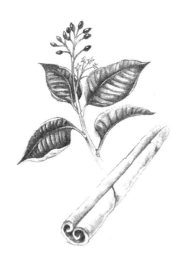

Parts Used

Bark.

Healing Properties

Actions: Carminative, diaphoretic, astringent, stimulant, antimicrobial.

Uses: Cinnamon is a warming carminative used to promote digestion and relieve nausea, vomiting and diarrhea. It is used for upset stomach and to treat irritable bowel syndrome (see page 62). Recent research has shown that cinnamon helps the body use insulin more efficiently, which may be helpful in the management of diabetes.

Availability

Dried rolled sticks are sold in 2- to 18-inch (5 to 45 cm) lengths. Powdered cinnamon and ground cinnamon, which is coarser, are widely available.

How to Use in Smoothies

Ground: Add up to $1/2$ tsp (2 mL) ground cinnamon to other ingredients before blending.

Infusion: In a teapot, pour $1/4$ cup (50 mL) boiling water over 1 tsp (5 mL) ground cinnamon (or one 1-inch/2.5 cm long stick cinnamon, broken into pieces). Cover and steep for 10 minutes. Strain, discard stick (if using) and let cool. Use to replace $1/4$ cup (50 mL) liquid in smoothie recipes.

Healing Smoothies

• Digestive Drink, page 227
• Flu Fighter #2, page 229
• Gas Guzzler, page 228
• Hot Flu Toddy, page 230

Clove

Syzygium aromaticus

The pink unopened flower buds of an evergreen tree native to Indonesia that's now grown in Zanzibar, Madagascar, the West Indies, Brazil, India and Sri Lanka.

Parts Used

Dried buds.

Healing Properties

Actions: Antioxidant, anesthetic, antiseptic, anti-inflammatory, anodyne, antispasmodic, carminative, stimulant, antiemetic, antihistamine, warming.

Uses: Cloves are used to treat asthma, bronchitis, nausea, vomiting, flatulence, diarrhea and hypothermia. Some studies indicate that cloves may have anticoagulant properties and may stimulate the production of enzymes that fight cancer. Clove oil is the active ingredient in some mouthwashes, toothpastes, soaps, insect repellents, perfumes, foods and veterinary medications, as well as many over-the-counter toothache remedies.

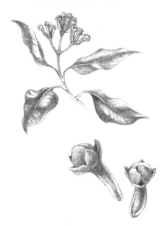

Availability

Whole and ground dried cloves are widely available.

How to Use in Smoothies

Ground: Use $1/4$ tsp (1 mL) for each smoothie recipe. Add to other ingredients before blending.

Infusion: In a teapot, pour $1/4$ cup (50 mL) boiling water over $1/4$ tsp (1 mL) lightly crushed whole cloves. Cover and steep for 10 minutes. Strain, discard cloves and let cool. Use to replace $1/4$ cup (50 mL) liquid in smoothie recipes.

Healing Smoothies
- Digestive Drink, page 227
- Herb-eze, page 223

Coriander Seeds

Coriandrum sativum

A hardy annual with slender, erect branched stems that bear aromatic pinnate parsley-like leaves. Small flat umbels of tiny white-to–pale mauve flowers yield round green berries (seeds) that ripen to a brownish yellow.

Parts Used
Seeds.

Healing Properties
Actions: Soothing digestive, appetite stimulant, improve digestion and nutrient absorption.
Uses: Digestive problems, flatulence.

Availability
Dried seeds are readily available in natural-food stores and Indian markets.

How to Use in Smoothies
Dried seeds: Crush to a powder. Add $1/2$ tsp (2 mL) to other ingredients before blending.

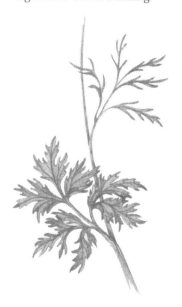

Infusion: In a teapot, pour $1/4$ cup (50 mL) boiling water over 1 tsp (5 mL) lightly crushed dried seeds. Cover and steep for 10 minutes. Strain, discard seeds and let cool. Use to replace $1/4$ cup (50 mL) liquid in smoothie recipes.

Cumin

Cuminum cyminum

A slender annual with dark green leaves found wild from the Mediterranean to Sudan in Africa and in central Asia. Umbels of tiny white or pink flowers are followed by bristly oval seeds.

Parts Used
Seeds.

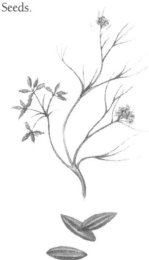

Healing Properties
Actions: Stimulant, soothing digestive, antispasmodic, diuretic, increases milk in breastfeeding.
Uses: Indigestion, flatulence.

Availability
Dried seeds are readily available in natural-food stores and Indian markets.

How to Use in Smoothies
Dried seeds: Crush to a powder. Add $1/2$ tsp (2 mL) to other ingredients before blending.

Infusion: In a teapot, pour $1/4$ cup (50 mL) boiling water over $1/2$ tsp (2 mL) lightly crushed dried seeds. Cover and steep for 10 minutes. Strain, discard seeds and let cool. Use to replace $1/4$ cup (50 mL) liquid in smoothie recipes.

Healing Smoothies
- Gas Guzzler, page 228

Dandelion

Taraxacum officinale

A hardy herbaceous perennial commonly found in most parts of North America.

Parts Used
Roots, stems, leaves and flowers.

Dandelion Leaf
Healing Properties
Actions: Diuretic, liver and digestive tonic.
Uses: Dandelion is used for liver, gallbladder, kidney and bladder ailments, including hepatitis and jaundice. It is also used as a diuretic. The leaves are used specifically to support the kidneys.

Availability
Whole plants are easily foraged from spring through fall. Look for fresh leaves in some supermarkets, farmer's markets and natural-food stores; chopped dried leaves are available in natural-food stores.

How to Use in Smoothies
Fresh leaves: Wash, pat dry and roughly chop before adding to the blender. Use 1 to 2 tbsp (15 to 25 mL) in each smoothie recipe.
Dried leaves: Crush to a powder. Use 1 tsp (5 mL) for each smoothie recipe. Add to other ingredients before blending.

Infusion: In a teapot, pour $\frac{1}{4}$ cup (50 mL) boiling water over 1 tbsp (15 mL) chopped fresh dandelion leaves (or 1 tsp/5 mL dried). Cover and steep for 10 minutes. Cool (no need to strain) and use to replace $\frac{1}{4}$ cup (50 mL) liquid in smoothie recipes.

Healing Smoothies
• Diuretic Tonic, page 225

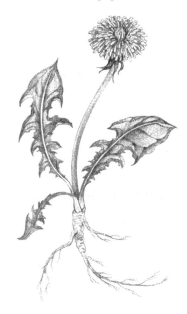

Dandelion Root
Healing Properties
Actions: Liver tonic, promotes bile flow, diuretic, mild laxative, antirheumatic.
Uses: Dandelion is used for liver, gallbladder, kidney and bladder ailments, including hepatitis and jaundice. It is also used as a diuretic. The root is used specifically to support the liver.

Availability
Dig fresh roots in the fall. Chopped dried roots and tinctures are available in alternative/health stores.

How to Use in Smoothies
Fresh root: Scrub, chop and add 1 tsp (15 mL) to other ingredients before blending.

Dried root: Crush to a fine powder. Use 1 tsp (5 mL) for each 1 cup (250 mL) of smoothie. Add to other ingredients before blending.
Decoction: In a small saucepan, gently simmer 1 tsp (5 mL) chopped dried root in $\frac{1}{4}$ cup (50 mL) water for 10 minutes. Strain, discard root and let cool. Use to replace $\frac{1}{4}$ cup (50 mL) liquid in smoothie recipes.
Tincture: Add 1 tsp (5 mL) tincture to each 1 cup (250 mL) of smoothie.

Healing Smoothies
• Popeye's Power, page 229
• Teenage Tonic, page 226

Dill
Anethum graveolens
A tall top-heavy annual with a long hollow stem growing out of a spindly taproot. Terminal flower heads, which grow out of the top of the stem, appear in a wide, flat umbel of numerous yellow flowers. Branches along the stem support feathery blue-green leaflets.

Parts Used
Seeds.

Healing Properties
Actions: Soothing digestive, antispasmodic, increases milk in breastfeeding.
Uses: Flatulence, infant colic, bad breath.

Availability
Easy to grow, dill seeds can be harvested from late summer through early fall. Dried seeds are readily available in natural-food stores and supermarkets.

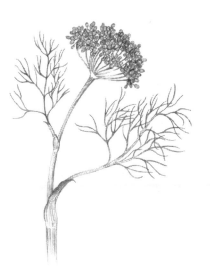

How to Use in Smoothies
Dried seeds: Crush to a powder. Add $\frac{1}{2}$ tsp (2 mL) to other ingredients before blending.
Infusion: In a teapot, pour $\frac{1}{4}$ cup (50 mL) boiling water over 1 tsp (5 mL) lightly crushed dried seeds. Cover and steep for 10 minutes. Strain, discard seeds and let cool. Use to replace $\frac{1}{4}$ cup (50 mL) liquid in smoothie recipes.

Healing Smoothies
• Turmeric Cocktail, page 241

Echinacea
Echinacea angustifolia,
E. pallida and *E. purpurea*
A hardy perennial also known as coneflower that is native to North America, with bright purple petals surrounding a brown cone.

Parts Used
Leaves, seeds, flowers, roots, stems.

Healing Properties
Actions: Immune modulating, anti-inflammatory, antibiotic, antimicrobial, antiseptic, analgesic, antiallergenic, lymphatic tonic.

Uses: Echinacea is used clinically to prevent and treat infections in the respiratory, urinary and digestive systems. It is useful in chronic candida and sinus infections and to support the health of patients undergoing chemotherapy. Externally, echinacea speeds healing of skin infections and wounds. Evidence shows that echinacea is effective because it increases the activity of phagocytes, which play an important role in preventing and overcoming bacterial, viral and fungal infections. Test-tube studies of its antiviral properties indicate that the above ground parts of *E. purpurea* may be effective in inhibiting the viruses that cause herpes, influenza and polio. The roots of *E. angustifolia*, *E. pallida* and *E. purpurea* may be effective in defending the body against the herpes simplex and influenza viruses.

Availability

Whole or chopped dried root, stems and leaves are available in alternative/health stores. Echinacea is also available in tincture and tablet form.

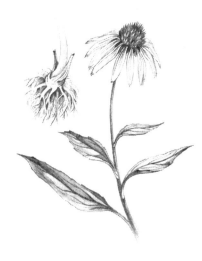

How to Use in Smoothies

Decoction: In a small saucepan, gently simmer 1 tsp (5 mL) chopped dried root in 1/4 cup (50 mL) water for 10 minutes. Strain, discard root and let cool. Use to replace 1/4 cup (50 mL) liquid in smoothie recipes.
Tincture: Add 1/2 tsp (2 mL) tincture to each 1 cup (250 mL) of smoothie.

Healing Smoothies

• Flu Fighter #2, page 229

Elder

Sambucus nigra
A fast-growing hardy perennial shrub common in many parts of North America.

Parts Used
Bark, flowers and berries.

Healing Properties
Actions: (Flowers) Expectorant, reduce phlegm, circulatory stimulant, diaphoretic, diuretic, topically anti-inflammatory. (Berries) Diaphoretic, diuretic, laxative. (Bark) Purgative, large doses are emetic, diuretic.
Uses: (Flowers) Elderflowers can be taken early in allergy season to strengthen the upper respiratory tract and help prevent hay fever. (Berries) Elderberries support detoxification by promoting bowel movements, urination, sweating and mucus secretion. Elderberries are effective in combating viruses, including those that cause colds and flu.

Availability
Fresh elderberries are found in season at farmer's markets. Dried flowers, fresh or dried berries and elder tinctures are available in alternative/health stores.

How to Use in Smoothies
Fresh flowers: Wash, pat dry and chop. Add 1 tbsp (15 mL) to other ingredients before blending.
Dried flowers: Add 1 tsp (5 mL) to other ingredients before blending.

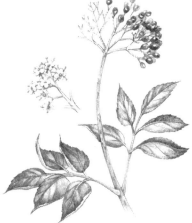

Infusion, flowers: In a teapot, pour 1/4 cup (50 mL) boiling water over 1 tbsp (15 mL) fresh elderflowers (or 1 tsp/5 mL dried). Cover and steep for 10 minutes if using dried flowers, or for 15 minutes if using fresh flowers. Cool (no need to strain) and use to replace 1/4 cup (50 mL) liquid in smoothie recipes.
Fresh berries: Add up to 1/4 cup (50 mL) fresh elderberries to other ingredients before blending.
Infusion, berries: Pour 1/4 cup (50 mL) boiling water over 1 tbsp (15 mL) fresh elderberries (or 1 tsp/5 mL lightly crushed dried elderberries). Cover and steep for 10 minutes. Cool (no need to strain) and use to replace 1/4 cup (50 mL) liquid in smoothie recipes.
Tincture: Add 1 tsp (5 mL) tincture to each 1 cup (250 mL) of smoothie.

Healing Smoothies
• Hot Flu Toddy, page 230

Evening Primrose

Oenothera biennis

An erect biennial with a rosette of basal leaves. In summer, yellow flowers open at night. Downy pods that contain tiny black seeds follow blooms.

Parts Used

Seed oil.

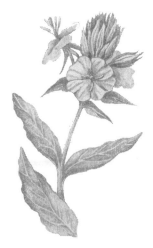

Healing Properties

Actions: Anticoagulant, anti-inflammatory, improves blood circulation, nutritive, the essential fatty acids in the seed oil help repair tissues.

Uses: Acne, anxiety, arthritis, asthma, breast tenderness, diabetes, dry skin, eczema, hangover, inflammation, high blood pressure, hyperactivity in children, migraines, multiple sclerosis, premenstrual syndrome.

Availability

Evening primrose oil is widely available in gel capsule form and sometimes in bulk in natural-food stores.

How to Use in Smoothies

Oil: If using capsules, slit open and collect oil in a measuring spoon. Add 1 tsp (5 mL) oil to other ingredients before blending.

Healing Smoothies

- Psoria-Smoothie, page 230
- The Regular, page 231

Fennel Seeds

Foeniculum vulgare

The fennel plant looks like a larger version of dill. Stout, solid stems support bright yellow, large umbel clusters of flowers. Thread-like, feathery green leaves alternately branch out from joints on the stem. Flowers appear in summer, followed by gray-brown seeds, which are used for medicinal purposes.

Parts Used

Seeds.

Healing Properties

Actions: Soothing diuretic, anti-inflammatory, antispasmodic, soothing digestive, increases milk in breastfeeding, mild expectorant.

Uses: Indigestion, flatulence, increases milk in breastfeeding, relieves colic in babies when taken by nursing mother. Fennel seed infusion is safe to treat colic and coughs in babies and children.

Caution

Avoid large doses if you are pregnant, as fennel seeds are a uterine stimulant.

Availability

Fennel grows wild in Mediterranean Europe and Asia and has become naturalized in many other parts of the world, where the fleshy bulb is harvested and used as a vegetable (see page 140). Harvest seeds in late summer and early fall. Dried seeds are readily available in natural-food stores and supermarkets.

How to Use in Smoothies

Dried seeds: Crush to a powder. Add $1/4$ tsp (1 mL) to other ingredients before blending.

Infusion: In a teapot, pour $1/4$ cup (50 mL) boiling water over $1/4$ to $1/2$ tsp (1 to 2 mL) lightly crushed dried seeds. Cover and steep for 15 minutes. Strain, discard seeds and let cool. Use to replace $1/4$ cup (50 mL) liquid in smoothie recipes.

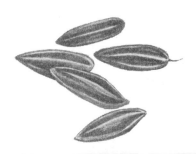

Healing Smoothies

- Anise Anise, page 235
- Aspirin in a Glass, page 235
- Digestive Drink, page 227
- Gas Guzzler, page 228
- Gout Gone, page 225
- Psoria-Smoothie, page 230

Fenugreek

Trigonella foenum-graecum

Grown as a fodder crop in southern and central Europe, fenugreek is widely naturalized from the Mediterranean to southern Africa to Australia. This annual has aromatic trifoliate leaves and solitary or paired yellow-white flowers, followed by beaked pods with yellow-brown seeds.

Parts Used

Aerial parts (stem, leaves and flowers) and seeds.

Healing Properties

Actions: Expectorant, soothing digestive, protects intestinal surfaces, reduces blood sugar level, increases milk in breastfeeding.
Uses: Bronchitis, coughs, diabetes, diverticular disease, ulcerative colitis, Crohn's disease, menstrual pain, peptic ulcers, stomach upsets.

Availability

Dried seeds are available in natural-food stores.

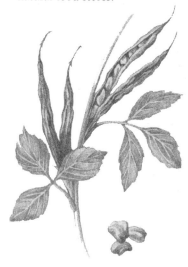

How to Use in Smoothies

Decoction: In a small saucepan, gently simmer 1 to 2 tsp (5 to 10 mL) lightly crushed dried seeds or aerial parts (stem, leaves and flowers) in 1 cup (250 mL) water for 10 minutes. Strain, discard solids and let cool. Use to replace up to 1 cup (250 mL) liquid in smoothie recipes.

Feverfew
Tanacetum parthenium

A perennial that appears throughout northern temperate regions. Bright green oblong leaves contain pungent volatile oils that may cause unpleasant reactions if handled or consumed in excess. Flowers are small and daisy-like.

Parts Used

Leaves.

Healing Properties

Actions: Anti-inflammatory, vasodilator, digestive.
Uses: Prevention of migraine headaches, inflammatory arthritis, menstrual pain.

Caution

Do not take feverfew if you are pregnant, since it stimulates the uterus. Fresh leaves may cause mouth ulcers in sensitive people.

Availability

Easily grown, fresh leaves may be harvested from June through late fall. Chopped dried leaves are available in natural-food stores.

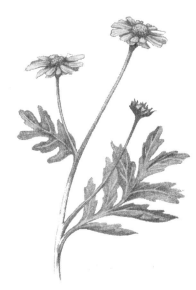

How to Use in Smoothies

Fresh leaves: Use 1 leaf in each smoothie recipe. Wash, pat dry and add to other ingredients before blending.
Dried leaves: Crush to a fine powder. Use 1 tsp (5 mL) for each 1 cup (250 mL) of smoothie. Add to other ingredients before blending.
Tincture: Add 5 to 20 drops tincture to 1 cup (250 mL) of smoothie.

Healing Smoothies

• Migraine Tonic, page 231

Garlic
Allium sativum

A hardy perennial with an onion-like bulb that's easily grown in North America.

Parts Used

Bulb or "bud" at the root of the plant.

Healing Properties

Actions: Antimicrobial, antibiotic, cardioprotective, hypotensive, anticancer, diaphoretic, anticoagulant, lowers blood cholesterol level, lowers blood sugar level, expectorant, digestive stimulant, diuretic, antihistamine, antiparasitic.
Uses: Research has shown that garlic inhibits cancer-cell formation and proliferation. It lowers total and low-density lipoprotein (LDL) cholesterol in humans and reduces blood clotting, thereby reducing the risks of blocked arteries and heart disease. Garlic is also an antioxidant and stimulates the immune system. It has strong antibiotic and anti-inflammatory properties, making it a good topical medicine. Garlic protects organs from damage inflicted by synthetic drugs, chemical pollutants and radiation.

Availability

Buy fresh whole organic bulbs at farmer's markets and supermarkets.

How to Use in Smoothies

Fresh cloves: Only fresh cloves of garlic have medicinal value. Add half to 1 whole fresh clove to other ingredients before blending.

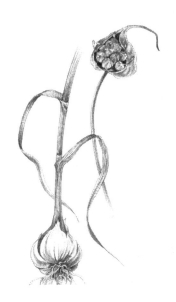

Healing Smoothies
• Allium Antioxidant, page 232

German Chamomile
Matricaria recutita
A low-growing hardy annual easily grown in North America. Flowers have daisy-like petals that surround rounded yellow centers.

Parts Used
Flower heads and petals.

Healing Properties
Actions: Gentle sedative, anti-inflammatory, mild antiseptic, antiemetic, antispasmodic, carminative, nervine, emmenagogue, mild pain reliever.
Uses: Anxiety, insomnia, indigestion, peptic ulcer, motion sickness, inflammation (such as gastritis) and menstrual cramps. Chamomile also reduces flatulence and gas pains.

Availability
Whole dried flower heads and tinctures are available in alternative/health stores.

How to Use in Smoothies
Fresh petals and flower heads: Add 1 tbsp (15 mL) to other ingredients before blending.
Infusion: In a teapot, pour ¼ cup (50 mL) boiling water over 1 tbsp (15 L) fresh flower heads (or 1 tsp/5 mL dried). Cover and steep for 10 minutes. Cool (no need to strain) and use to replace ¼ cup (50 mL) liquid in smoothie recipes.
Tincture: Add 1 tsp (5 mL) tincture to 1 cup (250 mL) of smoothie.

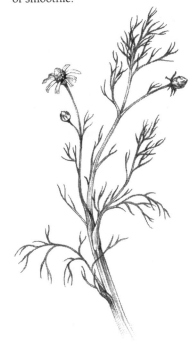

Healing Smoothies
• Calming Chamomile, page 232
• Hangover Remedy, page 240
• Sleepytime Smoothie, page 227
• Slippery Banana, page 240

Ginger
Zingiber officinale
A tender perennial edible rhizome native to Southeast Asia.

Parts Used
Root.

Healing Properties
Actions: Antinausea, relieves headaches and arthritis, anti-inflammatory, circulatory stimulant, expectorant, antispasmodic, antiseptic, diaphoretic, anticoagulant, peripheral vasodilator, antiemetic, carminative, antioxidant.
Uses: Gingerroot calms nausea and morning sickness and prevents vomiting. It is a cleansing, warming herb. Ginger stimulates blood flow to the digestive system and increases nutrient absorption. It increases the action of the gallbladder while protecting the liver against toxins and preventing the formation of ulcers. Studies show that ginger gives some relief from the pain and swelling of arthritis without side effects. Ginger is also used to control flatulence, circulation problems and impotence, and to prevent nausea after chemotherapy.

Caution
Ginger can be irritating to the intestinal mucosa and should be taken with or after meals. Ginger is contraindicated for people who are suffering from kidney disease.

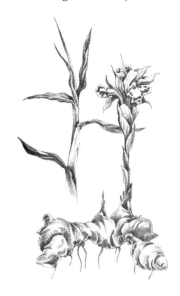

Availability

Fresh gingerroot and ground dried ginger are widely available in supermarkets, Asian and Indian markets, and natural-food stores.

How to Use in Smoothies

Fresh root: Fresh and clean-tasting with a hot bite, ginger blends well with most fruits in smoothies. Cut one ½-inch (1 cm) slice of fresh gingerroot and peel (if not organic). Cut into 4 pieces and add to other ingredients before blending.

Infusion: In a teapot, pour ¼ cup (50 mL) boiling water over 1 tsp (5 mL) grated peeled fresh gingerroot. Cover and steep for 10 minutes. Cool (no need to strain) and use the infusion to replace ¼ cup (50 mL) liquid in smoothie recipes.

Ground dried root: Add 1 tsp (5 mL) ground dried ginger to other ingredients before blending.

Healing Smoothies

- Cramp Crusher, page 224
- Flu Fighter, page 229
- Hangover Remedy, page 240
- Hot Flu Toddy, page 230
- Migraine Tonic, page 231
- Morning After, page 237
- Slippery Banana, page 240
- Woman's Smoothie, page 236

Ginkgo

Ginkgo biloba

A deciduous tree and one of the oldest trees to survive to the present day, ginkgo originated in central China but is grown as an ornamental in central North America. Light green fan-shaped leaves with two lobes turn yellow in autumn.

Parts Used

Leaves.

Healing Properties

Actions: Antioxidant, circulatory stimulant, increases blood flow to the brain, relieves bronchial spasms.

Uses: Asthma, tinnitus, cold hands and feet, varicose veins, hemorrhoids, headache, hangover, age-related memory loss, hearing loss, eyesight changes, Alzheimer's disease, Raynaud's disease, retinopathy, impotence.

Availability

Leaves can be gathered when yellow in the fall. Dried ginkgo leaves are available in natural-food stores.

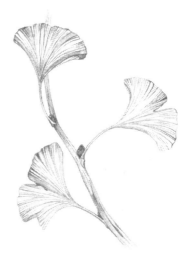

How to Use in Smoothies

Dried leaves: Crush to a fine powder. Use 1 tsp (5 mL) for each 1 cup (250 mL) of smoothie. Add to other ingredients before blending.

Infusion: In a teapot, pour ¼ cup (50 mL) boiling water over 1 tbsp (15 mL) chopped fresh leaves (or 1 tsp/5 mL dried). Cover and steep for 10 minutes. Cool (no need to strain) and use to replace ¼ cup (50 mL) liquid in smoothie recipes.

Liquid extract: Add 40 drops liquid extract to each 1 cup (250 mL) of smoothie.

Healing Smoothies

- Green Energy, page 232
- Smart Smoothie, page 239

Ginseng

Siberian
Eleutherococcus senticosus
North American
Panax quinquefolius
Asian
Panax ginseng

A hardy perennial native to cool wooded areas of eastern and central North America.

Parts Used

Root (from plants more than four years old) and leaves (if organic).

Healing Properties

Actions: Antioxidant, adaptogen, tonic, stimulant, regulates blood sugar and cholesterol levels, stimulates the immune system.

Uses: Ginseng helps the body resist and adapt to stress. It is a mild stimulant and, as a tonic, promotes long-term overall health. Along with increasing resistance to diabetes, cancer, heart disease and various infections, ginseng is also credited with improving memory, increasing fertility, protecting the liver against toxins and protecting the body against radiation. It is also used to treat impotence and depression.

Caution

Avoid ginseng if you have a fever, asthma, bronchitis, emphysema, high blood pressure or cardiac arrhythmia. Do not take ginseng if you are pregnant or if you drink coffee, and never give ginseng to a hyperactive child. Do not take continuously for a period of more than four weeks.

Availability

Whole or chopped dried root, tea, powdered and tinctures are all available in natural-food stores and Asian grocery stores. In its native North American woodlands, ginseng has been harvested to near extinction. Please do not collect it in the wild or purchase wildcrafted North American ginseng.

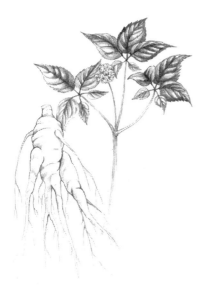

How to Use in Smoothies

Fresh root: Wash and chop one 1-inch (2.5 cm) long piece. Add to other ingredients before blending. Only use organic ginseng and leave the peel on.
Dried root: Grate finely. Add 1/4 tsp (1 mL) to each 1 cup (250 mL) of smoothie.
Decoction: In a small saucepan, gently simmer 1 tsp (5 mL) chopped dried root in 1/4 cup (50 mL) water for 10 minutes. Strain, discard root and let cool. Use to replace 1/4 cup (50 mL) liquid in smoothie recipes.
Tincture: Add 10 to 20 drops tincture to each 1 cup (250 mL) of smoothie.

Healing Smoothies

- Day Starter, page 233

Goldenrod
Solidago virgaurea

A perennial with upright stems, oval leaves and yellow flowers that appear in late summer. Goldenrod is indigenous to North America, with a long history of use by native peoples.

Parts Used

Aerial parts (stem, leaves and flowers).

Healing Properties

Actions: Anticatarrhal, anti-inflammatory, antiseptic to mucous membranes, urinary antiseptic, diuretic, diaphoretic.
Uses: Bronchitis, coughs, respiratory congestion, urethritis, tonsillitis, prostatitis, kidney and bladder problems.

Availability

Goldenrod is widely available in the wild and in waste lands. Harvest from July through fall. Chopped dried leaves, stems and flowers are available in alternative/health stores.

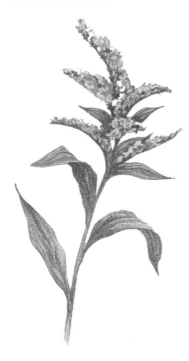

How to Use in Smoothies

Fresh sprigs: Use 1 sprig for each 1 cup (250 mL) of smoothie. Wash, pat dry and strip leaves and flowering tops off stem. Discard stem and coarsely chop leaves and flowering tops before adding to blender.
Dried leaves and flowers: Crush to a fine powder. Use 1/4 to 1/2 tsp (1 to 2 mL) for each 1 cup (250 mL) of smoothie. Add to other ingredients before blending.
Infusion: In a teapot, pour 1/4 cup (50 mL) boiling water over 1 tbsp (15 mL) fresh goldenrod (or 1 tsp/5 mL dried). Cover and steep for 10 minutes. Cool (no need to strain) and use to replace 1/4 cup (50 mL) liquid in smoothie recipes.

Green Tea
Camellia sinensis

Green and black tea come from a shrub or small tree indigenous to the wet forests of Asia. It is now cultivated commercially in Asia, Africa, South America and North America.

Parts Used

Leaves.

Healing Properties

Actions: Antioxidant, diuretic, recently found to have anticancer properties.
Uses: Cancer prevention, protection against radiation if taken daily at least a week before exposure.

Caution

Green tea contains caffeine, so minimize your intake of it if you have a health condition that is aggravated by caffeine.

Availability
Available dried in bulk in Asian grocery stores and natural-food stores, or individually wrapped in supermarkets.

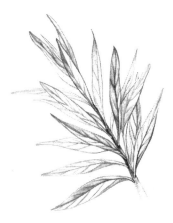

How to Use in Smoothies
Dried leaves: Crush to a fine powder. Use 1 tsp (5 mL) for each 1 cup (250 mL) of smoothie. Add to other ingredients before blending.
Infusion: In a teapot, pour $1/4$ cup (50 mL) boiling water over 1 tsp (5 mL) dried green tea leaves. Cover and steep for 10 minutes. Cool (no need to strain) and use to replace $1/4$ cup (50 mL) liquid in smoothie recipes.

Healing Smoothies
• Green Tea, page 233

Hawthorn
Crataegus monogyna and *C. oxyacanthoides*
A thorny shrub found throughout northern temperate regions, hawthorn grows wild in hedgerows in Europe and the northeastern United States and Canada. Scented white flowers bear dark red oval fruit with stony pits.

Parts Used
Flowering tops and fruit.

Healing Properties
Actions: Heart tonic, improves coronary circulation.
Uses: Angina, hypertension, poor circulation.

Caution
Consult your health-care practitioner before taking hawthorn if you are taking other heart medications.

Availability
Harvest flowering tops in the spring and fresh fruit in late summer and dry for medicinal use. Dried hawthorn "berries" are available in alternative/health stores.

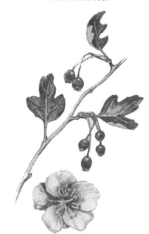

How to Use in Smoothies
Fresh berries: The pits in hawthorn berries make it difficult to remove the flesh for smoothies. If enough flesh can be separated (up to $1/2$ cup/125 mL), add to any fruit or berry smoothie for an excellent heart tonic.
Infusion: In a teapot, pour $1/4$ cup (50 mL) boiling water over 1 to 2 tsp (5 to 10 mL) bruised fresh or dried hawthorn blossoms or lightly crushed fresh or dried berries. Cover and steep for 10 minutes. Cool, strain and discard berries with pits (no need to strain blossoms). Use to replace $1/4$ cup (50 mL) liquid in smoothie recipes.

Tincture: Add 10 to 20 drops tincture to each 1 cup (250 mL) of smoothie.

Horse Chestnut
Aesculus hippocastanum
A large tree common in North America and southeastern Europe with palmate leaves and long spikes of white flowers that appear in the spring. Globular green-brown spiny fruits replace flowers in summer.

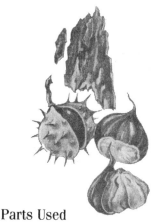

Parts Used
Bark and seeds.

Healing Properties
Actions: Astringent, anti-inflammatory, circulatory tonic, strengthens and tones veins.
Uses: Varicose veins, hemorrhoids, phlebitis. Horse chestnut tea can be used externally to treat bruises and leg ulcers.

Availability
Dried bark and seeds are available in alternative/health stores.

How to Use in Smoothies
Infusion: In a teapot, pour $1/4$ cup (50 mL) boiling water over $1/2$ tsp (2 mL) lightly crushed bark and seeds. Cover and steep for 15 minutes. Cool, strain and discard bark and seeds. Use to replace $1/4$ cup (50 mL) liquid in smoothie recipes.

Tincture: Add 30 drops tincture to each 1 cup (250 mL) of smoothie.

Hyssop
Hyssopus officinalis
A bushy evergreen woody perennial native to central and southern Europe, western Asia and northern Africa. The square, upright stems have linear opposite leaves and dense spikes at the tops that bear whorls of purple flowers.

Parts Used
Leaves and flowering tops.

Healing Properties
Actions: Antispasmodic, expectorant, diaphoretic, mild pain reliever, diuretic, antiviral against herpes simplex, reduces phlegm, soothing digestive.
Uses: Asthma, bronchitis, colds, coughs, influenza, fevers, flatulence.

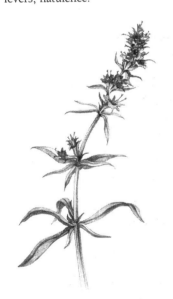

Availability
Hyssop is easy to grow and can be harvested from May through fall in central and northern North America. Dried leaves are available in alternative/health stores.

How to Use in Smoothies
Fresh sprigs: Use 1 to 3 leaves per smoothie recipe. Wash, pat dry, strip leaves and flowering tops off stems (discard stems if woody) and chop before adding to the blender.
Dried leaves and flowers: Crush to a fine powder. Use 1 tsp (5 mL) for each 1 cup (250 mL) of smoothie. Add to other ingredients before blending.
Infusion: In a teapot, pour $1/4$ cup (50 mL) boiling water over 1 tbsp (15 mL) chopped fresh hyssop (or 1 tsp/5 mL dried). Cover and steep for 10 minutes. Cool (no need to strain) and use to replace $1/4$ cup (50 mL) liquid in smoothie recipes.

Healing Smoothies
• Bronchial Aid, page 233

Kava Kava
Piper methysticum
An evergreen shrub grown and used in Polynesia that belongs to the pepper (*Piper*) genus of plants.

Parts Used
Root and rhizome.

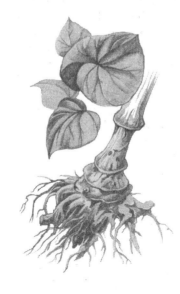

Healing Properties
Actions: Antimicrobial, especially to the genitourinary system; antispasmodic; nerve and muscle relaxant; diuretic; stimulant.
Uses: Stress; anxiety; chronic fatigue syndrome; fibromyalgia; insomnia; infections of the kidneys, bladder, vagina, prostate or urethra.

Caution
Do not use kava kava if you are pregnant or breastfeeding. Consult with your health-care practitioner before taking kava kava with other drugs that act on the nervous system. Do not take for a period of more than three months unless advised to do so by your health-care practitioner. Do not drive or operate heavy machinery while taking kava kava and do not use if you drink alcohol or take drugs that affect the liver.

Availability
Dried root and liquid extracts are available in alternative/health stores.

How to Use in Smoothies
Decoction: In a small saucepan, combine $1/2$ cup (125 mL) boiling water with 1 tsp (5 mL) dried root. Cover and simmer for 10 minutes or until light brown. Cool, strain and discard root. Use part to replace $1/4$ cup (50 mL) liquid in smoothie recipes.
Liquid extract: Add $1/2$ to 1 tsp (2 to 5 mL) to each 1 cup (250 mL) of smoothie.

Lavender
Lavandula spp
A shrub-like plant with dense, woody stems from which linear pine-like gray-green leaves grow. Whorls of tiny flowers grow on spikes that branch off the long stems.

Parts Used
Leaves, stems and flowering tops.

Healing Properties
Actions: Relaxant, antispasmodic, antidepressant, nervous system tonic, circulatory stimulant, antibacterial, antiseptic, carminative, promotes bile flow.
Uses: Colic, depression, exhaustion, indigestion, insomnia, stress, tension headaches.

Caution
Avoid large doses if you are pregnant because it is a uterine stimulant.

Availability
Easily grown in temperate climates, lavender can be harvested from June through fall. Dried flower buds are available at natural-food stores.

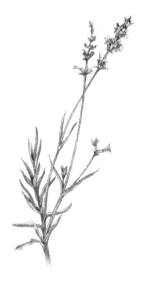

How to Use in Smoothies
Fresh sprigs: Use up to 1 tsp (5 mL) chopped fresh leaves and flowers per smoothie recipe. Start with a small amount because lavender has a distinctive taste. Wash, pat dry and strip leaves and flowers off stems. Discard stems and chop leaves and flowers before adding to the blender.

Dried flowers: Crush to a fine powder. Use $1/4$ to $1/2$ tsp (1 to 2 mL) per smoothie recipe. Add to other ingredients before blending.
Infusion: In a teapot, pour $1/4$ cup (50 mL) boiling water over 1 tsp (5 mL) chopped fresh lavender flowers (or $1/2$ tsp/2 mL dried). Cover and steep for 15 minutes. Cool (no need to strain) and use to replace $1/4$ cup (50 mL) liquid in smoothie recipes.

Healing Smoothies
• Lavender Smoothie, page 234

Lemon Balm
Melissa officinalis
A bushy perennial with strongly lemon-scented opposite oval leaves that grow on thin, square stems. White or yellow tubular flowers grow in clusters at the base of the leaves.

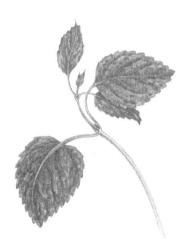

Parts Used
Leaves and flowering tops.

Healing Properties
Actions: Antioxidant, antihistamine, carminative, antispasmodic, antiviral, antibacterial, nerve relaxant, antidepressant, stimulates bile flow, hypotensive.

Uses: Anxiety, depression, stress, flatulence, indigestion, insomnia.

Availability
An easily grown perennial, lemon balm leaves and flowers can be harvested from June through autumn. Dried leaves are available in natural-food stores.

How to Use in Smoothies
Fresh sprigs: Use up to 3 leaves and/or flowers in each smoothie recipe. Wash, pat dry and strip leaves and flowers off stem. Discard stem and chop leaves and flowers. Add to other ingredients before blending.
Dried leaves and flowers: Crush to a fine powder. Use 1 tsp (5 mL) per smoothie recipe. Add to other ingredients before blending.
Infusion: In a teapot, pour $1/4$ cup (50 mL) boiling water over 1 tbsp (15 mL) chopped fresh leaves and flowers (or 1 tsp/5 mL dried). Cover and steep for 10 minutes. Cool (no need to strain) and use to replace $1/4$ cup (50 mL) liquid in smoothie recipes.

Healing Smoothies
• Anti-Depression Tonic, page 223
• Lavender Smoothie, page 234
• Lemon Lemon, page 234
• The Cool Down, page 235

Lemon Verbena
Aloysia triphylla
A fast-growing deciduous shrub native to South America that grows to a height of over six feet (180 cm) in zones 8 to 10. Long, pointed green leaves grow on erect stems that grow out of green-to-brown bark and turn woody when mature. Tiny lavender-colored flowers grow in spikes.

Parts Used
Leaves.

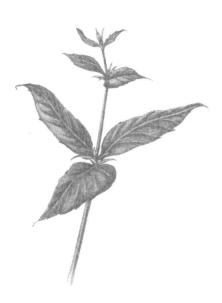

Licorice

Glycyrrhiza glabra
A tender perennial hardy in zones 7 to 9 that is native to the Mediterranean region and southwest Asia.

Parts Used
Root.

Healing Properties
Actions: Gentle laxative, tonic, anti-inflammatory, antibacterial, antiarthritic, soothes gastric and intestinal mucous membranes, expectorant.
Uses: Licorice root is considered one of the best tonic herbs because it provides nutrients to almost all body systems. It detoxifies, regulates blood sugar level and recharges depleted adrenal glands. It has also been shown to heal peptic ulcers, soothe irritated membranes and loosen and expel phlegm in the upper respiratory tract. It is also used to treat sore throats, urinary tract infections, coughs, bronchitis, gastritis and constipation.

Caution
Large amounts taken over long periods of time may cause fluid retention and lower blood potassium levels. Avoid if you have high blood pressure.

Availability
Whole or ground dried root is available in natural-food stores.
Note: Extracts lack the tonic action.

How to Use in Smoothies
Decoction: Gently simmer 1 tsp (5 mL) chopped dried root in 1/4 cup (50 mL) water for 10 minutes. Cool, strain and discard root. Use to replace 1/4 cup (50 mL) liquid in smoothie recipes.

Healing Properties
Actions: Antispasmodic, digestive.
Uses: Indigestion, flatulence.

Availability
Dried leaves may be available in natural-food stores.

How to Use in Smoothies
Fresh sprigs: Use up to 3 leaves in each smoothie recipe. Wash, pat dry and strip leaves off stem. Discard stem and chop leaves before adding to the blender.
Dried leaves: Crush to a fine powder. Use 1 tsp (5 mL) per smoothie recipe. Add to other ingredients before blending.
Infusion: In a teapot, pour 1/4 cup (50 mL) boiling water over 1 tbsp (15 mL) bruised fresh leaves (or 1 tsp/5 mL dried). Cover and steep for 10 minutes. Cool (no need to strain) and use to replace 1/4 cup (50 mL) liquid in smoothie recipes.

Healing Smoothies
• Lemon Lemon, page 234

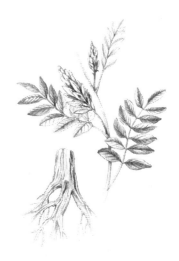

Healing Smoothies
• Anise Anise, page 235
• Bronchial Aid, page 233
• Flu Fighter #2, page 229

Linden Flower

Tilia x *europaea*
A deciduous tree with shiny dark green heart-shaped leaves and yellow-white flowers that appear in midsummer. Found throughout northern temperate regions, linden is often grown as an ornamental in North American cities.

Parts Used
Leaves and flowering tops.

Healing Properties
Actions: Antispasmodic, diaphoretic (hot tea), diuretic (warm tea), hypotensive, relaxant, mild astringent.
Uses: Linden flower tea is a pleasant-tasting, relaxing remedy for stress, anxiety, tension headache and insomnia. It relaxes and nourishes blood vessels, making it a useful treatment for high blood pressure and heart disease. Because it promotes sweating, it is helpful in treating colds, flu and fevers. The tea can be given to children as a calming remedy or to reduce fever.

Availability

Harvest flowers in mid-June and leaves from early summer through fall. Dried leaves and flowers are available in natural-food stores. Linden tea bags are often available in supermarkets.

How to Use in Smoothies

Fresh or dried leaves and flowers: Part of linden's actions are due to its essential oils, which are only released when exposed to heat. For this reason, fresh or dried linden is not added to smoothies except as a cooled tea (see Infusion, below).

Infusion: In a teapot, pour $1/4$ cup (50 mL) boiling water over 1 tbsp (15 mL) chopped fresh or dried leaves and flowers. Cover and steep for 10 minutes. Cool (no need to strain) and use to replace $1/4$ cup (50 mL) liquid in smoothie recipes.

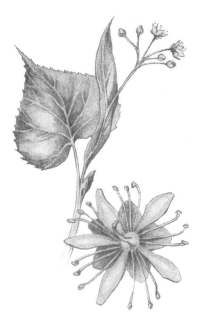

Healing Smoothies

• Lemon Lemon, page 234

Marshmallow
Althaea officinalis

A robust perennial with a fleshy taproot and upright stems that bear toothed oval leaves and pale pink flowers. Marshmallow is partial to wet ground and is often found in the wild in the United States, southern Canada, western Europe, central Asia and northern Africa. Hollyhock (*A. rosea*) is in the same genus.

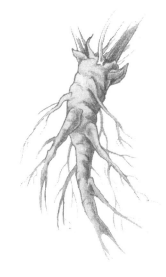

Parts Used

Flowers, leaves and root.

Healing Properties

Actions: (Root and leaves) Soothes mucous membranes; diuretic; expectorant; soothes, cleanses and heals external wounds. (Flower) Expectorant.

Uses: The high mucilage content of marshmallow root makes it useful for soothing inflammation in the digestive tract, kidneys and bladder; peptic ulcers; ulcerative colitis; Crohn's disease; urethritis; hiatal hernia; cystitis; diarrhea; and gastritis. Marshmallow leaves are used to treat bronchial inflammations, such as bronchitis, and in teas for internal ulcerative conditions. Marshmallow flower is used in expectorant cough syrups.

Availability

Gather leaves and flowers from mid-June through fall and harvest roots in the fall. Dried root is available in natural-food stores.

How to Use in Smoothies

Fresh sprigs: Use 1 or 2 leaves and/or flowers per smoothie recipe. Wash, pat dry and strip leaves and flowers off stem. Discard stem and chop leaves and flowers before adding to the blender.

Dried leaves and flowers: Crush to a fine powder. Use 1 tsp (5 mL) for each 1 cup (250 mL) of smoothie. Add to other ingredients before blending.

Infusion: In a teapot, pour $1/4$ cup (50 mL) boiling water over 1 tbsp (15 mL) chopped fresh leaves and flowers (or 1 tsp/5 mL dried). Cover and steep for 10 minutes. Cool (no need to strain) and use to replace $1/4$ cup (50 mL) liquid in smoothie recipes.

Fresh root: Scrub and chop. Use a $1/2$-inch (1 cm) piece for each 1 cup (250 mL) of smoothie. Add to other ingredients before blending.

Decoction: In a small saucepan, pour $1/4$ cup (50 mL) boiling water over 1 tsp (5 mL) chopped dried root. Cover and simmer for 10 minutes. Remove from heat; steep for 10 minutes. Cool, strain and discard root. Use to replace $1/4$ cup (50 mL) liquid in smoothie recipes.

Healing Smoothies

• Bronchial Aid, page 233

Meadowsweet
Filipendula ulmaria

A hardy herbaceous perennial found in moist or boggy soils throughout Europe, North America and temperate Asia. Toothed pinnate leaves grow on upright stems. Creamy white almond-scented flowers appear from midsummer to early autumn.

Parts Used

Aerial parts (stem, leaves and flowers).

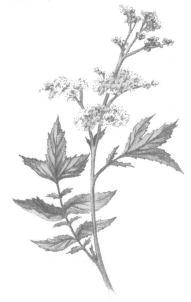

Healing Properties

Actions: Antacid, anti-inflammatory, anticoagulant, astringent, antirheumatic, diuretic, liver supportive, diaphoretic.
Uses: The anti-inflammatory and antacid actions of meadowsweet are useful in treating rheumatoid arthritis, cystitis, peptic ulcer, hyperacidity and gastric reflux. As an astringent, it is used to treat some types of diarrhea. Meadowsweet contains salicylic acid and can be used instead of Aspirin as an anti-inflammatory. Because it protects the mucous membranes of the digestive tract, unlike Aspirin, long-term use does not cause stomach bleeding.

Availability

Harvest leaves and flowers from mid-July through fall. Dried leaves and flowers are available in alternative/health stores.

How to Use in Smoothies

Dried leaves and flowers: Crush to a fine powder. Use 1 tsp (5 mL) for each 1 cup (250 mL) of smoothie. Add to other ingredients before blending.
Infusion: In a teapot, pour $1/4$ cup (50 mL) boiling water over 1 tbsp (15 mL) chopped fresh stem, leaves and flowers (or 1 tsp /5 mL dried). Cover and steep for 10 minutes. Cool (no need to strain) and use to replace $1/4$ cup (50 mL) liquid in smoothie recipes.
Tincture: Add 40 drops tincture to each 1 cup (250 mL) of smoothie.

Healing Smoothies

- Aspirin in a Glass, page 235

Milk Thistle

Silybum marianus

One of two species in this genus (Blessed Thistle is the other), milk thistle is a stout annual or biennial with large oblong leaves and purple flowers. Black seeds, each bearing a tuft of white hairs, appear in mid- to late summer.

Parts Used

Seeds.

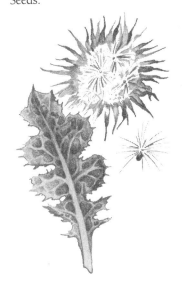

Healing Properties

Actions: Antioxidant, promotes bile production and flow, protects the liver by promoting development of new liver cells and repairing existing liver cells, detoxifies, increases milk in breastfeeding.
Uses: Milk thistle's strong liver-protective action is important in treating diseases such as alcoholism, cirrhosis and hepatitis, as well as in chronic conditions that cause liver congestion, such as constipation, bloating and premenstrual syndrome.

Availability

Seeds may be collected in the wild in midsummer but are widely available in alternative/health stores.

How to Use in Smoothies

Dried seeds: Crush to a fine powder. Use 1 tbsp (15 mL) for each 1 cup (250 mL) of smoothie. Add to other ingredients before blending.
Infusion: In a teapot, pour $1/4$ cup (50 mL) boiling water over 1 tsp (5 mL) ground dried seeds. Cover and steep for 15 minutes. Cool, strain and discard seeds. Use to replace $1/4$ cup (50 mL) liquid in smoothie recipes.
Tincture: Add 10 to 20 drops tincture to each 1 cup (250 mL) of smoothie.

Healing Smoothies

- Spa Special, page 236

Motherwort

Leonurus cardiaca

A strong-smelling perennial found throughout temperate Europe, Asia and North America. Deeply lobed palmate leaves grow out of purple stems. Mauve-pink to white flowers grow in whorls from single stems from midsummer to mid-autumn.

Parts Used

Aerial parts (stem, leaves and flowers).

Healing Properties

Actions: Antispasmodic, nerve and heart sedative, hypotensive, uterine stimulant.

Uses: Motherwort has long been used to ease menstrual pain. It eases hot flashes and other menopausal symptoms, as well as the anxiety associated with premenstrual syndrome. As a heart tonic, motherwort is especially useful for palpitations and other heart conditions in which anxiety and tension play a part. Its relaxing action makes it helpful in reducing withdrawal symptoms from antidepressant drugs.

Caution

Do not take if you are pregnant or during heavy menstrual bleeding.

Availability

Gather aerial parts (stem, leaves and flowers) from midsummer to mid-fall. Dried leaves and flowers are available in alternative/health stores.

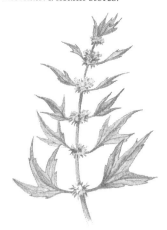

How to Use in Smoothies

Fresh leaves: Use up to 3 leaves in each smoothie recipe. Wash, pat dry and strip leaves off stem. Discard stem and chop leaves before adding to the blender.

Dried leaves and flowers: Crush to a fine powder. Use 1 tsp (5 mL) for each 1 cup (250 mL) of smoothie. Add to other ingredients before blending.

Infusion: In a teapot, pour 1/4 cup (50 mL) boiling water over 1 tbsp (15 mL) chopped fresh stem, leaves and flowers (or 1 tsp/5 mL dried). Cover and steep for 15 minutes. Cool (no need to strain) and use to replace 1/4 cup (50 mL) liquid in smoothie recipes.

Tincture: Add 1 tsp (5 mL) tincture to each 1 cup (250 mL) of smoothie.

Healing Smoothies

• Woman's Smoothie, page 236

Mustard

Brassica spp

A tall hearty annual indigenous to North America with bright green oval leaves. Yellow flowers appear in midsummer and seedpods develop in late summer to early fall.

Parts Used

Seeds (and cooked leaves; see Leafy Greens, page 140).

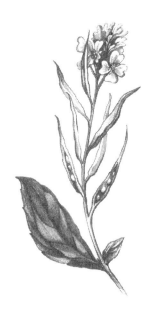

Healing Properties

Actions: Regulates blood cholesterol, blood sugar and heartbeat; reduces flatulence.

Uses: Mustard seeds are a good source of magnesium (1 tbsp/15 mL ground mustard seeds contains 33 mg of magnesium), which helps regulate cholesterol, blood sugar and heartbeat. North American First Peoples used mustard to treat asthma, bronchitis, congestion, constipation, dropsy, fever, indigestion, sore muscles and toothache. It has been found to give energy to people with chronic fatigue syndrome.

Availability

Yellow, white, black or brown dried mustard seeds are widely available in supermarkets, and plants are easy to grow from seed.

How to Use in Smoothies

Dried seeds: Crush to a fine powder. Use 1/2 tsp (2 mL) per smoothie recipe.

Healing Smoothies

• Gas Guzzler, page 228

Nutmeg

Myristica fragrans

A bushy evergreen tree native to the tropical rain forests in the Moluccas and the Banda Islands that is now grown commercially in Asia, Australia, Indonesia and Sri Lanka. Pale yellow flowers produced in axillary clusters are followed by fleshy yellow globe- to pear-shaped fruits (generally called seeds).

Parts Used

Dried kernel of the nutmeg fruit.

Healing Properties

Actions: Anti-inflammatory, antispasmodic, carminative, digestive stimulant, sedative.

Uses: Colic, diarrhea, flatulence, nausea, vomiting, muscle tension.

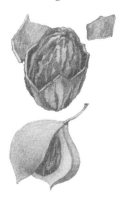

Caution
Do not use in medicinal doses if you are pregnant, as nutmeg has strong volatile oil components.

Availability
Whole, dried nutmeg seeds are available in natural-food stores, specialty stores and many supermarkets. Ground nutmeg is widely available.

How to Use in Smoothies
Dried seeds: Grate to a fine powder. Use $1/4$ tsp (1 mL) per smoothie recipe. Add to other ingredients before blending.

Healing Smoothies
• Slippery Banana, page 240

Oats
Avena sativa
A grain commonly grown throughout North America.

Parts Used
All, including seeds.

Healing Properties
Actions: Antioxidant, nerve restorative, antidepressant, nourishes brain and nerves, improves stamina, can increase libido if taken regularly.

Uses: Anxiety, depression, stress, withdrawal from alcohol and antidepressant drugs.

Availability
Oat seeds, oat straw and oatmeal are available at natural-food stores. Oatmeal is available in supermarkets.

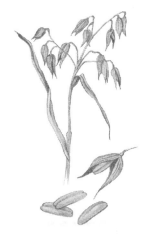

How to Use in Smoothies
Dried seeds, leaves and straw: Crush to a fine powder. Use 1 tsp (5 mL) per smoothie recipe. Add to other ingredients before blending.
Infusion: In a teapot, pour $1/4$ cup (50 mL) boiling water over 1 tsp (5 mL) dried oat straw or seeds. Cover and steep for 10 minutes. Cool, strain and discard straw or seeds. Use to replace $1/4$ cup (50 mL) liquid in smoothie recipes.

Oregon Grape
Mahonia aquifolium
Also called mountain grape, Oregon grape is the state flower of Oregon. It bears holly-like leaves and bright yellow flowers that mature into grape-like berry clusters. It grows in the mountainous regions of the West Coast of the United States and southern British Columbia.

Parts Used
Root and rhizome.

Healing Properties
Actions: Laxative; blood tonic; increases bile flow; liver stimulant; digestive; antimicrobial in the digestive tract; stimulates salivary and stomach secretions, including hydrochloric acid.
Uses: Eczema, psoriasis, constipation, indigestion, liver and gallbladder problems, gum and tooth problems.

Availability
Dried root and powdered dried root are available in alternative/health stores or by mail order.

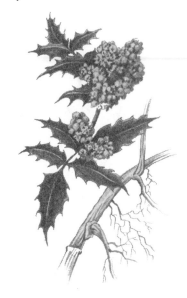

How to Use in Smoothies
Powdered dried root: Add $1/4$ to $1/2$ tsp (1 to 2 mL) ground dried root to other ingredients before blending.
Decoction: In a small saucepan, combine $1/4$ cup (50 mL) boiling water and 1 tsp (5 mL) chopped dried root. Cover and steep for 10 minutes. Cool, strain and discard root. Use to replace $1/4$ cup (50 mL) liquid in smoothie recipes.

Parsley

Petroselinum crispum

A hardy biennial native to the Mediterranean and grown as an annual in colder climates.

Parts Used

Leaves, stems and root.

Healing Properties

Actions: Antioxidant, tonic, digestive, diuretic.

Uses: As a diuretic, parsley helps the body expel excess water and flush the kidneys. Always look for and treat underlying causes of water retention. Parsley is one of the richest food sources of vitamin C.

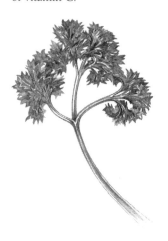

Caution

Do not take large doses of parsley if you are pregnant because it is a uterine stimulant. Parsley is also contraindicated if you are suffering from kidney inflammation.

Availability

Fresh sprigs are available in most supermarkets year-round.

How to Use in Smoothies

Fresh sprigs: Use 1 or 2 sprigs for each 1 cup (250 mL) of smoothie. Wash, pat dry and chop before adding to the blender.

Dried leaves: Add 1 tsp (5 mL) ground leaves to other ingredients before blending.

Infusion: In a teapot, pour ¼ cup (50 mL) boiling water over 1 tbsp (15 mL) chopped fresh parsley (or 1 tsp/5 mL dried). Cover and steep for 10 minutes. Cool (no need to strain) and use to replace ¼ cup (50 mL) liquid in smoothie recipes.

Healing Smoothies

- Bronchial Aid, page 233
- Diuretic Tonic, page 225
- Gout Gone, page 225
- Green Tea Smoothie, page 233
- Migraine Tonic, page 231
- Morning After, page 237

Passionflower

Passiflora incarnata

A perennial climbing vine with deeply lobed leaves and showy, fragrant, white-to-purple flowers. Some 350 species of passionflower are native to the southeastern United States and Mexico. Other species grow in tropical Asia and Australia.

Parts Used

Leaves and flowers.

Healing Properties

Actions: Antispasmodic, mild sedative, mild pain reliever, central nervous system relaxant.

Uses: Anxiety, asthma, insomnia, restlessness, headache, Parkinson's disease, withdrawal from antidepressant drugs and alcohol.

Availability

Passionflower can be harvested from May through July in the wild or in cultivated gardens. Dried passionflower is available in alternative/health stores.

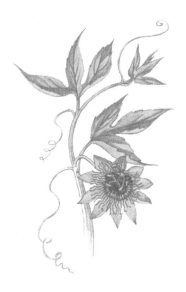

Folklore

The distinctive flower is said to symbolize the Passion of Christ by representing the elements of the Crucifixion.

How to Use in Smoothies

Dried leaves and flowers: Crush to a fine powder. Use ¼ tsp (1 mL) for each 1 cup (250 mL) of smoothie. Add to other ingredients before blending.

Infusion: In a teapot, pour ¼ cup (50 mL) boiling water over 1 tbsp (15 mL) chopped fresh passionflower (or ½ tsp/2 mL dried). Cover and steep for 15 minutes. Cool (no need to strain) and use to replace ¼ cup (50 mL) liquid in smoothie recipes.

Tincture: Add 40 drops tincture to each 1 cup (250 mL) of smoothie.

Peppermint

Mentha piperita

An invasive hardy perennial native to Europe and Asia but easily grown in North America. It has aromatic bright green oval leaves on purple stems and small pink, white or purple flowers in elongated conical spikes at the tops of the stems.

Parts Used

Leaves and flowers.

Healing Properties

Actions: Antispasmodic, digestive tonic, antiemetic, carminative, peripheral vasodilator, diaphoretic, promotes bile flow, analgesic.

Uses: Taking peppermint before eating helps stimulate the liver and gallbladder by increasing bile flow to the liver and intestines. It is well known for its ability to quell nausea and vomiting. Peppermint is used to treat ulcerative colitis, Crohn's disease, diverticular disease, motion sickness, fevers, colds and flu, and to improve appetite.

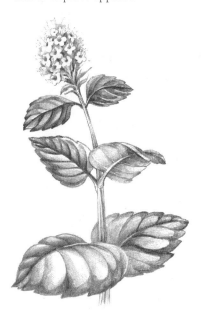

Caution

Do not use if you are pregnant or give to a child.

Availability

Fresh sprigs appear in some farmer's markets and supermarkets year-round. Dried leaves are available in alternative/health stores. Peppermint tea in bulk and bags is widely available.

How to Use in Smoothies

Fresh leaves: Use 3 to 4 leaves for each 1 cup (250 mL) of smoothie. Wash, pat dry and strip leaves and flowers off stem. Discard stem and chop leaves and flowers. Add to other ingredients before blending.

Dried leaves: Add 1 tsp (5 mL) ground dried leaves to each smoothie recipe.

Infusion: In a teapot, pour 1/4 cup (50 mL) boiling water over 1 tbsp (15 mL) chopped fresh peppermint (or 1 tsp/5 mL dried). Cover and steep for 10 minutes. Cool (no need to strain) and use to replace 1/4 cup (50 mL) liquid in smoothie recipes.

Healing Smoothies

• Peppermint Aperitif, page 237

Plantain

Plantago major and *P. lanceolata*

Broad-leaved plantain and narrow-leaved plantain are common weeds found in waste areas throughout North America. Leaves grow in a basal rosette, and flowers top long cylindrical spikes that grow up to six inches (15 cm) above leaves.

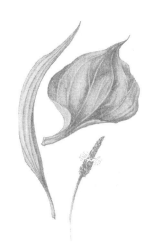

Parts Used

Leaves.

Healing Properties

Actions: Antibacterial, soothing expectorant, provides mucilage-rich protection to digestive tract, nutrient, antihistamine, astringent.

Uses: Coughs, bronchitis, allergies, irritable bowel syndrome, gastric ulcers.

Availability

The leaves can be collected throughout the summer. Dried leaves are available in alternative/health stores.

Folklore

Fresh plantain leaves have traditionally been rubbed on insect bites to soothe inflammation.

How to Use in Smoothies

Fresh leaves: Use 1 leaf per smoothie recipe. Wash, pat dry and chop before adding to the blender.

Infusion: In a teapot, pour 1/4 cup (50 mL) boiling water over 1 tbsp (15 mL) chopped fresh plantain leaves (or 1 tsp/5 mL dried). Cover and steep for 10 minutes. Cool (no need to strain) and use to replace 1/4 cup (50 mL) liquid in smoothie recipes.

Red Clover

Trifolium pratense

A perennial with tubular pink-to-red flowers throughout the summer, red clover grows in fields throughout North America. Its three long oval leaflets distinguish it as a clover.

Parts Used

Flowering tops.

Healing Properties

Actions: Antispasmodic, expectorant, balances hormones, nutritive, anticoagulant, lymphatic cleanser.
Uses: Coughs, bronchitis, whooping cough, menstrual problems.

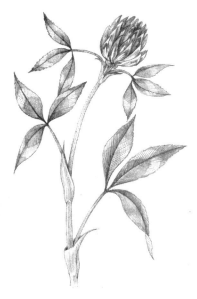

Caution

Because it helps thin the blood, don't use red clover during heavy menstrual flow.

Availability

The flowering tops can be harvested from May through September in the wild or in cultivated gardens. Dried flowers are available in alternative/health stores. Dried clover that has turned brown is of little use; be sure that the flowers are still pink.

How to Use in Smoothies

Fresh sprigs: Use 1 or 2 sprigs per smoothie recipe. Wash, pat dry and strip leaves and flowers off stems. Discard stems and green centers of flowers and chop leaves and petals before adding to blender.

Dried leaves and flowers: Crush to a fine powder. Use 1 tsp (5 mL) for each 1 cup (250 mL) of smoothie. Add to other ingredients before blending.
Infusion: In a teapot, pour $\frac{1}{4}$ cup (50 mL) boiling water over 1 tbsp (15 mL) chopped fresh red clover (or 1 tsp/5 mL dried). Cover and steep for 15 minutes. Cool (no need to strain) and use to replace $\frac{1}{4}$ cup (50 mL) liquid in smoothie recipes.

Healing Smoothies

• Woman's Smoothie, page 236

Red Raspberry
Rubus idaeus

A deciduous shrub with prickly stems and pinnately divided leaves that is widespread in Europe, Asia and North America. Small white flowers appear in clusters, and aromatic, juicy red fruit follow in early summer.

Parts Used

Leaves.

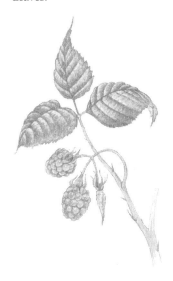

Healing Properties

Actions: Antispasmodic, astringent, increases milk in breastfeeding.

Uses: Red raspberry leaves have long been used to tone the uterus during pregnancy and labor, resulting in less risk of miscarriage, relief of morning sickness and safer, easier birth. As an astringent, raspberry leaves ease sore throat and diarrhea.

Availability

Harvest leaves from early summer through fall. Dried leaves are available in alternative/health stores.

How to Use in Smoothies

Fresh leaves: Use 1 or 2 leaves per smoothie recipe. Wash, pat dry and chop before adding to the blender.
Dried leaves: Crush to a fine powder. Use 1 tsp (5 mL) for each 1 cup (250 mL) of smoothie. Add to other ingredients before blending.
Infusion: In a teapot, pour $\frac{1}{4}$ cup (50 mL) boiling water over 1 tbsp (15 mL) chopped fresh leaves (or 2 tsp/10 mL dried). Cover and steep for 15 minutes. Cool (no need to strain) and use to replace $\frac{1}{4}$ cup (50 mL) liquid in smoothie recipes.

Healing Smoothies

• Raspberry Raspberry, page 237

Rose
Rosa spp

Cultivation of roses dates back thousands of years, with *R. rugosa, R. gallica, R. rubra* and *R. damascena* being among the oldest varieties. *R. rugosa* is a deciduous shrub with thorny stems and dark green oval leaves; dark pink or white flowers appear in summer and are followed by large globular bright red rose hips (fruit). Wild roses (including *R. canina* of North America) grow in northern temperate regions throughout the world.

Parts Used
Petals and hips.

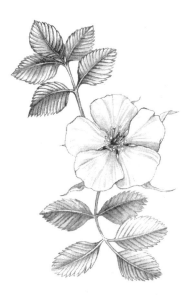

Healing Properties
Actions: (Rose hips from *R. canina*) Contain vitamin C, diuretic, astringent, mild laxative. (Rose petals from *R. gallica*, *R. damascena*, *R. centifolia*, *R. rugosa*) Antidepressant, anti-inflammatory, astringent, blood tonic.
Uses: (Rose hips) The nutrient value of rose hips makes them useful in preventing the common cold. A tasty addition to herbal teas, rose hips improve immune function. As an astringent, they are used to treat diarrhea. (Rose petals) Add them to teas for their relaxing and uplifting fragrance. Used in baths, they ease the pain of rheumatoid arthritis.

Availability
Harvest petals from midsummer through fall and hips in the fall.

How to Use in Smoothies
Dried flowers or hips: Crush to a fine powder. Use $1/2$ tsp (2 mL) for each 1 cup (250 mL) of smoothie. Add to other ingredients before blending.

Infusion: In a teapot, pour $1/4$ cup (50 mL) boiling water over 1 tbsp (15 mL) fresh rose petals or chopped fresh rose hips (or 1 tsp/5 mL dried petals or crushed dried hips). Cover and steep for 10 minutes. Cool (no need to strain) and use to replace $1/4$ cup (50 mL) liquid in smoothie recipes.

Healing Smoothies
• Rose Smoothie, page 238

Rosemary
Rosmarinus officinalis
An evergreen shrub native to the Mediterranean that grows to a height of six feet (180 cm) in warm climates.

Parts Used
Leaves and flowers.

Healing Properties
Actions: Antioxidant, anti-inflammatory, astringent, nervine, carminative, antiseptic, diuretic, diaphoretic, promotes bile flow, antidepressant, circulatory stimulant, antispasmodic, nervous system and cardiac tonic.
Uses: An effective food preservative, rosemary may help prevent breast cancer and fight the deterioration of brain function. It is also useful in treating migraine and tension headaches, nervous tension, flatulence, depression, chronic fatigue syndrome and joint pain.

Caution
Do not take large amounts if you are pregnant, as rosemary contains strong volatile oil components.

Availability
Look for fresh sprigs in markets and supermarkets year-round. Dried whole and ground leaves are widely found in supermarkets and natural-food stores.

How to Use in Smoothies
Fresh sprigs: Use $1/2$ tsp (2 mL) chopped fresh rosemary leaves and flowers per smoothie recipe. Wash, pat dry and strip leaves and flowers off stem. Discard stem and chop leaves and flowers before adding to the blender.
Infusion: In a teapot, pour $1/4$ cup (50 mL) boiling water over 1 tbsp (15 mL) chopped fresh rosemary (or 1 tsp/5 mL dried). Cover and steep for 10 minutes. Cool (no need to strain) and use to replace $1/4$ cup (50 mL) liquid in smoothie recipes.

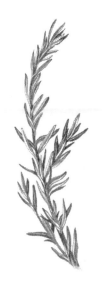

Healing Smoothies
• Migraine Tonic, page 231
• Thyme in a Glass, page 241

Sage
Salvia officinalis
A hardy evergreen woody perennial shrub native to the western United States and Mexico, with wrinkled gray-green oval leaves and purple, pink or white flowers.

Parts Used
Leaves and flowers.

Healing Properties

Actions: Antioxidant, antimicrobial, antibiotic, antiseptic, carminative, antispasmodic, anti-inflammatory, circulatory stimulant, estrogenic, peripheral vasodilator, reduces perspiration, uterine stimulant.
Uses: Sage's volatile oil kills bacteria and fungi — even those that are resistant to penicillin. It makes a very good gargle for sore throats, laryngitis and mouth ulcers. It is also used to reduce breast milk production and to relieve night sweats and hot flashes during menopause.

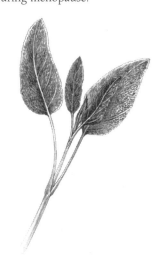

Caution

Sage can cause convulsions in very large doses. Do not use if you have high blood pressure or epilepsy or if you are pregnant.

Availability

Fresh sprigs can be found at some supermarkets and farmer's markets. Whole, rubbed or ground dried sage is available at most supermarkets.

How to Use in Smoothies

Fresh leaves: Use 1 leaf per smoothie recipe. Wash, pat dry and strip leaves off stem (discard stem if woody). Chop before adding to the blender.

Dried leaves and flowers: Crush to a fine powder. Use $^1/_2$ tsp (2 mL) for each 1 cup (250 mL) of smoothie. Add to other ingredients before blending.
Infusion: In a teapot, pour $^1/_4$ cup (50 mL) boiling water over 1 tbsp (15 mL) chopped fresh sage (or 1 tsp/5 mL dried). Cover and steep for 10 minutes. Cool (no need to strain) and use to replace $^1/_4$ cup (50 mL) liquid in smoothie recipes.

Healing Smoothies

• Sage Relief, page 238

Saw Palmetto

Seranoa serrulata

A clump-forming evergreen palm with long blue-green leaves and blue-black berries. It grows mainly along coastal areas of southeastern North America and forms dense thickets along the Atlantic coasts of Georgia and Florida.

Parts Used

Berries.

Healing Properties

Actions: Diuretic, urinary antiseptic, stimulates the hormone-secreting glands.
Uses: Benign prostate enlargement, low libido.

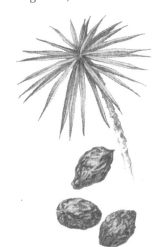

Availability

The berries can be harvested from September though January. Dried berries are available ground and in tablet form in alternative/health stores.

How to Use in Smoothies

Ground dried berries: Use $^1/_4$ tsp (1 mL) per smoothie recipe. Add to other ingredients before blending.
Infusion: In a teapot, pour $^1/_4$ cup (50 mL) boiling water over 1 tsp (5 mL) crushed fresh berries (or $^1/_2$ tsp/2 mL crushed dried). Cover and steep for 10 minutes. Cool, strain and discard berries. Use to replace $^1/_4$ cup (50 mL) liquid in smoothie recipes.
Liquid extract: Add 10 to 25 drops liquid extract to each 1 cup (250 mL) of smoothie.

Healing Smoothies

• Prostate Power, page 239

Skullcap

Scutellaria laterifolia

A perennial member of the mint family that features hooded violet-blue flowers. It grows in wooded areas in most of the United States and southern Canada, except along the West Coast.

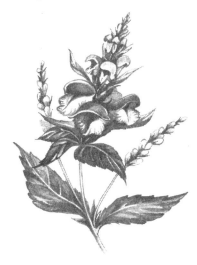

Parts Used

Aerial parts (stem, leaves and flowers).

Healing Properties

Actions: Antispasmodic, nourishes central nervous system, relaxant, sedative.
Uses: Drug addiction withdrawal, premenstrual tension, headaches, migraines, mental exhaustion, insomnia, stress.

Availability

Aerial parts (stem, leaves and flowers) can be collected while the plant is in flower. Dried skullcap is available in natural-food stores.

How to Use in Smoothies

Fresh sprigs: Use 1 leaf and/or flower per smoothie recipe. Wash, pat dry and strip leaves and flowers off stem. Discard stem and chop leaves and flowers before adding to the blender.
Dried leaves and flowers: Crush to a fine powder. Use 1 tsp (5 mL) for each 1 cup (250 mL) of smoothie. Add to other ingredients before blending.
Infusion: In a teapot, pour $1/4$ cup (50 mL) boiling water over 1 tbsp (15 mL) chopped fresh skullcap (or 1 tsp/5 mL dried). Cover and steep for 10 minutes. Cool (no need to strain) and use to replace $1/4$ cup (50 mL) liquid in smoothie recipes.
Tincture: Add 40 drops tincture to each 1 cup (250 mL) of smoothie.

Healing Smoothies

• Smart Smoothie, page 239

Slippery Elm
Ulmus fulva

A deciduous tree found in moist woods in the eastern and midwestern United States and southeastern Canada.

Parts Used

Dried inner bark.

Healing Properties

Actions: Soothing digestive, antacid, nutritive, provides mucilage-rich protection to the digestive tract.
Uses: Peptic ulcers, indigestion, heartburn, hiatal hernia, Crohn's disease, ulcerative colitis, irritable bowel syndrome, diarrhea. A paste of slippery elm bark powder can be used to soothe and heal wounds and burns. It is one of the most useful herbs in herbal medicine.

Availability

Ground dried inner bark and lozenges are available in alternative/health stores.

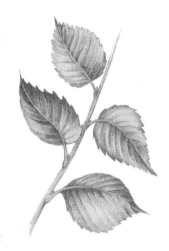

How to Use in Smoothies

Smoothies are a great medium in which to take slippery elm, which is so soothing for the bowel but so difficult to consume because the powder doesn't dissolve in or mix with liquids.
Ground dried bark: Add 1 tsp (5 mL) to each 1 cup (250 mL) of smoothie.

Healing Smoothies

• Hangover Remedy, page 240
• Muscle Relief, page 228
• Peptic Tonic, page 226
• Slippery Banana, page 240

Spearmint
Mentha spicata

A hardy invasive perennial found in wet soil in most of North America. Like all mints, it has a square stem with bright green lanceolate leaves and lilac, pink, or white flowers that form in a terminal, cylindrical spike.

Parts Used

Leaves and flowering tops.

Healing Properties

Actions: Antispasmodic, digestive, diaphoretic.
Uses: Common cold, influenza, indigestion, flatulence, lack of appetite. Spearmint is milder than peppermint, so it is often used to treat children's colds and flus.

Availability

The leaves are best harvested just before the flowers open. Dried leaves are available in natural-food stores.

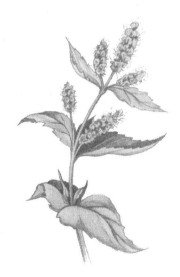

How to Use in Smoothies

Fresh sprigs: Use 2 to 3 leaves per smoothie recipe. Wash, pat dry and strip leaves and flowers off stems. Discard stems and chop leaves and flowers before adding to the blender.

Dried leaves and flowers: Crush to a fine powder. Use $1/2$ tsp (2 mL) for each 1 cup (250 mL) of smoothie. Add to other ingredients before blending.
Infusion: In a teapot, pour $1/4$ cup (50 mL) boiling water over 1 tbsp (15 mL) chopped fresh spearmint (or 1 tsp/5 mL dried). Cover and steep for 10 minutes. Cool (no need to strain) and use to replace $1/4$ cup (50 mL) liquid in smoothie recipes.

Healing Smoothies

• Mint Julep, page 241

St. John's Wort

Hypericum perforatum

A perennial native of woodlands in Europe and temperate Asia that has also naturalized in temperate areas of the United States and Canada. It is an upright plant with straight stems that are woody at the base and has five-petaled yellow flowers growing from the tips of the branched stems. When rubbed, the yellow petals stain the fingers red.

Parts Used

Flowering tops.

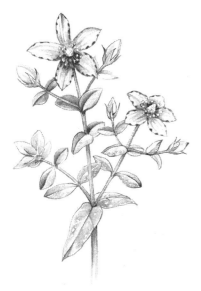

Healing Properties

Actions: Astringent, antiviral, anti-inflammatory, antidepressant, nervous system tonic, sedative.
Uses: St. John's wort is widely used as an antidepressant. It has become popular because of its effectiveness and lack of side effects. As a sedative and nervous-system tonic, it is useful in treating neuralgia, shingles, sciatica, tension, anxiety, and emotional instability in premenstrual syndrome and menopause.

Caution

Recent studies suggest that St. John's wort increases the metabolism of certain drugs, reducing their effectiveness. If you are taking prescription drugs, consult with your herbalist, doctor or pharmacist about possible drug interactions before taking St. John's wort. Of particular concern are oral contraceptives, anticonvulsants, antidepressants (especially selective serotonin reuptake inhibitors), HIV drugs, anticoagulants (warfarin), cyclosporine (an immunosuppressant drug given after transplants) and digoxin.

Availability

Harvest flowering tops for two to three weeks in midsummer. Dried aerial parts (stem, leaves and flowers) and tinctures are available in alternative/health stores.

How to Use in Smoothies

Dried leaves and flowers: Crush to a fine powder. Use 1 tsp (5 mL) for each 1 cup (250 mL) of smoothie. Add to other ingredients before blending.
Infusion: In a teapot, pour $1/4$ cup (50 mL) boiling water over 1 tbsp (15 mL) chopped fresh flowers (or 1 tsp/5 mL dried). Cover and steep for 15 minutes. Cool (no need to strain) and use to replace $1/4$ cup (50 mL) liquid in smoothie recipes.

Tincture: Add 20 to 40 drops tincture to each 1 cup (250 mL) of smoothie.

Stevia

Stevia rebaudiana

A small tender shrub native to northeastern Paraguay and adjacent areas of Brazil.

Parts Used

Leaves.

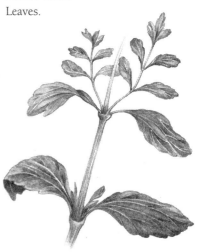

Healing Properties

Actions: Energy booster, natural sweetener (without calories), tonic, digestive, diuretic.
Uses: Stevia's main benefit is that it is a safe sweetener and sugar alternative. With its powerful sweet licorice flavor (stevia is 200 to 300 times sweeter than sugar), it prevents cavities and does not trigger a rise in blood sugar. It increases energy and improves digestion by stimulating the pancreas without feeding yeast or fungi.

Availability

Cut and dried ground leaves and liquid extracts are available in alternative/health stores.

How to Use in Smoothies

Fresh leaves: Use 1 leaf per smoothie. Wash, pat dry and strip leaves off stem. Discard stem and chop leaves before adding to the blender.

Dried leaves: Crush to a fine powder. Use $1/8$ tsp (0.5 mL) for each 1 cup (250 mL) of smoothie. Add to other ingredients before blending.

Infusion: In a teapot, pour $1/4$ cup (50 mL) boiling water over 1 tsp (5 mL) chopped fresh leaves (or $1/4$ tsp/1 mL dried). Cover and steep for 10 minutes. Cool (no need to strain) and use to replace $1/4$ cup (50 mL) liquid in smoothie recipes.

Liquid extract: Add 1 or 2 drops liquid extract to each 1 cup (250 mL) of smoothie.

Stinging Nettle
Urtica dioica

A perennial widespread in temperate regions of Europe, North America and Eurasia with bristly stinging hairs on the stems and toothed ovate leaves that cause minor skin irritation when touched. Minute green flowers appear in clusters during the summer.

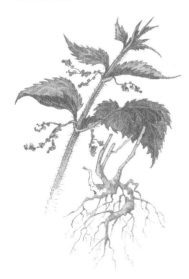

Parts Used

Leaves, root and seeds.

Healing Properties

Actions: (Leaves and flowers) Astringent, blood tonic, circulatory stimulant, diuretic, eliminates uric acid from the body, nutritive (high in iron, chlorophyll and vitamin C), increases milk in breastfeeding. (Fresh root) Astringent, diuretic.

Uses: (Leaves and flowers) A valuable herb, stinging nettle is useful as a general, everyday nourishing tonic, as well as for treatment of iron-deficiency anemia, gout, arthritis and kidney stones. It is also a good blood tonic to take during pregnancy or if you have diabetes, poor circulation or a chronic skin disease, such as eczema. (Fresh root) Fresh stinging nettle root has a strong effect on the urinary system. It is useful in treating water retention, kidney stones, urinary tract infections, cystitis, prostatitis and prostate enlargement.

Availability

Gather leaves and flowers while flowering in summer and root in fall. Use gloves to protect your hands from its uric acid, which dissipates with drying or cooking. Dried leaves and flowers are available in alternative/health stores.

Folklore

A common remedy for arthritis is flailing the affected joints with fresh stinging nettle leaves. The sting brings healing blood flow to the area.

How to Use in Smoothies

Infusion: In a teapot, pour $1/4$ cup (50 mL) boiling water over 1 tbsp (15 mL) chopped fresh leaves (or 1 tsp/5 mL dried). Cover and steep for 15 minutes. Cool (no need to strain) and use to replace $1/4$ cup (50 mL) liquid in smoothie recipes.

Tincture: Add 1 tsp (5 mL) tincture to each 1 cup (250 mL) of smoothie.

Thyme
Thymus vulgaris

A bushy low-growing shrub easily grown in North America.

Parts Used

Leaves and flowers.

Healing Properties

Actions: Antioxidant, expectorant, antiseptic, antispasmodic, astringent, tonic, antimicrobial, antibiotic, heals wounds, carminative, calms coughs, nervine.

Uses: Thyme is ideal for deep-seated chest infections, such as chronic coughs and bronchitis. It is also used to treat sinusitis, laryngitis, asthma and irritable bowel syndrome.

Caution

Do not take if you are pregnant. Children under two years of age and people with thyroid problems should not take thyme.

Availability

Fresh sprigs are available in season at farmer's markets and most supermarkets year-round. Dried whole leaves can be found in natural-food stores.

How to Use in Smoothies

Fresh sprigs: Use 1 sprig per smoothie recipe. Wash, pat dry and strip leaves and flowers off stem (discard stem if woody). Chop before adding to the blender.

Dried leaves and flowers: Add 1 tsp (5 mL) dried leaves and crushed flowers to each 1 cup (250 mL) of smoothie.

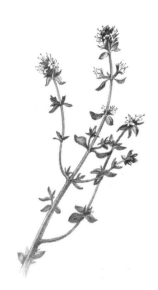

Infusion: In a teapot, pour $1/4$ cup (50 mL) boiling water over 1 tbsp (15 mL) chopped fresh thyme (or 1 tsp/5 mL dried). Cover and steep for 15 minutes. Cool (no need to strain) and use to replace $1/4$ cup (50 mL) liquid in smoothie recipes.

Healing Smoothies
• Thyme in a Glass, page 241

Turmeric

Curcuma longa

A deciduous tender perennial in the ginger family native to southeast Asia that is hardy to zone 10. The long rhizome resembles ginger but is thinner and rounder, with brilliant orange flesh.

Parts Used
Root.

Healing Properties

Actions: Antioxidant, anti-inflammatory, antimicrobial, antibacterial, antifungal, antiviral, anticoagulant, analgesic, lowers blood cholesterol, reduces postexercise pain, heals wounds, antispasmodic, protects liver cells, increases bile production and flow.

Uses: Turmeric appears to inhibit colon and breast cancer and is used to treat hepatitis, nausea and digestive disturbances. It also helps people whose gallbladders have been removed. It boosts insulin activity and reduces the risk of stroke. Turmeric is also used to treat rheumatoid arthritis, cancer, candida, AIDS, Crohn's disease and eczema.

Availability

Asian stores stock fresh, frozen or dried whole rhizomes. Alternative/health stores offer dried whole rhizomes, and supermarkets sell ground turmeric.

How to Use in Smoothies

Fresh root: Use one $1/2$- to 1-inch (1 to 2.5 cm) long piece per smoothie recipe. Scrub, peel (if not organic) and cut into quarters before adding to the blender.
Ground dried root: Use 1 tsp (5 mL) ground dried root for each 1 cup (250 mL) of smoothie. Add to other ingredients before blending.
Infusion: In a teapot, pour $1/4$ cup (50 mL) boiling water over 1 tbsp (15 mL) freshly grated turmeric (or 1 tsp/5 mL chopped or ground dried root). Cover and steep for 10 minutes. Cool, strain and discard root. Use to replace $1/4$ cup (50 mL) liquid in smoothie recipes.

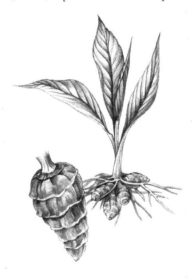

Healing Smoothies
• Turmeric Cocktail, page 241

Valerian

Valeriana officinalis

A tall hardy perennial with strong-smelling white clustered flowers that grows wild in eastern Canada and the northeastern United States.

Parts Used
Root.

Healing Properties

Actions: Sedative, relaxant, antispasmodic.
Uses: High blood pressure, insomnia, anxiety, tension headaches, muscle cramps, migraines.

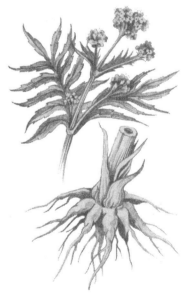

Caution

Some people experience adverse reactions to valerian.

Availability

Roots can be harvested in late fall in the wild or in cultivated gardens. Dried roots and tinctures are available in alternative/health stores.

How to Use in Smoothies

Fresh root: Valerian roots are a mass of thin rootlets. After digging up, immerse in water to remove loose soil, then scrub and chop. Wrap fresh root in a towel and store in the refrigerator for one to two weeks. Dry chopped root to store longer. Use 2 tsp (10 mL) chopped fresh root per smoothie recipe.

Decoction: In a small saucepan, pour $\frac{1}{4}$ cup (50 mL) boiling water over 1 tbsp (15 mL) chopped fresh root (or 1 tsp/5 mL chopped dried). Cover and simmer for 10 minutes. Cool, strain and discard root. Use to replace $\frac{1}{4}$ cup (50 mL) liquid in smoothie recipes.

Tincture: Add 20 to 40 drops tincture to each 1 cup (250 mL) of smoothie.

Healing Smoothies
• Sleepytime Smoothie, page 227

Wild Lettuce

Lactuca virosa
A tall biennial with lanceolate leaves and dandelion-like flowers that grows easily from seed.

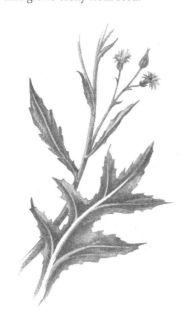

Parts Used
Leaves and flowers.

Healing Properties
Actions: Nerve relaxant, mild sedative, mild pain reliever.
Uses: Anxiety, insomnia, hyperactivity in children.

Availability
Gather leaves in June and July, otherwise not widely available.

How to Use in Smoothies
Dried leaves and flowers: Crush to a fine powder. Use 1 tsp (5 mL) for each 1 cup (250 mL) of smoothie. Add to other ingredients before blending.
Infusion: In a teapot, pour $\frac{1}{4}$ cup (50 mL) boiling water over 1 tbsp (15 mL) chopped fresh leaves (or 1 tsp/5 mL ground dried leaves). Cover and steep for 10 minutes. Cool (no need to strain) and use to replace $\frac{1}{4}$ cup (50 mL) liquid in smoothie recipes.

Yarrow

Achillea millefolium
A one- to three-foot (30 to 90 cm) tall hardy perennial with feathery leaves and white (occasionally pink) flowers that grows wild in fields throughout North America and is easily grown in the garden.

Parts Used
Stem, leaves and flowers.

Healing Properties
Actions: Anti-inflammatory, bitter, promotes bile flow, diaphoretic, digestive, relaxant, promotes blood circulation, heals wounds.
Uses: High blood pressure, colds, fevers, influenza, varicose veins.

Caution
Large doses of yarrow are toxic if taken over a long period of time.

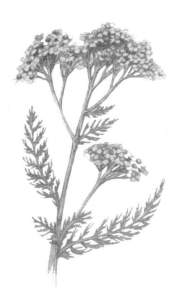

Availability
Harvest aboveground parts while flowering in the wild from June through September. Dried stems, leaves and flowers and tinctures are available in alternative/health stores.

How to Use in Smoothies
Dried stems, leaves and flowers: Crush to a fine powder. Use 1 tsp (5 mL) for each 1 cup (250 mL) of smoothie. Add to other ingredients before blending.
Infusion: In a teapot, pour $\frac{1}{4}$ cup (50 mL) boiling water over 1 tbsp (15 mL) chopped fresh flowers (or 1 tsp/5 mL dried). Cover and steep for 10 minutes. Cool (no need to strain) and use to replace $\frac{1}{4}$ cup (50 mL) liquid in smoothie recipes.
Tincture: Add 40 drops tincture to each 1 cup (250 mL) of smoothie.

Yellow Dock

Rumex crispus
A large one- to five-foot (30 to 150 cm) tall perennial with small green-to-red flowers that grows in waste areas throughout North America.

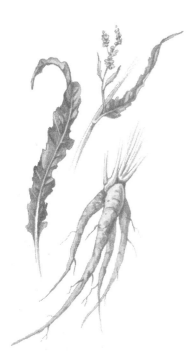

Parts Used
Root.

Healing Properties
Actions: Bitter, laxative, lymphatic, increases bile flow.
Uses: Fresh roots are rich in iron and can be used to treat iron-deficiency anemia. Yellow dock also helps cleanse the body by supporting liver function and eliminating toxins through the bile. It is an especially helpful cleanser for skin diseases, rheumatoid arthritis, swollen lymph glands and constipation.

Availability
The root can be harvested in the wild from September through November. Dried root is available in alternative/health stores.

How to Use in Smoothies
Fresh root: Immerse root in water to remove loose soil, then scrub and chop (leave skin on if it has been wildcrafted and you are certain is has not been contaminated by pesticides or waste). Wrap fresh root in a towel and store in the refrigerator for one to two weeks. Dry chopped root to store longer. Use 2 tsp (10 mL) fresh chopped root per smoothie recipe.
Ground dried root: Add 1 tsp (5 mL) ground dried root to each 1 cup (250 mL) of smoothie.
Decoction: In a small saucepan, pour ¼ cup (50 mL) boiling water over 1 tbsp (15 mL) chopped fresh root (or 1 tsp/5 mL chopped dried). Cover and simmer for 10 minutes. Cool, strain and discard root. Use to replace ¼ cup (50 mL) liquid in smoothie recipes.

Fruit Profiles

Apples
Actions: Tonic, digestive, diuretic, detoxifying, laxative, antiseptic, lower blood cholesterol, antirheumatic, liver stimulant.
Uses: Fresh apples help cleanse the system, lower blood cholesterol levels, keep blood sugar level up and aid digestion. The French use the peels in preparations for rheumatism and gout, as well as in urinary tract remedies. Apples are also very useful components in cleansing fasts because they help eliminate toxins. Apples are good sources of vitamin A. They also contain some vitamins B and C and riboflavin and are high in two important phytochemicals: pectin and boron.

Buying and storing: Look for blemish-free apples with firm, crisp flesh and smooth, tight skin. Because of the widespread use of pesticides on apples, choose organic whenever possible or peel before using. Apples will keep in a cool, dark, dry place (or the crisper drawer of your refrigerator) for one month or more.
For smoothies: Apples can be blended with any fruit or vegetable. They lend a natural sweetness and an abundance of fiber and texture. The greener the apple the sharper its taste. Wash, peel (if not organic) and core, if desired, but do not use the seeds. One apple, peeled and cored, yields approximately 1 cup (250 mL) roughly chopped. Homemade or commercially packaged applesauce may also be used in smoothies.

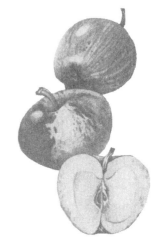

Apple Smoothies
- Apple Crisp, page 156
- Apple Currant, page 156
- Apple Fresh, page 156
- Apple Mint, page 157
- Apple Pear, page 184
- Apple Pie, page 157
- Apple Spice Cocktail, page 158

Apricots

Actions: Antioxidant, anticancer.
Uses: Apricots are very high in beta-carotene, a precursor of vitamin A, which may prevent the formation of cholesterol deposits in the arteries, thus preventing heart disease (three small fresh apricots deliver 2,770 IU of vitamin A; $1/2$ cup/125 mL dried apricots contain 8,175 IU). Apricots are also high in vitamin B2, potassium, boron, iron, magnesium and fiber. Apricots help normalize blood pressure and heart function and maintain normal body fluids. They contain virtually no sodium or fat, so fresh or dried apricots are especially recommended for women because they are good sources of calcium and excellent sources of vitamin A.
Buying and storing: Choose firm, fresh apricots that range in color from dark yellow to orange. Keep in a cool, dry place for up to one week.

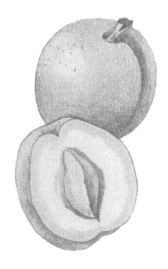

For smoothies: Wash and peel fresh apricots (if not organic) but do not use the pits. Dried apricots may be used to add extra sweetness to smoothies. Look for unsulphured dried apricots (especially if you have allergies) and substitute two dried apricot halves for one fresh apricot. Canned apricots and their juices may also be used in smoothies. You can also make Apricot Milk (see page 247) to use as a liquid in smoothies.

Apricot Smoothies
- Apricot Apricot, page 158
- Apricot Explosion, page 158
- Apricot Peach, page 159
- Triple A, page 159

Bananas

Actions: Antiulcer, antibacterial, boost immunity, lower blood cholesterol levels.
Uses: Due to their ability to strengthen the surface cells of the stomach lining and protect them against acids, bananas are recommended when ulcers or the risk of ulcers is present. High in potassium and vitamin B6, bananas help prevent heart attacks, strokes and other cardiovascular problems.
Buying and storing: Look for ripe bananas: they are soft, yellow and slightly speckled with brown. Store in a cool, dark, dry place.
For smoothies: Used often in fruit smoothies, bananas thicken the mixture and add a fresh fruit flavor. Peel and cut a banana into four pieces before adding to the blender. Use one fresh or frozen whole banana for every 2 cups (500 mL) of smoothie.
To freeze bananas: Choose fully yellow bananas with no bruises or brown spots. Peel and cut each into four chunks and arrange on a baking sheet. Freeze in the coldest part of the freezer for 30 minutes. Place the chunks in one large or several individual freezer bags. Seal and store the chunks in the freezer for four to six months. Four frozen chunks equal one whole fresh banana.

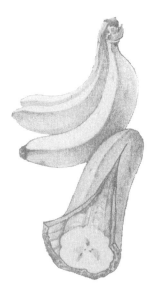

Banana Smoothies
- Almond Banana, page 159
- Bananarama, page 160
- Banana Nut, page 160
- Banana Mango, page 160

Blackberries

Actions: Antioxidant.
Uses: Blackberries are an excellent source of vitamin C and fiber and have high levels of potassium, iron, calcium and manganese.
Buying and storing: Choose plump, richly colored berries with firm flesh. They're best used immediately (if necessary, store for one day only in the refrigerator). Wash just before using.

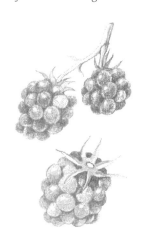

For smoothies: Blackberries add a dark blue color and sweet-to-slightly-tart flavor to smoothies. Use fresh, frozen or canned blackberries in blended drinks.

Blackberry Smoothies
- Berry Blast, page 161
- Black Belt, page 161
- Black Pineapple, page 161

Black Currants

Actions: Antioxidant, antibacterial, antidiarrheal, anticancer, boost immunity, promote healing.
Uses: Black currant flesh is extremely high in vitamin C — 200 mg in 3 oz (90 g). Black-currant skins and the outer layers of flesh closest to the skin contain anthocyanins, which have been proven to prevent the growth of bacteria such as *E. coli.* Black currants (especially the seeds) are high in gamma linolenic acid (GLA) ,which is important for heart health and a number of bodily functions. For these reasons, whole currants are used in smoothies more often than their juice. Although red currants are not as common, they have similar properties and may be substituted for black.
Buying and storing: Currants are not widely available but are sometimes found at farmer's markets. While not as fragile as blackberries or raspberries, fresh currants must be stored in the refrigerator, where they will keep for up to one week. Wash just before using.
For smoothies: Use fresh, dried or frozen currants, including the seeds. They are tart and sharp, so blend them with sweeter fruits, such as apples, pineapples or bananas.

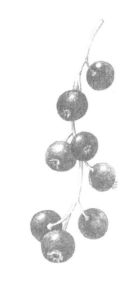

Black Currant Smoothies
- Apple Currant, page 156
- Black Currant, page 162
- Red, Black and Blue, page 162

Blueberries

Actions: Antidiarrheal, antioxidant, antibacterial, antiviral.

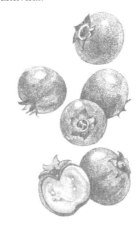

Uses: High concentrations of tannins are found in blueberries. They kill bacteria and viruses and help prevent (or relieve) bladder infections. Anthocyanins protect blood vessels against cholesterol buildup. High in pectin, vitamin C, potassium and natural acetylsalicylic acid, blueberries also add extra fiber to smoothies.

Buying and storing: A silvery "bloom" on blueberries indicates freshness. Choose plump, firm, dark blue berries with smooth skin. Pick over and discard split or soft berries. Blueberries are best used immediately but can be stored in the refrigerator for up to three days. Wash just before using.
For smoothies: As the flavor can be tart, especially in wild varieties, treat in the same way you would black currants: blend with sweeter fruits, such as apples, apricots and bananas. Frozen, canned or dried blueberries can be used if fresh are not available.
To prevent bladder infections: Add at least $1/2$ cup (125 mL) to other ingredients before blending and take daily for a minimum of three weeks.

Blueberry Smoothies
- Blueberry, page 162
- Blue Cherry, page 163
- Blue Water, page 163
- Pump It Up, page 163
- Red, Black and Blue, page 162

Cantaloupes
See Melons

Cherries

Actions: Antibacterial, antioxidant, anticancer.
Uses: Cherries are high in ellagic acid (a potent anticancer agent), vitamins A and C, biotin and potassium. Black cherry juice protects against tooth decay.
Buying and storing: Choose sweet varieties and look for dark red, firm, plump, tight-skinned fruit with the stems attached. Whole ripe cherries are best used immediately but will keep in the refrigerator for up to two days.

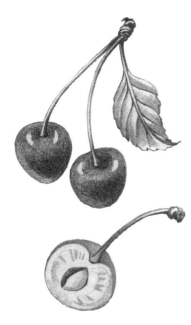

For smoothies: Wash, cut in half and remove pits. When fresh cherries are not available, use pitted frozen, dried or canned cherries in smoothies.

Cherry Smoothies
- Cherries Jubilee, page 164
- Cherry Berry, page 164
- Cherry Sunrise, page 164
- Cran-Cherry, page 165
- Eye Opener, page 165

Citrus Fruits
Oranges, lemons, limes, grapefruit and tangerines

Actions: Antioxidant, anticancer.
Uses: All citrus fruits are high in vitamin C and limonene, which is thought to inhibit breast cancer. Red grapefruit is high in cancer-fighting lycopene. Oranges are a good source of choline, which improves mental function. The combination of carotenoids, flavonoids, terpenes, limonoids and coumarins makes citrus fruits an excellent all-around cancer-fighting package.

Buying and storing: Purchase plump, juicy fruits that are heavy for their size and yield slightly to pressure. Although citrus fruits will keep for at least a couple of weeks if kept moist in the refrigerator, they are best if used within one week. Organic is preferable — you can be certain the fruits are not injected with gas for transportation.

For smoothies: Make fresh citrus juice with a citrus press or juicing machine, or use the fruit whole. To use whole citrus fruits, remove the peel, pith and seeds (they contain bitter elements), chop and add to other ingredients before blending. Canned oranges or grapefruit may be used if fresh are not available.

Lemon or lime juice adds a fresh, sharp edge that tones down the cloying sweetness of many fruits. One-half of a lemon or lime produces about 3 tbsp (45 mL) juice.

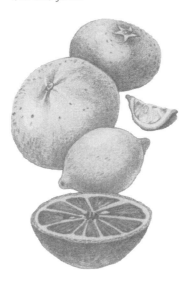

Citrus Smoothies
- C-Blend, page 166
- C-Blitz, page 166
- Citrus Cocktail, page 165
- Mellow Mandarin, page 167
- Mellow Yellow, page 167
- Tangerine, page 167

Cranberries

Actions: Antibacterial, antiviral, antioxidant, anticancer.
Uses: Cranberries are extremely useful in treating urinary tract and bladder infections. They work like elderberries, preventing the hooks on the bacteria from attaching to the cells of the bladder or urinary tract, rendering them ineffective. Best used as a preventive step against urinary tract and bladder infections, cranberry juice does not take the place of antibiotic drugs, which are more effective in eliminating bacteria once an infection has taken hold. High in vitamins A and C, iodine and calcium, cranberries also prevent kidney stones and deodorize the urine.

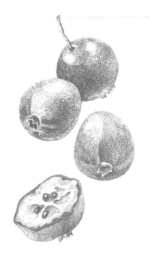

Buying and storing: Choose bright red, plump cranberries that bounce. Keep in the crisper drawer of your refrigerator for two to three weeks.

For smoothies: Use fresh, canned, dried or frozen whole cranberries or cranberry sauce for smoothies. Cranberries are in season during the fall. Fresh cranberries freeze very well and can be added frozen to smoothies. Wash just before using.

Unless used in small quantities or combined with very sweet fruits, fresh cranberries' tartness makes it appropriate to cook them with sugar, honey or stevia and a small amount of water or juice before combining with other fruits for smoothies.

To prevent bladder infections: Add at least 1/2 cup (125 mL) cranberries per smoothie recipe and take daily for a minimum of three weeks.

Cranberry Smoothies
- Cran-Apple, page 168
- Cran-Orange, page 168
- Cranberry Pineapple, page 168
- Fruit Explosion, page 169
- Fruit Splash, page 169

Crenshaw Melons

See Melons

Dates

Actions: Boost estrogen levels, laxative.

Uses: Dates are good sources of boron, which prevents calcium loss. They also contain vitamins A, B1, B2, C and D and valuable mineral salts, as well as fiber.

Caution: Dates may trigger headaches in some people.

Buying and storing: Dried dates are widely available and keep at room temperature for a couple of months. Fresh dates may be found in season in Middle Eastern grocery stores. Buy firm, plump, fresh dates with dark, shiny skins. Fresh dates will keep for several days in the refrigerator.

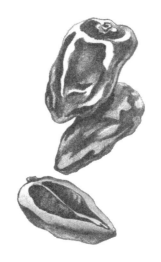

For smoothies: High in sugar (60% in fresh and 70% in dried), dates sweeten and add fiber to blended drinks. Small amounts can even be used in vegetable smoothies. Pitted dates are often sold in a block. Chop before adding to smoothies. Pit whole dates and cut in half before adding to blender. Date Milk (see page 247) can be used as a liquid in smoothies.

Date Smoothies
- Date and Nut, page 169
- Date Time, page 170
- Special Date, page 170

Elderberries

Actions: Diuretic, laxative, diaphoretic.

Uses: Elderberries support detoxification by promoting bowel movements, urination, sweating and mucus secretion. They are effective in combating viruses, such as those that cause colds and flu.

Buying and storing: Elderberries are still mainly harvested in the wild (although some are now grown commercially in the United States and Canada). They are usually available at farmer's markets from mid- to late

summer. Look for plump deep purple–black berries with tight, shiny skin and firm flesh. Use immediately or, if necessary, store for one day in the refrigerator. Wash just before using.

For smoothies: Elderberries add a dark blue color and a sweet-to-slightly-tart taste to smoothies. Use fresh or frozen elderberries, about 1/2 cup (125 mL) per smoothie recipe or 1 to 2 tbsp (15 to 25 mL) elderberry syrup or jam per smoothie.

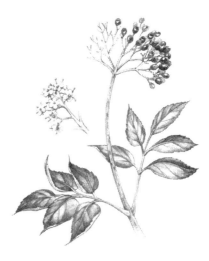

Elderberry Smoothies
- Berry Bonanza, page 170
- Flu Fighter #1, page 171

Figs

Actions: Antibacterial, anticancer, antiulcer, digestive, demulcent, laxative.

Uses: Figs contain benzaldehyde, a cancer-fighting agent. They are also high in potassium, B vitamins, calcium and magnesium.

Caution: Figs can trigger headaches in some people.

Buying and storing: Dried figs are readily available in supermarkets throughout the year. In summer and early fall, some supermarkets and most Middle Eastern grocery stores carry fresh figs. When purchasing fresh figs, choose soft, plump, dark brown fruit with thin skins.

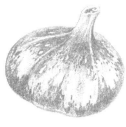

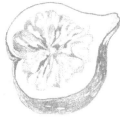

For smoothies: Fresh figs contain 12% sugar (dried contain approximately 50%) and can be used to sweeten and thicken smoothies. Remove the skin of fresh figs before adding to the blender. You can also substitute fresh or dried figs for fresh or dried apricots in smoothie recipes. Fig Milk (see page 248) can be used as a liquid in smoothies.

Fig Smoothies
- Figgy Duff, page 171
- Fruity Fig, page 171

Gooseberries

Actions: Protect skin and gums, laxative.
Uses: High in vitamin C, potassium and pectin, gooseberries are often added to jams to make them set.
Buying and storing: Once found in many home gardens, gooseberries are now rather scarce. They can sometimes be found at farmer's markets in early summer. Be sure to use dessert varieties (early-ripening amber

and yellow gooseberries). If amber or yellow are unavailable, use green gooseberries, which are the most common in some parts of North America, but be aware that they are not the best variety to use raw. Look for plump, almost transparent berries with tight, shiny skin and firm flesh. Red-skinned gooseberries are too tart for smoothies. Use immediately or, if necessary, store for one day in the refrigerator. Wash just before using.

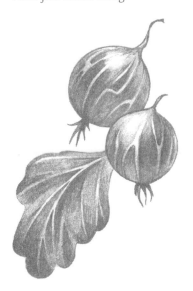

For smoothies: Refreshingly sweet-tart, gooseberries add depth to the sweetness of seasonal berries and bananas.

Gooseberry Smoothies
- Gooseberry Fool, page 172
- Loosey-Goosey, page 172

Grapefruit
See Citrus Fruits

Grapes
Actions: Antioxidant, antiviral, anticancer.

Uses: Grapes contain large amounts of ellagic and caffeic acids, which deactivate carcinogens, and are a good source of potassium. The flavonoids in grape juice protect the heart, and the resveratrol found in red wine and red grape juice has a protective effect on the cardiovascular system. Grapes also contain boron, which helps maintain estrogen levels (thus preventing calcium loss) and may be instrumental in preventing osteoporosis.

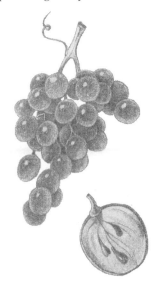

Buying and storing: Organic grapes are preferable due to the large amounts of pesticides used on non-organic crops. When purchasing grapes, always look for bright color, firm flesh and unwrinkled skin. Wash in food-grade hydrogen peroxide (or other produce cleaner) and store in the crisper drawer of your refrigerator for three or four days.
For smoothies: Grapes are sweet, and their mild taste blends nicely with most fruits in smoothies. Thompson seedless and Concord (red or green) seedless are common varieties used in smoothies. Use with the skin but wash thoroughly and cut in half before blending.

Raisins are dried grapes and are a good source of fiber, boron and natural sweetness — add $\frac{1}{4}$ cup (50 mL) to any smoothie recipe. Golden sultanas are the best raisins to use because they are light and plump. Look for unsulphured raisins that have not been sprayed with mineral oils.

Grape Smoothies
- Grape Glacé, page 172
- Grape Heart, page 173
- Raisin Pie, page 173
- Sunrise Supreme, page 173

Honeydew Melons
See Melons

Kiwis
Actions: Antioxidant, anticancer, aid digestion.
Uses: Kiwis are often used as part of cleansing regimens or to aid digestion. They are high in vitamins C and E (they are one of the few fruits that contain vitamin E), which act as an antioxidant and protect cells from free-radical damage. Kiwis are also high in potassium and contain some calcium.

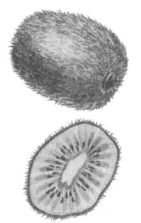

Buying and storing: Choose ripe fruits that yield to gentle pressure. Kiwis will ripen in a brown paper bag at room temperature after two or three days. They will keep for at least one week in the crisper drawer of the refrigerator.
For smoothies: Use fresh; peel and cut into cubes before blending.

Kiwi Smoothies
- Ki-Lime, page 174
- Pineapple Kiwi, page 174
- Sher-Lime, page 174
- Tropics, page 175

Lemons
See Citrus Fruits

Limes
See Citrus Fruits

Mangoes
Actions: Antioxidant, anticancer.
Uses: High in vitamin A (there are 8,000 IU of beta-carotene in one mango), vitamin C, potassium, niacin and fiber, mangoes help protect against cancer and arteriosclerosis. They also help the body fight infection and maintain bowel regularity.

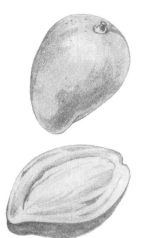

Buying and storing: Choose large, firm, unblemished yellow to yellow-red fruit with flesh that gives slightly when gently squeezed. Store in the crisper drawer of your refrigerator for three or four days.
For smoothies: Mangoes are fibrous (which makes smoothies thick), with a sweet, banana-pineapple flavor. Remove the peel and handle it carefully, as it contains a skin-irritating sap. Slice the flesh off the fibrous pit. Discard the pit and chop the flesh before adding to the blender. Use dried mangoes sparingly — they are intensely sweet — and look for ones that are unsulphured (it will be noted on the package).

Mango Smoothies
- Breakfast Cocktail, page 175
- Mango Madness, page 175
- Mango Mango, page 176
- Mango Tango, page 176
- Tropi-Cocktail, page 177

Melons
Cantaloupe, honeydew, Crenshaw, Spanish and musk
Actions: Antioxidant, anticancer, anticoagulant (cantaloupe and honeydew).
Uses: Adenosine is an anticoagulant chemical found in melons that lessens the risks of heart attack and stroke. Melons are a good source of vitamin A and contain vitamin C and calcium.
Buying and storing: Ripe melons are heavy for their size and give off a full, sweet perfume. Avoid soft, blemished fruit.
For smoothies: Cut a melon in half. Leave the seeds and rind on one half. Cut the other half into four wedges. Peel the wedges and remove and discard the seeds.

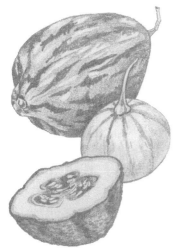

Store unused wedges and half in perforated plastic bags in the refrigerator. Use one or two wedges per smoothie recipe and chop the flesh before adding to the blender.

Melon Smoothies
- Berry Best, page 177
- Beta Blast, page 177
- Green Goddess, page 178
- Mega Melon Supreme, page 178
- Melon Morning Cocktail, page 178

Musk Melons
See Melons

Nectarines
Actions: Antioxidant, anticancer.
Uses: A good source of vitamins A and C and potassium, nectarines are an ancient fruit and not, as many people think, a cross between a peach and a plum.
Buying and storing: Choose fruit with some bright red areas that are smooth and tight, with no soft patches. Nectarines should be heavy for their size (which means they are full of juice) and firm when pressed. They should not be hard.

For smoothies: Wash, cut in half and remove the pit. Peel (if not organic) and chop before adding to the blender. Nectarines are usually sweeter than peaches, for which they can be substituted in smoothie recipes.

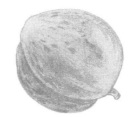

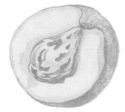

Nectarine Smoothies
- Nectar of the Gods, page 179
- Nectarine on Ice, page 179
- Nectarlicious, page 179
- Orange Aid, page 180

Oranges
See Citrus Fruits

Papayas
Actions: Antioxidant, anticancer, aid digestion.
Uses: High in vitamins A and C and potassium.
Buying and storing: Choose large, firm, unblemished yellow fruit with flesh that gives slightly when gently squeezed. Store in the crisper drawer of your refrigerator for three or four days.
For smoothies: Peel and cut into pieces before adding to the blender (the seeds contain protein and may be used if desired). Papayas sweeten and blend well with other fruits and add a creamy texture to smoothies.

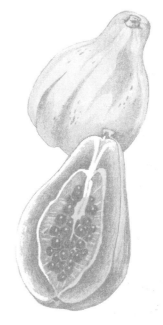

Papaya Smoothies
- Fruity Twist, page 180
- Hawaiian Silk, page 181
- Papaya Passion, page 180
- Taste of the Tropics, page 181

Peaches
Actions: Antioxidant, anticancer.
Uses: Rich in vitamin A and potassium, peaches contain boron, niacin, some iron and vitamin C. They help protect against cancer, osteoporosis and heart disease, and their sugar content is low (about 9%).
Buying and storing: Fruit that is full and heavy for its size, with fuzzy down and lightly firm flesh, is preferable. Store in the crisper drawer of your refrigerator for up to four days. Freestone varieties (such as Loring and Redhaven) are easier to pit than clingstone varieties.
For smoothies: Use fresh, dried, frozen or canned peaches in smoothies. Wash fresh peaches, then cut in half and remove and discard the pit. Peel (if not organic) and chop before adding to the blender.

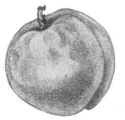

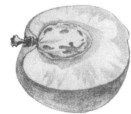

Peach Smoothies
- Minty Peach, page 181
- Peach Bliss, page 182
- Peach Cobbler, page 182
- Peach Paradise, page 183
- Peaches and Cream, page 183
- Peachy Melon, page 183

Pears

Actions: Protect the colon.
Uses: Perhaps one of the oldest cultivated fruits, pears are a good source of vitamin C, boron and potassium. Pears are also a sweet source of fiber.

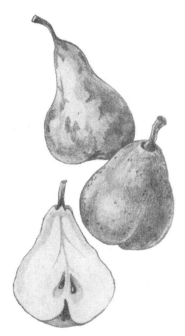

Buying and storing: Pears should be lightly firm, unblemished and sweetly pear-scented. They are often available before they are fully ripe, in which case they can be ripened in a brown paper bag at room temperature for one to three days. Ripe pears can be stored in the crisper drawer of your refrigerator for three or four days.
For smoothies: Use fresh, frozen, dried or canned pears for smoothies. Juicy varieties, such as Bartlett, Comice, Seckel and Bosc, are best. Wash, peel (if not organic) and core. Chop before adding to the blender.

Pear Smoothies
- Apple Pear, page 184
- Autumn Refresher, page 184
- Pear Fennel, page 184
- Pear Pineapple, page 185
- Pear Raspberry, page 185

Pineapples

Actions: Aid digestion.
Uses: Pineapples are a good source of potassium and contain some vitamin C and iron.
Buying and storing: Choose large, firm fruits (heaviness indicates juiciness) that are yellow all over.
For smoothies: Pineapples add a fresh, sweet taste to smoothies. Cut off the base and top leaves, cut in half and use one half at a time. Slice one half into four wedges. Remove the skin from each wedge (remove the core only if woody) and chop the flesh before adding to the blender. One fresh wedge of pineapple equals approximately 1 cup (250 mL) chopped. Frozen, canned or dried pineapple may be substituted for fresh in smoothies.

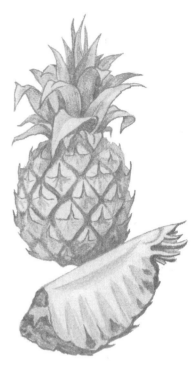

Pineapple Smoothies
- B-Vitamin, page 187
- Liquid Gold, page 185
- Pine-Berry, page 186
- Pineapple Citrus, page 186
- Pineapple Soy, page 186

Plums

Actions: Antibacterial, antioxidant.
Uses: A good source of vitamin A, plums contain calcium and a small amount of vitamin C.
Buying and storing: Ripe plums are firm, with no soft spots or splits. Look for brightly colored (yellow, black or red) plums with tight skins that are heavy for their size and smell sweet. Keep in the crisper drawer of your refrigerator for up to four days.
For smoothies: Wash, peel (if not organic) and remove pit. Canned and frozen plums may be substituted for fresh.

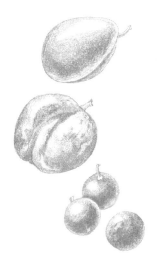

Prunes are dried plums and are high in pectin and other insoluble fiber, and low in sugar. They act as a natural laxative, and the pectin in them fights colon cancer. Use two or three pitted prunes per smoothie recipe.
To treat constipation: Use four to six prunes for each 1 cup (250 mL) of smoothie.

Plum Smoothies
- Plum Berry, page 187
- Plum Lico, page 188
- Plums Up, page 188
- Prune, page 188

Raspberries
Actions: Enhance immunity.
Uses: Raspberries are rich in potassium and niacin and also contain iron and some vitamin C (see also Red Raspberry, page 116).
Buying and storing: Buy or pick in peak season and choose whole, plump, brightly colored berries. Sort and discard soft or broken berries. Store in the crisper drawer of your refrigerator for one day. Wash just before using.

For smoothies: Raspberries blend well with other berries in smoothies, and their flavor is enhanced by a small amount of citrus juice. You can substitute frozen, dried or canned raspberries for fresh. You can also add up to $1/4$ cup (50 mL) raspberry jam to smoothies.

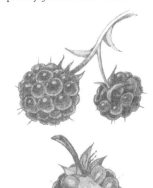

Raspberry Smoothies
- Berry Fine Cocktail, page 189
- Raspberry, page 189
- Razzy Orange, page 190
- Real Raspberry, page 189

Rhubarb
Actions: Laxative.
Uses: Rhubarb is actually a vegetable that is almost always identified as a fruit. It is high in potassium and contains a fair amount of iron. The calcium in 1 cup (250 mL) of cooked rhubarb is twice that of the same amount of milk.
Caution: Never use rhubarb leaves, which are toxic and inedible due to their high concentration of oxalic acid.
Buying and storing: If you do not have a rhubarb patch in your garden, look for rhubarb in farmer's markets in the spring.

Choose thin, firm stalks that are at least 90% red. Rhubarb should snap when bent. Store in a cool, dry place or the crisper drawer of your refrigerator for no longer than two days.
For smoothies: Use only one raw ripe stalk in smoothies. Cooking mellows the tart taste and softens the laxative effect. In a medium saucepan, combine 1 cup (250 mL) chopped fresh rhubarb, 1 cup (250 mL) chopped seeded peeled apple and $1/4$ cup (50 mL) sugar or honey (or 2 tsp/10 mL stevia). Cover with water or apple juice and simmer until soft. Use up to $1/2$ cup (125 mL) of this mixture per smoothie recipe. Cooked frozen or canned rhubarb may also be used in smoothies.

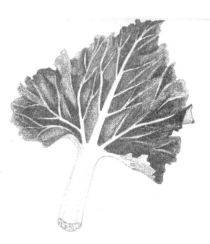

Rhubarb Smoothies
- Rhubarb Apple, page 190
- Rhubarb Pineapple, page 190

Spanish Melons
See Melons

Strawberries
Actions: Antioxidant, antiviral, anticancer.

Uses: Effective against kidney stones, gout, rheumatism and arthritis, strawberries are also used in cleansing juices and as a mild tonic for the liver. Strawberries are high in cancer-fighting ellagic acid and vitamin C. They are also a good source of vitamin A and potassium, and contain some iron. Both the leaves and the fruit are used medicinally. Strawberry leaf tea can be used to treat diarrhea and dysentery.

Buying and storing: Pick your own or choose brightly colored firm berries with the hulls attached. They are best used immediately but may be stored for no more than two days in the refrigerator. Wash just before using.

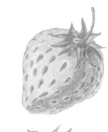
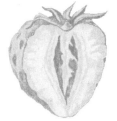

For smoothies: You can substitute frozen strawberries for fresh. Hull and cut fresh strawberries in half before adding to the blender. Strawberries add a sweet, powerful flavor to smoothies and are best blended with only one or two other fruits, especially bananas and other berries. Their flavor is enhanced by a bit of lemon or lime juice.

Strawberry Smoothies

- Best Berries, page 191
- Pineapple-C, page 191
- Sea-Straw, page 191
- Strawberry Blush, page 192
- Strawberry Swirl, page 192

Tangerines

See Citrus Fruits

Watermelons

Actions: Antibacterial, anticancer.
Uses: Watermelons contain vitamins A and C, iron and potassium. Their high water content makes them good summer refreshments.
Buying and storing: A watermelon should have a bright green rind and firm flesh (no blemishes or soft spots) and feel heavy for its size. Store in a cool dark place or in the refrigerator for two or three days.

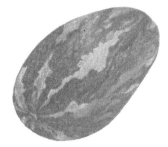
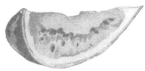

For smoothies: Watermelon blends well with other fruits to make a sweet thirst quencher. Cut in half lengthwise and use one half at a time. With the cut side of one half facing up, slice and discard one round end. Move the knife over 1 to 1 1/2 inches (2.5 to 4 cm) and cut a slice. Remove and discard the rind and seeds, then chop the flesh before adding it to the blender. This-size slice yields approximately 1 cup (250 mL) of chopped fruit. Wrap the remainder in plastic wrap and store in the refrigerator.

Watermelon Smoothies

- Perfect in Pink, page 192
- Watermelon, page 193
- Watermelon-Strawberry Splash, page 193
- Watermelon Wave, page 193

Vegetable Profiles

Asparagus

Actions: Antioxidant, anticancer, anti-cataracts, diuretic, promotes healing.
Uses: Asparagus is one of only four vegetables that are high in vitamin E. It is also a source of vitamins A and C, as well as potassium, niacin and some iron.

Buying and storing: Look for tight buds at the tips and smooth green stalks with some white at the very bottoms. Fresh asparagus will snap at the point where the tender stalk meets the tougher end. Store stalks upright in 1/2 inch (1 cm) of water in the refrigerator for up to two days.

For smoothies: Wash, snap off tough stems and cook in boiling water for three minutes. Drain, cool to room temperature and chop before adding to smoothies. Frozen or canned asparagus with juices may be substituted when fresh is not available.

134   Ingredient Profiles

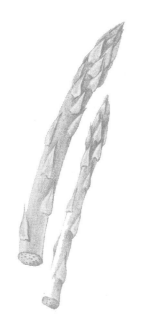

Asparagus Smoothies
• Spring Celebration, page 197

Avocados

Actions: Antioxidant.

Uses: Avocados (which are technically fruits) contain more potassium than many other fruits and vegetables (bananas are just slightly higher). High in essential fatty acids, avocados also contain 17 vitamins and minerals, including vitamins A, C and E; all the B vitamins, except B12, and including riboflavin; iron; calcium; copper; phosphorus; zinc; niacin; and magnesium. They also have the largest amount of protein of any fruit. One avocado blended into a smoothie adds creamy texture and exceptional nutritional value.

Buying and storing: Look for ripe, heavy avocados that have dull dark green skin with no dents. Ripe avocados give slightly when gently squeezed. Avocados are often sold unripe, but you can ripen them in a paper bag at room temperature and store them in the refrigerator for just over one week once ripe.

For smoothies: Peel, cut in half, remove pit and cut into pieces. Brush the flesh with lemon juice to keep it from turning brown. Avocados thicken smoothies (in much the same way that bananas do) because of their relatively low water content. Up to 30% of an avocado's weight may be oil, and, for this reason, they should be used sparingly.

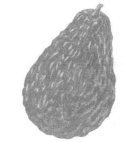

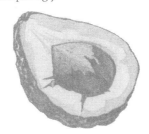

Avocado Smoothies
• Avocado Orange, page 197
• Avocado Pineapple, page 197

Beans

Fresh green, yellow wax, Italian, snap and string beans; green peas; snow peas; and legumes (dried peas, lentils and beans)

Actions: Improve memory, antioxidant.

Uses: Green beans and peas are the same botanically as dry beans because they are all leguminous plants, meaning that they produce their seeds in pods. However, fresh beans have lower nutrient levels than dried legumes. A good source of choline, which improves mental function, beans also

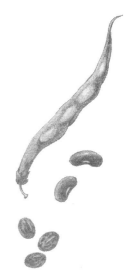

contain vitamin A and potassium, as well as some protein, iron, calcium and vitamins B and C. The amino acids in beans and peas make them a valuable food for vegetarians.

Buying and storing: Buy fresh peas and beans with firm pods that show no signs of wilting. The bigger the pea or bean inside the pod the older the vegetable. Fresh yellow or green beans should be pliant but still snap when bent. Store unwashed fresh peas (in their pods) and beans in a plastic bag in the refrigerator for two or three days. Parboiled fresh beans and peas freeze well.

For smoothies: Fresh or frozen beans and peas can be cooked and used in smoothies, as can the canned varieties. Dried peas, beans and lentils can also be used, after they are soaked and cooked, in vegetable smoothies. The fiber in legumes adds texture to smoothies, which means that additional liquid is required. Lima and black beans, split peas and chickpeas are the most popular legumes used in smoothies.

Bean Smoothies
• Creamy Chickpea, page 198
• Lima Curry, page 199
• Peas Please, page 199
• Pease Porridge, page 200

Beets

Actions: Antibacterial, antioxidant, tonic, cleansing, laxative.

Uses: Beets (the root of the beet plant) are high in vitamin A and the enzyme betaine, which nourishes and strengthens the liver and gallbladder. Beets are also an excellent source of potassium and are cleansing for the liver, kidneys and gallbladder.

Buying and storing: Bright, glossy, crisp beet greens indicate fresh beets (see Leafy Greens, page 140, for how to use beet greens in smoothies). Buy firm unblemished small beets with greens intact, if possible. To store, cut off tops and treat as leafy greens. Store unwashed beets in a plastic bag in the refrigerator. Beets will keep for up to $1^1/_2$ weeks. Wash just before cooking.

For smoothies: Use cooked fresh, frozen or canned beets with juices.

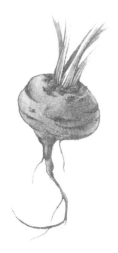

Beet Smoothies
- Apple Beet Pear, page 200
- Beet, page 201
- Blazing Beets, page 201
- Clam Beet, page 201

Broccoli

Actions: Antioxidant, anticancer, promotes healing, anti-cataracts.

Uses: Broccoli is one of only four vegetables that are high in vitamin E. It is also high in cancer-fighting indoles and glucosinolates and has fair amounts of vitamins A, B and C.

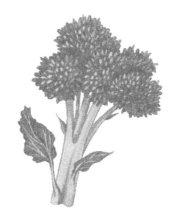

Buying and storing: Broccoli yellows as it ages, so deep green color and firm tight buds are signs of freshness. Thin stalks are more tender than thick or hollow ones. Store in a vented plastic bag in the crisper drawer of the refrigerator for up to three days.

For smoothies: Use cooked fresh, frozen or canned broccoli with juices.

Broccoli Smoothies
- Brocco-Carrot, page 202
- Cheesy Broccoli, page 202

Brussels Sprouts
See Cabbage

Cabbage
Green, red, Savoy, bok choy and Chinese cabbage; kohlrabi; and Brussels sprouts

Actions: Antibacterial, anticancer, helps memory, antioxidant, detoxifying, diuretic, anti-inflammatory, tonic, antiseptic, restorative, antiulcer, boosts immunity, anti-cataracts, promotes healing.

Uses: High in cancer-fighting indoles and a good source of choline, which improves mental function, cabbage is one of only four vegetables that are high in vitamin E. An excellent remedy for anemia, cabbage has also been used as a nutritive tonic to restore strength in cases of debility and during convalescence. Beneficial to the liver, cabbage is also effective in preventing colon cancer and may be of help to diabetics by reducing blood sugar levels. Cabbage juice is especially effective in preventing and healing ulcers.

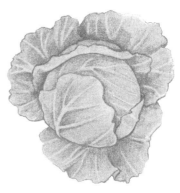

Buying and storing: Fresh cabbage has loose outer leaves around a firm center head. Stored cabbage does not have the outer wrapper leaves and tends to be paler in color. Cabbage will keep for up to two weeks in a plastic bag in the refrigerator. Wash and cut or slice just before using.

For smoothies: Wash, shred or cut fresh or frozen cabbage into chunks for smoothies.

Cabbage Smoothies
- Cabbage Cocktail, page 203
- Minestrone, page 203
- Red Rocket, page 204

Carrots

Actions: Antioxidant, anticancer, protect arteries, expectorant, antiseptic, diuretic, boost immunity, antibacterial, lower blood cholesterol levels, prevent constipation.

Uses: Carrots are extremely nutritious and rich in vitamins A, B and C; iron; calcium; potassium; and sodium. They have a cleansing effect on the liver and digestive system, help prevent the formation of kidney stones and relieve arthritis and gout. Their antioxidant properties come from carotenoids (including beta-carotene), which have been shown to cut cancer risk, protect against arterial and cardiac disease, and lower blood cholesterol. Carrots enhance mental function and decrease the risk of cataracts and macular degeneration.

Buying and storing: The green tops continue to draw nutrients out of the carrot, so choose fresh carrots that are sold loose without the tops, or remove the tops immediately after purchase. Choose firm well-shaped carrots with no cracks. If stored unwashed in a cold, moist place, carrots should not shrivel. Keep for up to two weeks in a vented plastic bag in the crisper drawer of your refrigerator.

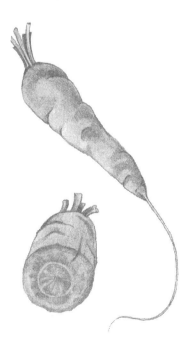

For smoothies: Carrots are versatile vegetables that are naturally sweet. They can be used in almost any smoothie recipe. The deeper the color the higher the concentration of beta carotene. Do not use carrot greens in smoothies. Carrots may be used raw, but cooking frees up carotenes (precursors to vitamin A), the anticancer agents in carrots. Steam or simmer carrots just until tender, then add to the blender along with other fruits or vegetables.

Carrot Smoothies
- Carrot Raisin Cooler, page 204
- Orange Zinger, page 204
- Rustproofer #1, page 205
- Spiced Carrot, page 205

Cauliflower

Actions: Antioxidant, anticancer.
Uses: Like all cruciferous vegetables (cabbage, Brussels sprouts, broccoli, collard greens, kohlrabi), cauliflower is rich in cancer-fighting indoles. Cauliflower contains vitamin C and potassium, as well as some protein and iron.
Buying and storing: Fresh cauliflower has dense, tightly packed florets, and the head is surrounded by crisp green leaves. Keep loosely covered in a perforated plastic bag in the refrigerator for no longer than one week.

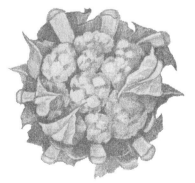

For smoothies: Cut into pieces and cook before using. Use some of the core if it is not woody.

Cauliflower Smoothies
- Cauliflower Cocktail, page 206
- Herbed Cauliflower, page 206

Celery and Celeriac

Actions: Mild diuretic, anticancer.
Uses: Sometimes used as a treatment for high blood pressure (two to four stalks per day), celery also helps detoxify carcinogens (see also Celery Seeds, page 95, for their healing properties).
Buying and storing: Fresh celery has crisp green leaves and firm, crisp ribs. (The leaves are removed from older stalks.) Store for up to two weeks in a vented plastic bag in the refrigerator.

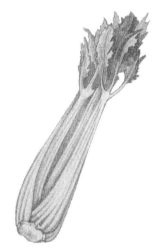

For smoothies: Use celery stalks and leaves in vegetable cocktails to add natural saltiness. Scrub and cut celery into pieces before adding to the blender. Celeriac, the root of a different variety of celery than common table celery, adds a stronger celery flavor to smoothies. Peel off the tough outer skin, then slice and chop before adding to the blender.

Celery Smoothies
• Celery Cream, page 207

Chile Peppers

Actions: Stimulant, tonic, diaphoretic, rubefacient, carminative, antiseptic, antibacterial, expectorant, anti-bronchitis, anti-emphysema, decongestant, blood thinner.
Uses: Chiles are hot peppers that contain the active element capsaicin. They are high in vitamin A and contain some vitamin C, calcium, iron, magnesium, phosphorus and potassium. Chile peppers help people with bronchitis and related problems by irritating the bronchial tubes and sinuses, causing the secretion of fluid that thins the constricting mucus and helps move it out of the body. Capsaicin also blocks pain messages from the brain, making it an effective pain reliever. In addition, it also helps prevent heart attacks (if taken on a consistent basis), as it has clot-dissolving properties. Cayenne (see page 95) is a variety of chile. It appears in the Herb Profiles section because it is used medicinally, as well as in cooking.
Buying and storing: Look for firm, crisp chile peppers with smooth skin and no blemishes. Store in a paper bag in the crisper drawer of your refrigerator for up to four days. Peppers freeze well and may be added frozen to smoothies. When purchasing

---

Trial by Fire
Common Chile Peppers

There are five cultivated species of the *Capsicum* genus — *C. annuum, C. frutescens, C. chinense, C. baccatum* and *C. pubescens* — and over 20 wild varieties. Color does not help in identifying chiles because the same fresh peppers can be either picked green or allowed to ripen and turn red. Most are dried, some are smoked and many are canned. And, to confuse matters even more, chiles change their names with different preserving methods.

Around the turn of the 20th century, Wilbur Scoville, a Detroit pharmacist, developed the Scoville Organoleptic Test to determine the heat of different varieties of chile pepper. Listed in order from mild to hot, the following are just a few of the hundreds of varieties enjoyed today.

New Mexico chiles (often called Anaheim) are mildly flavored and long and green when fresh. Left on the bush, they turn red in the fall, and the dried versions are a rich shade of oxblood, with an enchanting smoky taste. Milder than most, New Mexico chiles are used in most classic Tex-Mex dishes and are a good choice for beginning chile users.

Poblano/ancho chiles are big, flat, relatively mild peppers. They are the widest chiles (hence the name *ancho*, which means "wide" in Spanish). They are known as poblanos when fresh and anchos when dried. In their dried form, they acquire a nutty taste and raisin-like appearance. They are the most commonly used variety in Mexico.

Jalapeño peppers are probably the most common and widely available chiles in North America and are at the halfway point on the Scoville Heat Unit Scale. Jalapeños lend a meaty texture and rich flavor to dishes. Their thick flesh makes them excellent for use in smoothies. When smoked and dried, jalapeños are called chipotles.

Serrano chiles are very hot to fiery with a slightly fruity taste. More flavorful than jalapeños, they originated in the Hidalgo and Puebla regions of central Mexico, and the word *serrano* means "from the mountains." They are the most popular choice for fresh salsas, stews and moles (spicy chocolate sauces usually served with meat).

Cayenne peppers are grown commercially in New Mexico, Africa, India, Japan and Mexico and are commonly available in dried form. A favorite in African and Cajun dishes, ground dried cayenne pepper is a major ingredient in barbecue rubs and powders. They are often used in Italian cooking as well and are the source of the hot pepper flakes that people often sprinkle over pasta or pizza. Ground cayenne is used extensively in cooking but has healing properties, too (see Cayenne, page 95).

Habanero chiles are small round peppers that are almost identical to Scotch Bonnet peppers (they can be used interchangeably) and are reputedly the hottest chiles. They are rated a blazing 10-plus on the Scoville Heat Unit Scale and really pack a punch in hot-pepper and Caribbean jerk sauces, to which they also impart a unique fruity undertone.

dried chile peppers, make sure they are clean and fully dried. Store them in a cool, dry place.

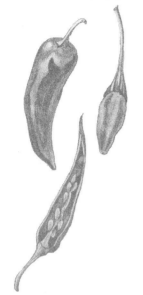

For smoothies: Wash and handle chiles carefully and wash your hands thoroughly after handling, as capsaicin will irritate your skin and eyes. Wash fresh chiles, remove the stems and coarsely chop. The hot, irritating component, capsaicin, is concentrated in the ribs of the flesh, not the seeds (as commonly thought), so the seeds may be left intact. When first using chiles, add half the recommended amount to the blender. Taste, add more, if desired, and blend. Use fresh, reconstituted dried or canned chiles in smoothies. You may also add hot sauce or powdered cayenne to smoothies as a substitute for chiles. Adding yogurt to chile drinks helps extinguish the fire.

Chile Smoothies
- Cajun Cocktail, page 207

Collard Greens
See Leafy Greens

Corn
Actions: Anticancer, antiviral, raises estrogen level, neutralizes stomach acid, high fiber helps with kidney stones and water retention.

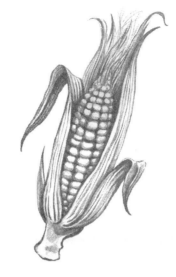

Uses: Used in moderation, corn adds fiber to the diet.
Caution: Corn and corn products (cereals, corn chips or foods made with cornstarch) may trigger food intolerances that lead to chronic conditions, including rheumatoid arthritis, headaches and irritable bowel syndrome.
Buying and storing: Fresh corn is best if cooked within minutes of picking. When that is not possible, buy corn that has been kept cold and use as soon as possible.
For smoothies: Use leftover cooked fresh corn by slicing kernels off the cob with a sharp knife. Frozen or canned whole-kernel corn packed in water can be used when fresh is not available.

Corn Smoothies
- Corn Chowder, page 208

Cucumbers
Actions: Diuretic.
Uses: Moderate sources of vitamin A, iron and potassium, cucumbers are high in water, making them good vegetables for smoothies. Cucumbers contain sterols, which may help the heart by reducing cholesterol.
Buying and storing: Choose shiny, bright green, firm cucumbers. Avoid those with yellow spots (although this is a sign of ripeness, the seeds will be bitter and the flesh too soft) and wax on the skin (which is not good to eat and usually a sign of age). Store in the crisper drawer of the refrigerator for four or five days.
For smoothies: Wash before using, peel (especially if the skin has been waxed or if not organic) and cut into cubes, leaving the seeds intact.

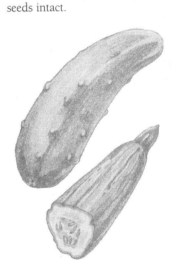

Cucumber Smoothies
- Flaming Antibiotic, page 208
- Gazpacho, page 209

Eggplants
Actions: Antibacterial, diuretic, may lower blood cholesterol levels, may prevent cancer.

Uses: Now used topically to treat skin cancer, the terpenes in eggplants may also work internally to deactivate steroidal hormones that promote certain cancers. Eggplants contain a fair amount of potassium, which normalizes blood pressure. They are also low in fat and calories.

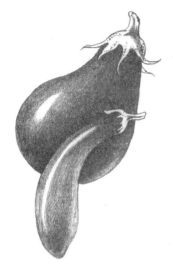

Buying and storing: Choose small deep-purple eggplants with firm, smooth skin that has no scrapes, cuts or bruises. Use immediately or keep for one or two days in the crisper drawer of the refrigerator.
For smoothies: Wash before using, peel (if not organic) and cut into cubes, leaving the seeds intact. One slice of fresh eggplant can be used in any vegetable smoothie. It adds fiber, which thickens drinks without changing the taste of the main ingredients.

Eggplant Smoothies
• Roasted Eggplant, page 209

Fennel
Actions: Antioxidant, seeds are digestive.
Uses: A bulb-like vegetable similar to celery but with a distinctly sweet anise taste, fennel is a good source of vitamin A.

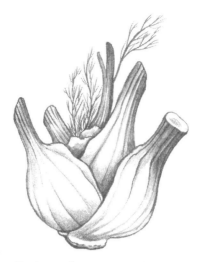

Buying and storing: Avoid wilted or browning stalks on fennel. The bulb should be firm and white with a light green tinge. Remove leaves and keep for up to one week in the refrigerator.
For smoothies: Cut fennel bulb in half and cut one of the halves in half again. Use one quarter at a time in any vegetable smoothie. Wash and chop (use the leaves if they are attached to the stalks) before adding to the blender. Fennel may be used raw, cooked or frozen in smoothies. One-quarter of a fennel bulb makes about 1 cup (250 mL) chopped.

Fennel Smoothies
• Anise Anise, page 235
• Creamy Fennel, page 210

Garlic
See Herb Profiles, page 102

Kale
See Leafy Greens

Kohlrabi
See Cabbage

Leafy Greens
Kale, Swiss chard, collard greens, mustard greens, turnip greens and lettuce
Actions: Antioxidant, anticancer.
Uses: Excellent sources of vitamin A and chlorophyll, leafy greens are also good sources of vitamin C, with some calcium, iron, folic acid and potassium, as well.
Buying and storing: Buy bright green, crisp (not wilted) greens and store unwashed in a vented plastic bag in the crisper drawer of your refrigerator. Leafy greens are very tender and will sag and yellow (or brown) when not stored or handled properly. Store away from fruits.
For smoothies: Wash, remove tough ribs and stems, then shred or chop before adding to the blender.

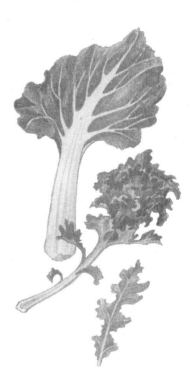

Leafy Greens Smoothies
• Garden Goodness, page 210
• Leafy Luxury, page 210

Leeks

Actions: Expectorant, diuretic, relaxant, laxative, antiseptic, digestive, hypotensive.

Uses: Easily digested, leeks are used in tonics, especially during convalescence from illness. They can be blended into toddies for relief from sore throats, thanks to their warming, expectorant and stimulating qualities.

Buying and storing: Bright green ends showing no signs of slime or wilt, with crisp white roots intact, means that leeks are fresh. Unwashed and kept in a vented plastic bag in the refrigerator, leeks should last for one to two weeks.

For smoothies: Leeks can be gritty, so it is important to clean them thoroughly before using. Trim the white roots and outer green leaves off, split lengthwise and wash the inner layers well. Cut into chunks. Leeks may be used raw but mellow and soften when cooked.

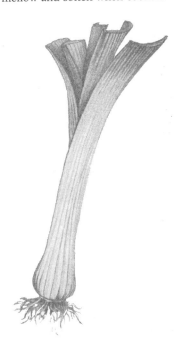

Leek Smoothies
- Quick Vichyssoise, page 211
- Vichyssoise, page 211

Legumes
See Beans

Lettuce
See Leafy Greens

Mustard Greens
See Leafy Greens

Onions

Actions: Antibacterial, anticancer, antioxidant, circulatory and digestive stimulant, antiseptic, detoxifying, lower blood cholesterol levels, hypotensive, lower blood sugar level, diuretic, cardioprotective.

Uses: Onions help prevent thrombosis, reduce high blood pressure, lower blood sugar, prevent inflammatory responses and prohibit the growth of cancer cells. Shallots and yellow or red onions are the richest dietary sources of quercetin, a potent antioxidant and cancer-inhibiting phytochemical.

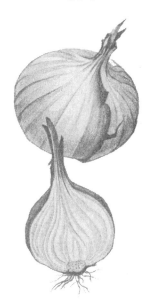

Buying and storing: Examine each onion to make sure it has dry, tight skin and is firm. Avoid onions with woody centers in the neck and black powdery patches. If stored in a cool, dry place with good air circulation, onions will keep for up to two weeks (one month or more in the refrigerator).

For smoothies: Vidalia or red onions are preferable for smoothies because they are milder in flavor. Peel and chop before adding to the blender.

Onion Smoothies
- Allium Antioxidant, page 232
- Creamed Onions, page 212

Parsnips

Actions: Anti-inflammatory, anticancer.

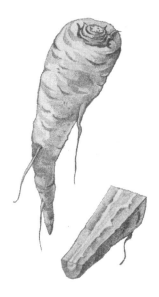

Uses: Parsnips are best fresh after frost has concentrated their carbohydrates into sugar, making them sweeter. Good sources of vitamins C and E and potassium, they also contain some protein, iron and calcium. Parsnips, like other root vegetables, keep well and are excellent in winter smoothies.

Buying and storing: Look for firm flesh with no evidence of shriveling, soft spots or cuts. Parsnips should snap when bent. Small thin parsnips with tops still intact are preferable. Keep them in a plastic bag in the refrigerator for up to 1½ weeks.
For smoothies: Small fresh parsnips are surprisingly sweet. Pair older parsnips with apples and/or carrots to sweeten them up. Peel (if not organic) and roughly chop parsnips. Place in a small saucepan, cover with water and simmer until soft.

Parsnip Smoothies
• Parsnip, page 212

Peas
See Beans

Peppers
Green, yellow, orange, purple and red bell peppers
Actions: Antioxidant, anticancer, cardioprotective.
Uses: Use green, yellow, orange, purple and red peppers in vegetable cocktails and blended drinks — they are all high in vitamins A and C and contain some potassium.
Buying and storing: Firm, crisp peppers with smooth skins and no blemishes are preferable. Avoid waxed peppers because the wax keeps the skin from breathing and prevents air from circulating, which can accelerate bacteria growth. Store peppers in a paper bag in the crisper drawer of the refrigerator for up to four days. Peppers freeze well and may be added to smoothies without thawing.

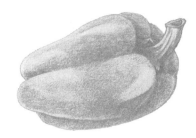

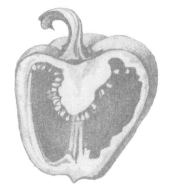

For smoothies: Wash and cut into pieces, leaving the seeds intact and discarding the stems. Frozen, canned or reconstituted dried peppers may be used in smoothies.

Pepper Smoothies
• Peppery Tomato Cocktail, page 213

Potatoes
Actions: Anticancer, cardioprotective.

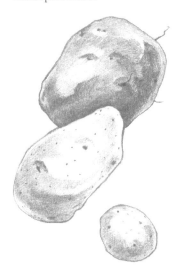

Uses: Potatoes are high in potassium, which may help prevent high blood pressure and strokes. They are a good source of B vitamins (except B12), vitamin C and fiber, and make satisfying low-fat additions to drinks.
Buying and storing: Select clean, smooth, well-shaped potatoes. Avoid those with wrinkled skin, soft spots or bruises. One medium potato weighs about 8 oz (250 g) and makes about 1 cup (250 mL) diced. If kept in a cool, dry place (for example, a cellar or porch), potatoes will last for up to one month. Keep covered with brown paper or burlap, as light causes potatoes to turn green.
For smoothies: Cook potatoes before adding to smoothies. You can also use canned or leftover cooked potatoes.

Potato Smoothies
• Peppered Potato, page 213

Spinach
Actions: Anticancer, improves memory, antioxidant, promotes healing, anti-cataracts, antianemia.

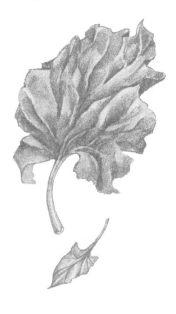

Uses: A good source of choline, which improves mental function, and folic acid, a heart protector, spinach is one of only four vegetables that are high in vitamin E. It is also high in cancer-fighting lutein, chlorophyll and vitamins A and C, and is a good source of calcium, iron, protein and potassium.

Buying and storing: Choose loose spinach, which is fresher than prepackaged, when available. However, be sure to wash it thoroughly, as it tends to be gritty. Look for broad, crisp, deep green leaves with no signs of yellowing, wilting or softness. Spinach keeps for up to three days in a perforated plastic bag in the crisper drawer of the refrigerator. Pick over and remove yellow or wilted leaves of prepackaged spinach before using.

For smoothies: Use fresh, frozen or canned spinach. Wash fresh leaves well, remove tough ribs and stems, and coarsely chop the leaves before adding to the blender. To measure, pack chopped spinach tightly into a dry measuring cup.

Spinach Smoothies

Squash
Acorn, butternut, Hubbard, pumpkin and turban

Actions: Antioxidant, anticancer.

Uses: Squash is a good winter vegetable that is high in vitamin A.

Buying and storing: Summer squash are small and tender, with pliable skins and seeds. Winter squash have been allowed to mature on the vine, and their rinds and seeds are tough and woody. Keep whole squash in a cold, moist place or in a perforated plastic bag in the refrigerator. Winter squash may keep for up to one month if stored properly. Cooked squash freezes well for use in smoothies.

For smoothies: Frozen, canned or leftover cooked squash is easiest to use in smoothies. Use one-quarter or less of a fresh squash at a time and cook before using in smoothies. Peel, chop and place in a medium saucepan. Cover with water and simmer until soft.

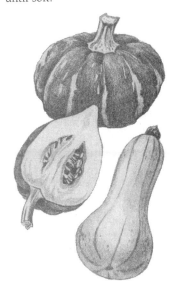

Squash Smoothies

Swiss Chard
See Leafy Greens

Tomatoes

Actions: Antioxidant, anticancer.

Uses: High in lycopene and glutathione, two powerful antioxidants, tomatoes are thought to reduce the risk of many cancers. Lycopene is also thought to help maintain mental and physical functions and is absorbed by the body more efficiently when tomatoes are juiced (or cooked). Tomatoes also contain glutamic acid, which is converted in the body to gamma-aminobutyric acid (GABA), a calming agent known to be effective in reducing kidney hypertension. Drink tomato juice or smoothies made with tomatoes to relax after a stressful day.

Buying and storing: Vine-ripened heritage varieties are the most flavorful. Tomatoes are best bought fresh only when in season (use canned or reconstituted dried at other times). Local tomatoes are not treated with ethylene gas to force reddening. Plump, heavy, firm-skinned, bright red tomatoes keep for two or three days at room temperature. When almost overripe, store tomatoes in the refrigerator for only one or two more days.

For smoothies: Skin and seeds may be used. If seeds are not desired, peel ripe tomatoes and press flesh through a sieve, catching the juice in a bowl.

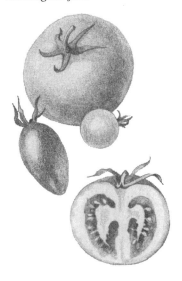

Tomato Smoothies

Turnips

Actions: Tonic, decongestant, antibacterial, anticancer, diuretic.
Uses: Turnips have a beneficial effect on the urinary system, purify the blood and aid in the elimination of toxins. For this reason, they make a good addition to cleansing smoothies. Both the root and the green tops (see Leafy Greens, page 140) are high in glucosinolates, which are thought to block the development of cancer. Good sources of calcium, iron and protein, small tender turnips are available in the spring and sometimes in the fall.
Buying and storing: Small firm white turnips with dark green leaves that show no signs of wilting or yellowing are best. Turnips will keep for up to one week in a plastic bag in the refrigerator.
For smoothies: Fresh cooked spring turnip is a pleasant addition to smoothies. Treat young turnips the same way you would parsnips. Their taste can be hot and peppery.

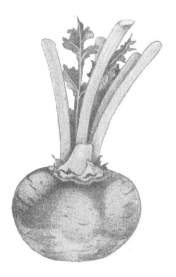

Turnip Smoothies
- Turnip Parsnip Carrot, page 218
- Turnip-Tomato Tango, page 218

Watercress

Actions: Antioxidant, diuretic, anticancer, tonic, antibiotic, cleansing.
Uses: High in fiber and vitamin C and a good source of vitamin A, watercress grows wild around streams and wet areas. Be careful not to harvest it in areas where fields drain directly into streams, because watercress takes in chemical runoff and the by-products of animal feces through its roots.

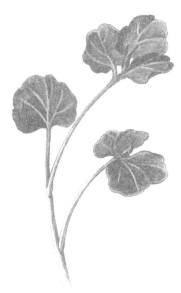

Buying and storing: Pick watercress just before using. If purchasing, choose crisp bright green sprigs with intact leaves. Sort through and remove any yellow or wilted stems. Watercress is fragile and should be used immediately. Wrapped in a towel in the crisper drawer of the refrigerator, it will keep for one or two days.
For smoothies: Wash well and chop. Watercress adds a peppery bite to smoothies. Use sparingly (only three to four sprigs per recipe).

Watercress Smoothies
- Watercress, page 219

Wild Greens

Dandelion, mustard, sorrel, turnip, wild garlic and wild leek (ramp)
See Leafy Greens

Zucchinis

Italian, yellow straightneck and yellow crookneck
Actions: Antioxidant.
Uses: A good source of vitamins A and C, potassium and niacin, zucchinis are mild tasting and blend well with stronger vegetables.

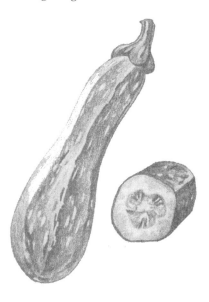

Buying and storing: Although zucchinis grow quite large, the smaller they are, the more tender. Look for soft thin skin with no cuts or bruises, and intact stem ends.
For smoothies: Choose small, firm zucchinis. Scrub well, trim off blossom ends, peel (if not organic) and chop before adding to the blender.

Zucchini Smoothies
- Zuke and Cuke, page 219

Blackstrap Molasses

Molasses is a thick syrup by-product of sugar refining, in which the sucrose (sugar) is separated from the liquid and nutrients from the raw cane plant. Several grades of molasses are available, but blackstrap contains the least sugar and the most nutrients: iron, six of the B vitamins, calcium, phosphorous and potassium.

For smoothies: Use sparingly — 1 to 2 tsp (5 to 10 mL) per 1 cup (250 mL) of smoothie — in drinks that require additional sweetening. Blackstrap molasses adds its own distinct flavor.

Carob

Carob, which is powdered carob beans, is used as a substitute for cocoa and chocolate. Carob is healthier than chocolate because, unlike cocoa (which chocolate is made from), it has no caffeine, does not need extra sugar, is lower in fat and provides some calcium and phosphorus. It is available in baking chips, which can be used in hot drinks, as well as in powdered form, which can be blended into smoothies (see also Coconut Carob Milk, page 250).

For smoothies: Carob tastes similar to cocoa and will add sweetness to blended drinks. Add 1 tbsp (15 mL) at a time and taste after each addition.

Cereal Grasses
Wheat and barley

Wheat and barley grass are grown from the seeds, or "berries," of the wheat or barley plant. Harvested when five to six inches (12.5 to 15 cm) tall, the fresh grass is then eaten or juiced. It can also be dried and used in powdered form or pressed into pills. High in chlorophyll, a powerful healing agent and infection fighter, as well as beta-carotene and vitamins C and E, these green foods are easily added to juices and smoothies. They have high levels of protein — even higher than those of soy products and legumes — making them the best plant sources of this nutrient.

Actions: Antioxidant, anti-inflammatory, anticancer, antibiotic, blood cleanser, protect against radiation.

For smoothies: Whisk 1 or 2 tsp (5 or 10 mL) powdered wheat or barley grass into 1 or 2 cups (250 or 500 mL) of smoothie.

Cider Vinegar

Distilled white vinegar is a mixture of acetic acid and water. It is useful as a disinfectant and cleaning agent but is not valuable as a food. Naturally fermented vinegar made from wine or fruit juice, such as the cider vinegar widely available in grocery stores, contains some nutrients. However, the most nutritious cider vinegar is available at natural-food stores. It is made from juice extracted from certified organic apples that is naturally fermented (without heat or the addition of clarifiers, enzymes or preservatives). This process yields a natural cider vinegar that contains some pectin and trace minerals, as well as beneficial bacteria and enzymes.

For smoothies: Add 1 tsp (5 mL) natural apple cider vinegar per smoothie recipe to enhance overall health.

Cheese

Cheese contains almost all of the nutrients in milk in concentrated form. People with milk intolerances cannot eat cheese made from cow's milk. While hard cheeses usually cannot be blended into drinks, soft and semisoft cheeses — such as feta, blue, cream and cottage cheeses, among many others — can be added to smoothies. Because softer cheeses are usually higher in fat, they should be used sparingly.

For smoothies: When using semisoft cheese, bring it to room temperature, remove the rind, if necessary, and chop before adding to the blender. The amount varies with the cheese, but a good rule of thumb is to add no more than $1/4$ cup (50 mL) per smoothie recipe.

Flax Seeds

Actions: Flaxseed oil is the best vegetable source of essential omega-3 fatty acids, which help lubricate the joints and prevent absorption of toxins by stimulating digestion.

For smoothies: Add 1 tbsp (15 mL) whole flax seeds to other ingredients before blending, or whisk 1 tbsp (15 mL) flaxseed oil into up to 2 cups (500 mL) of smoothie.

Grains

Buckwheat, oats, wheat, rye, spelt, amaranth and quinoa

Unrefined whole grains, which contain both the bran and the germ layers usually removed in refining, are nutritious because they retain all the nutritional value of the bran and the germ. Whole grains provide protein, carbohydrates, phytates, vitamin E, fiber (including lignins), some B vitamins (thiamin, riboflavin, niacin and folic acid), iron, zinc and magnesium.

Actions: Anticancer, antioxidant, fight heart disease, antiobesity, lower blood sugar level.

For smoothies: Add 2 to 3 tbsp (25 to 45 mL) steel-cut or rolled oats, spelt flakes or unprocessed oat bran to smoothie ingredients before blending. To use whole wheat berries in smoothies, soak 2 tbsp (25 mL) in 3 tbsp (45 mL) water overnight, then add to smoothie ingredients before blending. To use bulgur (steamed dried wheat) in smoothies, soak 2 tbsp (25 mL) in 2 tbsp (25 mL) hot water for 10 to 15 minutes, then add to smoothie ingredients before blending. To add buckwheat to smoothies, use kasha (roasted buckwheat kernels) and soak 2 tbsp (25 mL) in 3 tbsp (45 mL) hot water for one hour or until soft, then add to smoothie ingredients before blending. To use amaranth in smoothies, add 2 tbsp (25 mL) to smoothie ingredients before blending. To use quinoa in smoothies, thoroughly rinse 2 tbsp (25 mL) to smoothie ingredients before blending.

Green Algae

Chlorella and spirulina

Rich in carotenoids and chlorophyll, these microscopic single-celled green algae have been shown to be effective in reducing the effects of radiation and may be helpful in treating HIV infections. Available in capsules or bulk loose powder.

Actions: Antioxidant, anticancer, boosts immunity, reduces heavy-metal toxicity, hypotensive.

For smoothies: Add 2 tsp (10 mL) per smoothie recipe.

Hemp

Hemp seeds are high in protein and contain about 30% oil, which is high in essential fatty acids — omega-3 and omega-6, as well as gamma linolenic acid (GLA). Hemp nuts, the hulled seeds of the hemp plant, can be used in nut butters, baked products, dips and spreads, and incorporated into blended drinks.

For smoothies: Add 2 to 3 tbsp (25 to 45 mL) hemp nuts or 1 to 2 tsp (5 to 10 mL) hemp oil to each smoothie recipe.

Honey

Honey is almost as sweet as granulated white sugar. The difference is that honey has small amounts of B vitamins, calcium, iron, zinc, potassium and phosphorous. It also acts as a potent bacteria killer. One tbsp (15 mL) contains just under 2% of the recommended daily intake of vitamins A and C, iron and calcium. Generally, the darker the honey the higher its antioxidant value.

Actions: Antioxidant, antibacterial, antimicrobial, calms nerves, antidiarrheal.

Caution: The National Honey Board, along with other health organizations, recommends that you never feed honey to children under one year of age, because most unpasteurized honeys contain yeasts from nectar and pollen that can ferment.

For smoothies: Use honey as a sweetener for bitter vegetable smoothies or add to hot toddies and cold remedies to soothe a sore throat. Liquid and creamed honeys are the best types to use in smoothies.

Bee pollen is made from the seeds of flower blossoms that stick to the legs of bees as they go from flower to flower. When the bees return to the hive, they clean themselves and mix these seeds with nectar and their own enzymes to form the pollen. Bee pollen contains proteins; vitamins A, B, C and E; calcium; magnesium; selenium; nucleic acids; and lecithin. Add 1 tbsp (15 mL) bee pollen to up to 2 cups (500 mL) of smoothie.

Royal jelly is a milky product that is fed exclusively to the queen bee. It is rich in B vitamins, as well as vitamins A, C, D and E. Refrigerate fresh royal jelly or purchase freeze-dried to use in blended drinks. Add 1 tbsp (15 mL) royal jelly to up to 2 cups (500 mL) of smoothie.

Propolis is a protective antibiotic substance made by bees. They collect a sticky resinous substance from coniferous trees and mix it with their own secretions to form propolis. For humans, it supports the immune system and can be used as a tonic. Add 1 tsp (5 mL) propolis to each 1 cup (250 mL) of smoothie.

Ice Cream

Ice cream is a fundamental ingredient in milk shakes, which are one of the earliest blended drinks. By the late 1800s, milk shakes had become a favorite treat served at local drugstores and ice-cream parlors. Made from milk, flavored syrup and ice cream, the earliest versions were shaken by hand or using a hand-cranked device. Once electric milk-shake machines were developed, they quickly became popular. Since children and teenagers burn up more energy and have higher daily requirements for calcium than adults, homemade milk shakes are an acceptable snack once or twice a week. Use homemade ice cream when making the milk shakes in this book because it is a healthier choice: although it still contains sugar, it has none of the harmful additives or preservatives found in commercial ice cream.

Caution: The ice-cream smoothies in this book (see pages 256 to 260) contain sugar and extra calories, so use sparingly and only if an active lifestyle allows.

Maple Syrup

The sap from sugar maples (*Acer saccharum*), red maples (*A. rubrum*) and silver maples (*A. saccharinum*) is collected in the spring when it is flowing from the roots back into the aerial parts of the tree to provide energy for growth. The sap is 95 to 97% water, but when it is boiled down, a thick, sweet syrup composed of 65% sucrose is left behind. The syrup also contains organic acids, minerals (mainly potassium and calcium) and traces of amino acids and vitamins. One-quarter cup (50 mL) maple syrup provides 6% of the recommended daily intake of calcium and thiamin, and 2% of magnesium and riboflavin.

For smoothies: Stir 1 to 2 tbsp (15 to 25 mL) pure maple syrup (avoid maple-flavored syrup, which is primarily corn syrup with artificial flavoring) into 1 to 2 cups (250 to 500 mL) of vegetable smoothie when a sweetener is required. Maple sap — a thin, watery, clear liquid that is not as sweet as maple syrup — may be used as a liquid in smoothies.

Lecithin

Lecithin is one of the best sources of choline, which is known to improve memory by strengthening neurons in the brain's memory centers. Lecithin is available in natural-food stores in capsule or granular form. Add two capsules or 1 tbsp (15 mL) lecithin granules to 1 to 2 cups (250 to 500 mL) of smoothie.

Nuts

All nuts — including peanuts, which are technically legumes — contain large amounts of protein, vitamin E, fiber and protease inhibitors, which are known to prevent cancer in laboratory animals. Although nuts are extremely high in fat, their oils are polyunsaturated and, as such, reduce blood cholesterol levels. Nuts also contain essential fatty acids, which are necessary for healthy skin, hair, glands, mucous membranes, nerves and arteries, as well as being helpful in preventing cardiovascular disease. Nuts allow a slow, steady rise in blood sugar and insulin, making them good foods for people with diabetes (see also Nut Milks, page 246).

Actions: Anticancer, lower blood cholesterol levels, regulate blood sugar level.

Caution: Some nuts cause extreme allergic reactions in some people. Peanuts and peanut butter may be contaminated by aflatoxin, a carcinogen.

For smoothies: Use up to 3 tbsp (45 mL) chopped nuts per smoothie recipe. Add to other ingredients before blending.

Protein Powder

Soy protein (the protein extracted from soybeans) is believed to help reduce the risk of cancers of the breast, endometrium and prostate if it contains isoflavones. Isoflavones mimic the action of estrogen and thus reduce the symptoms of menopause and help prevent the loss of calcium, which is linked to osteoporosis. Research has shown that soy protein reduces both the overall cholesterol level and the low-density lipoprotein (LDL), or "bad," cholesterol level. Choose raw soy protein powder made from soybeans that are water-washed (not washed in alcohol), organically grown and specifically tested for high isoflavone levels.

For smoothies: Add up to 3 tbsp (45 mL) protein powder to each smoothie recipe. Add to other ingredients before blending.

Psyllium Seeds

Psyllium seeds, which are widely available in pharmacies and natural-food stores, are a good natural laxative. Mucilage-rich, they add bulk to the stool, which causes it to press against the bowel wall, triggering the contractions that lead to a bowel movement. Psyllium seeds are useful in treating constipation, irritable bowel syndrome, diverticular disease and obesity. When taking psyllium seeds, you need to drink at least eight glasses of water a day to avoid bowel obstruction. A diet high in fresh whole fruits and vegetables will soon take over their job.

Dose: Mix 1 tsp to 1 tbsp (5 to 15 mL) psyllium seeds into a smoothie and follow with a large glass of water. Take first thing in the morning for one week. You must drink at least eight glasses of water a day if you are taking psyllium seeds.

Caution: Psyllium can cause allergic reactions in sensitive individuals and should be avoided if you have asthma. If you experience an allergic reaction, discontinue use immediately. Psyllium should never be taken in cases of bowel obstruction.

Pumpkin Seeds

Pumpkin seeds are important to men because they contain high concentrations of amino acids that can reduce the symptoms of prostate enlargement.

For smoothies: Add 2 tbsp (25 mL) hulled fresh pumpkin seeds to ingredients before blending.

Ready-to-Use Juices

See Fruit Juices, page 154, or Liquids for Vegetable Smoothies, page 196.

Sea Herbs

(Sea vegetables or seaweed)
Arame, dulse, hijiki, nori, wakame and kelp
Their high concentrations of vitamin A, protein, calcium, iron

and other minerals make sea herbs important to overall health.
Actions: Anticancer, diuretic, antibacterial, boost immune function.

For smoothies: The salty taste of sea herbs blends well in vegetable smoothies. Available in dried form, sea herbs can be crushed and added dry to recipes. They can also be covered in hot water and allowed to soak for 10 to 20 minutes before using. Add 1 to 2 tbsp (15 to 25 mL) dried or 1/4 cup (50 mL) soaked sea herbs and the soaking water to other ingredients before blending.

Sesame Seeds

High in calcium and a good source of incomplete protein, sesame seeds lend a light, nutty taste to juices and blended drinks. Sesame seed oil is exceptionally stable and is a source of vitamin E and coenzyme Q10, an essential coenzyme for metabolism, or the rate at which the body produces energy (or burns calories).
Actions: Emollient, laxative, antioxidant.

For smoothies: Use plain or toasted sesame seeds and add 1 tbsp (15 mL) per smoothie recipe. Add to other ingredients before blending or use with nuts to make nut milks (see pages 248 to 250).

Soy Products

Soybeans are the only known plant source of complete protein, meaning that they contain all of the essential amino acids in the appropriate proportions that are essential for the growth and maintenance of cells. Because soy products are often rich in isoflavones, diets high in soy were once thought to prevent cancers of the prostate, breast, uterus,

lungs, colon, stomach, liver, pancreas, bladder and skin. However, recent studies have shown conflicting conclusions.
Actions: May be anticancer, lower blood cholesterol level, boost immunity.
Caution: Due to new research and the effects of genetic modification and heavy chemical use on soybeans, buy only organic fresh or dried soybeans and soy products.
Availability: Available raw, dried or canned whole, or in paste (miso), soy milk, tofu and tempeh.
For smoothies: Soy milk (see page 245) and tofu are often added to smoothies.

Tofu is a curd made from soybeans that is high in B vitamins, potassium and iron, as well as calcium, so long as that mineral has been used as the curdling agent (check the label). Tofu thickens and "smoothes" the taste of blended drinks. Silken tofu works best in smoothies. Add 1/4 to 1/2 cup (50 to 125 mL) to any smoothie recipe.

Tempeh, a mild, firm cake made from fermented cooked soybeans, may also be used in smoothies. It is usually sold frozen. Add 1/4 cup (50 mL) crumbled tempeh to any smoothie recipe.

Canned soybeans or cooked reconstituted dried soybeans are also good in smoothies and produce a thicker result. Add 1/2 cup (125 mL) canned or cooked soybeans per smoothie recipe.

Sprouts

A good source of B vitamins (except B12), sprouts also contain vitamins A and C, as well as bioflavonoids and enzymes.

They add a green, living nutritional boost to juices and blended drinks. Alfalfa (and other grains), bean, pea and herb seeds are easy to sprout in a warm, moist environment and offer a concentrated blast of the nutrients found in the mature plants. Grow sprouts in the winter months, when fresh leafy greens are not at their best.

Caution: The safety of seed sprouts depends upon the quality of the water in which they are grown. Some sprouts have been linked with harmful bacteria, and water is the culprit in generating that bacteria. The best source for sprouts is to grow them from clean, organic seeds in water that has been boiled or that is known to be free of contaminants.

Buying and storing: For reasons stated above, grow your own or purchase sprouts from reliable growers. Look for moist, crisp sprouts with no evidence of slime or wilting. Store in the refrigerator for up to one week.

For smoothies: Add up to 1/2 cup (125 mL) sprouts per smoothie recipe.

Sunflower Seeds

A good source of vitamin E and zinc, sunflower seeds may be added to other ingredients before blending into smoothies.

For smoothies: Add 2 tbsp (25 mL) shelled seeds to up to 2 cups (500 mL) of smoothie.

Tofu
See Soy Products

Wheat Germ

A good source of vitamin E and thiamin, wheat germ may be added to other ingredients before blending.

For smoothies: Use 2 tbsp (25 mL) per smoothie recipe.

Wheat Grass
See Cereal Grasses

Yogurt Products

Yogurt cheese: If you prefer a thicker smoothie, a cheese made from yogurt may be added. Use up to 1/4 cup (50 mL) per smoothie recipe.

To make yogurt cheese, suspend a strainer, sieve or colander lined with three layers of cheesecloth over a medium to large bowl. Empty a 16-oz (500 g) or larger container of plain yogurt into the strainer and cover with plastic wrap. Refrigerate for at least three

hours or overnight. Remove from refrigerator, drain and discard liquid (or save for use in stocks). Cover and store yogurt cheese in the refrigerator for up to one week. Makes 3/4 to 1 cup (175 to 250 mL) yogurt cheese.

Frozen yogurt: Use frozen yogurt as you would ice cream. Add up to 1/2 cup (125 mL) per smoothie recipe. Add to other ingredients before blending. Frozen yogurt thickens smoothies and may require the addition of extra liquid. Although most commercial frozen yogurts are low in fat, they are very high in sugar — use them sparingly or substitute homemade unsweetened frozen yogurt cubes.

Frozen yogurt cubes: Drain and discard liquid from a 16-oz (500 g) container of plain yogurt. Spoon into ice-cube trays and freeze. Use in smoothies where frozen yogurt is called for. Use six frozen yogurt cubes to replace one scoop or 1/2 cup (125 mL) frozen yogurt.

The Recipes

Smoothie Tips and Techniques

- Measure the ingredients into the blender jug in the order listed in the recipe, pouring liquid into the jug first. This is essential for the blender to work properly.
- Blend on the Low or Mix setting for 10 to 30 seconds, then increase the speed to the High, Puree or Liquefy setting for another 10 to 30 seconds. This allows the blades to chop the bigger chunks finely before they spin faster and lift the mixture up and out of range. This method actually shortens the time needed to liquefy the ingredients for drinking.
- Always chop ice with some liquid in the jug.
- Smoothie too thin? Add a couple of ice cubes, a banana or frozen fruit.
- Smoothie too thick? Add more liquid — juice, soy milk, milk or water.
- Smoothie too sweet? Add lemon juice, 1 tbsp (15 mL) at a time, until taste is corrected.
- Smoothie too sour? Add chopped sweet fruit (banana, apple, grapes, pineapple or dried apricots or dates), in $1/4$-cup (50 mL) increments, until desired sweetness is achieved.
- Blend, drink and enjoy — every day!

Fruit Smoothies

BURSTING WITH FLAVORFUL SWEETNESS AND NUTRITION, smoothies made from fruit are the most popular variety. Filled with healthful antioxidants and other vital phytochemicals, they are a great way to start the day. If you make them with milk, yogurt, tofu or fortified soy milk, they also add bone-building calcium to your diet.

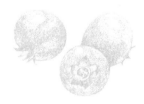

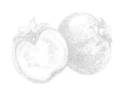

Sugar Alert

Fruits are high in natural sugar, which the body uses for fuel. However, people with diabetes and those who are prone to yeast infections and hypoglycemia must limit their consumption of fruits and fruit juices. Overconsumption can cause a rapid rise in blood sugar.

Most juices, particularly those made from concentrated fruit, contain a lot of natural sugar — 1 cup (250 mL) unsweetened apple juice contains, on average, 25 g sugar — and sugar is often added to commercially prepared juices.

Enjoy Fresh Seasonal Fruits

Smoothies are the perfect way to enjoy seasonal fruits when they are widely available from local growers and at the pinnacle of freshness. Fresh fruits picked at their peak, stored properly and consumed raw provide maximum vitamins, minerals, enzymes and phytonutrients. Buy organic fruit whenever possible to reduce your intake of potentially harmful chemicals. Look for smooth, blemish-free skins and choose fruit at the peak of ripeness. Underripe fruit produces smoothies that are chalky, lumpy and somewhat bitter — and they may cause diarrhea or stomach cramps. Overripe fruit may start to ferment and can cause the same symptoms.

To ripen soft-fleshed fruits (peaches, apricots, pears, plums and avocados), place the fruit in a brown paper bag and keep at room temperature for two or three days or until it is ripe. Store ripened fruit in the refrigerator.

Frozen Fruit Works, Too

Smoothies are colder, thicker and smoother when they're made with frozen fruits. In fact, combining fresh and frozen fruit in the same drink is ideal. To make the most-economical use of your blender, purchase large quantities of fresh seasonal produce and freeze it in individual servings. A more expensive but more convenient option is to use commercially frozen fruit, especially in winter, when fresh fruits are out of season. Look for frozen fruit that has no added sugar and avoid packages that are stained or show evidence of leakage, which are both indications that the contents have thawed and refrozen.

Freezing fresh fruit: Peel, seed or pit, and cut fruit in chunks. (If using berries, pick them over, discarding any wrinkled, split or soft berries, then wash and pat dry.) Arrange the pieces in a single layer on a baking sheet and freeze until hard. Transfer to a resealable plastic freezer bag, then seal and label. Use three or four frozen pieces of fruit or $1/2$ cup (125 mL) frozen berries (no need to thaw) in smoothies. Frozen fruit will keep for up to six months in the freezer.

NUTRITION IN A GLASS

Fruit smoothies supply the body with important vitamins, minerals, enzymes, fiber, water and essential phytonutrients. Unlike juices, which lack insoluble fiber, smoothies deliver all the natural fiber that's present in whole raw fruits.

Fruit Juices

Fruit juices are often used as liquids in smoothies. The best possible juice is made from fresh organic fruit and should be consumed immediately. When it is not possible to make your own juice, commercially prepared unsweetened organic juice is the next best choice. For convenience, keep a variety of frozen concentrated juices on hand. Look for unsweetened concentrates made from organic fruit.

Canned Fruit Is an Alternative

When fresh fruits are not in season, keeping a variety of canned fruits on hand is a convenient way to make a variety of flavorful smoothies. Studies show that canned fruits are very nutritious. When Ken Sammonds, an associate professor of human nutrition at the University of Massachusetts, compared two versions of the same fruit smoothie recipe — one made with canned fruit, the other made with fresh fruit — he found that many vitamin levels were comparable. "The ingredients you choose, not the form of the ingredients, are what really determine a recipe's nutrient content," he concluded. However, commercially processed fruits may contain additives, pesticide residues or large amounts of sugar. Organic fruit packed in its own juice or water with no sugar added (available at natural-food stores) is preferable.

To substitute canned fruit for fresh, use one 14-oz (398 mL) can for each 1 cup (250 mL) sliced or chopped fresh fruit. Use the liquid in the can (if it is not a heavy sugar syrup) but reduce the amount of other liquids in the recipe by $^1/_4$ cup (50 mL).

Using Dried Fruit

Dried fruit may also be used in smoothies, either as is or in fruit milks (see pages 247 to 250). Drying concentrates the sugars (glucose, fructose and sucrose) and fiber in fruits. This means that smoothies made with dried fruit are sweeter than those made with fresh and have more cleansing power because they are higher in fiber. (That's why prunes are a more effective laxative than fresh plums.) Fresh apricots, for example, are approximately 2% fiber, but dried apricots are about 20% fiber.

Substituting dried fruit: When substituting dried fruit for fresh, frozen or canned, add $^1/_4$ cup (50 mL) extra liquid to the recipe, or reconstitute the dried fruit before using.

Reconstituting dried fruit: Measure whole, sliced or halved dried fruit into a small bowl and pour boiling water over it to cover. Steep for 30 minutes to one hour or until fruit is plump and soft. Drain (reserve liquid to add to other liquid in recipe) and chop fruit before adding to the blender.

WATCH FOR SULPHUR

Commercially dried fruits (except dates and figs) are usually fumigated with sulphur dioxide, a gas that is poisonous and destroys B vitamins. Buy unsulphured fruits whenever possible, especially if you are feeding them to children, and wash thoroughly before using. To make your own dried fruit, buy organic fruit in season and dry in the oven or using a food dehydrator.

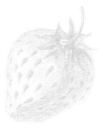

Apple Fresh

¾ cup	apple juice	175 mL
2	apples, peeled, cored and chopped	2
1 cup	seedless red grapes	250 mL
Half	lemon, peeled, seeded and chopped	Half
½ tsp	powdered ginseng (optional)	2 mL

In blender, combine apple juice, apples, grapes, lemon, and ginseng (if using). Process as directed until smooth.

SERVES 3

Apple Crisp

TIP
You can use fresh and frozen fruit interchangeably in most smoothies, although the results will differ. Frozen fruit not only chills a smoothie, it thickens it as well.

¾ cup	apple juice	175 mL
2	apples, peeled, cored and chopped	2
½ cup	frozen raspberries	125 mL
¼ cup	cranberry sauce	50 mL
Half	ripe banana, peeled and chopped	Half
1 tbsp	steel-cut or rolled oats	15 mL
¼ tsp	ground cinnamon	1 mL
Pinch	ground nutmeg	Pinch

In blender, combine apple juice, apples, raspberries, cranberry sauce, banana, oats, cinnamon and nutmeg. Process as directed until smooth.

SERVES 4

Apple Currant

⅔ cup	apple juice	150 mL
½ cup	black currants	125 mL
1	apple, peeled, cored and chopped	1
½ cup	applesauce	125 mL

In blender, combine apple juice, black currants, chopped apple and applesauce. Process as directed until smooth.

SERVES 1 OR 2

Apple Mint

½ cup	cooled peppermint infusion (see page 115)	125 mL
¼ cup	plain or frozen yogurt	50 mL
1	apple, peeled, cored and chopped	1
1	kiwi, peeled and chopped	1
1 tbsp	chopped fresh peppermint leaves	15 mL
¼ tsp	fennel seeds	1 mL
¼ cup	applesauce	50 mL

In blender, combine infusion, yogurt, apple, kiwi, peppermint, fennel seeds and applesauce. Process as directed until smooth.

SERVES 3 OR 4

TIP
The sweetness of this smoothie will increase significantly if you use sweetened frozen yogurt rather than plain yogurt.

Apple Pie

¼ cup	apple cider	50 mL
½ cup	silken tofu	125 mL
2	apples, peeled, cored and chopped	2
2 tbsp	spelt flakes (optional)	25 mL
¼ tsp	ground cinnamon	1 mL
⅛ tsp	ground cloves	0.5 mL
⅛ tsp	ground nutmeg	0.5 mL
Pinch	ground ginger (optional)	Pinch
½ cup	applesauce	125 mL

In blender, combine cider, tofu, apples, spelt flakes (if using), cinnamon, cloves, nutmeg, ginger (if using), and applesauce. Process as directed until smooth.

SERVES 2

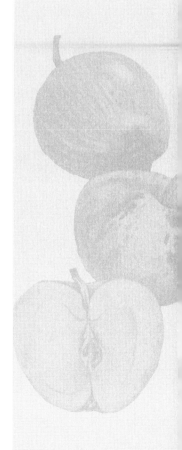

General Directions
Always place the lid securely on the blender before processing. Blend on Low for 30 seconds. Gradually (if possible) increase speed to High and blend an additional 30 seconds or until smooth.

Apple Spice Cocktail

¾ cup	apple juice	175 mL
3	apples, peeled, cored and chopped	3
1	piece (½ inch/1 cm) gingerroot, peeled and chopped	1
⅛ tsp	ground cardamom (optional)	0.5 mL
⅛ tsp	ground nutmeg	0.5 mL
¼ cup	cranberry sauce	50 mL

In blender, combine apple juice, apples, gingerroot, cardamom (if using), nutmeg and cranberry sauce. Process as directed until smooth.

SERVES 2

Apricot Apricot

¼ cup	orange or carrot juice	50 mL
1	can (14 oz/398 mL) apricots in juice	1
½ cup	chopped dried apricots	125 mL
1	ripe banana, peeled and chopped	1

In blender, combine orange juice, canned apricots with juice, dried apricots and banana. Process as directed until smooth.

SERVES 2

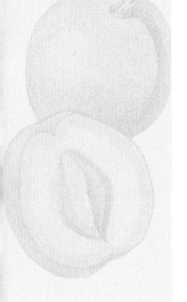

Apricot Explosion

½ cup	pineapple juice	125 mL
2	apricots, peeled, pitted and chopped	2
1	wedge pineapple, peeled and chopped	1
¼ cup	apricot or peach-flavored frozen yogurt	50 mL

In blender, combine pineapple juice, apricots, chopped pineapple and frozen yogurt. Process as directed until smooth.

SERVES 1 OR 2

Apricot Peach

½ cup	orange juice	125 mL
2	apricots, peeled, pitted and chopped	2
2	peaches, peeled, pitted and chopped	2
½ cup	green grapes	125 mL

In blender, combine orange juice, apricots, peaches and grapes. Process as directed until smooth.

SERVES 1 OR 2

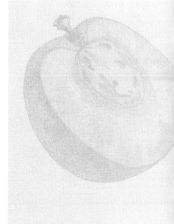

Triple A

½ cup	apricot or peach nectar or Apricot Milk (recipe, page 247)	125 mL
2	apricots, peeled, pitted and chopped	2
1	apple, peeled, cored and chopped	1
2 tbsp	chopped almonds	25 mL
¼ tsp	almond extract (optional)	1 mL

In blender, combine apricot nectar, chopped apricots, apple, almonds, and almond extract (if using). Process as directed until smooth.

SERVES 1 OR 2

Almond Banana

1 cup	plain soy milk or Almond Milk (recipe, page 248)	250 mL
3 tbsp	chopped almonds	45 mL
2	ripe bananas, peeled and chopped	2
Pinch	ground nutmeg	Pinch

In blender, combine soy milk, almonds, bananas and nutmeg. Process as directed until smooth.

SERVES 1 OR 2

TIP
Although many of the recipes call for plain soy milk, some flavored soy milks work equally well in fruit smoothies. Feel free to substitute your favorite flavor.

TIP
Use plain soy milk in place of the pineapple juice to reduce the sweetness of this smoothie.

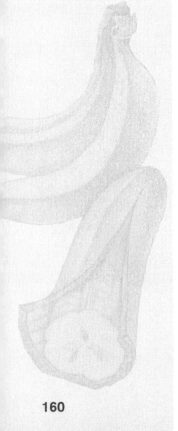

Bananarama

⅔ cup	pear nectar	150 mL
2 tbsp	lemon juice	25 mL
1	frozen ripe banana, peeled and chopped	1
1	pear, peeled, cored and chopped	1

In blender, combine pear nectar, lemon juice, banana and chopped pear. Process as directed until smooth.

SERVES 1

Banana Nut

½ cup	pineapple juice	125 mL
3 tbsp	chopped almonds	45 mL
2	wedges pineapple, peeled and chopped	2
1	ripe banana, peeled and chopped	1
¼ cup	banana-flavored frozen yogurt	50 mL
⅛ tsp	ground cinnamon	0.5 mL
Pinch	ground nutmeg	Pinch

In blender, combine pineapple juice, almonds, pineapple wedges, chopped banana, frozen yogurt, cinnamon and nutmeg. Process as directed until smooth.

SERVES 3

Banana Mango

½ cup	mango, apricot or peach nectar	125 mL
⅓ cup	silken tofu	75 mL
1	ripe banana, peeled and chopped	1
1	mango, peeled, pitted and chopped	1
½ cup	chopped pitted peeled apricots	125 mL

In blender, combine mango nectar, tofu, banana, chopped mango and apricots. Process as directed until smooth.

SERVES 2 OR 3

Berry Blast

¾ cup	raspberry juice	175 mL
2 tbsp	lemon juice	25 mL
6	frozen strawberries	6
6	frozen raspberries	6
½ cup	blackberries	125 mL
½ cup	blueberries	125 mL

In blender, combine raspberry juice, lemon juice, strawberries, raspberries, blackberries and blueberries. Process as directed until smooth.

SERVES 2 OR 3

TIP
Replacing fresh berries with frozen (or frozen with fresh) is fine in smoothie recipes. Keep in mind that if you use all frozen berries, the smoothie will be colder and thicker.

Black Belt

¾ cup	orange juice	175 mL
½ cup	frozen blackberries	125 mL
¼ cup	frozen blueberries	50 mL
1	frozen ripe banana, peeled and chopped	1

In blender, combine orange juice, blackberries, blueberries and banana. Process as directed until smooth.

SERVES 2

Black Pineapple

1 cup	pineapple juice	250 mL
2 tbsp	lemon juice	25 mL
½ cup	blackberries	125 mL
½ cup	blueberries	125 mL
½ cup	raspberries	125 mL
1 tbsp	chopped fresh parsley*	15 mL

* If you are pregnant, limit your intake of parsley to ½ tsp (2 mL) dried or one sprig fresh per day. Do not take parsley if you are suffering from kidney inflammation.

In blender, combine pineapple juice, lemon juice, blackberries, blueberries, raspberries and parsley. Process as directed until smooth.

SERVES 3

Fruit Smoothies

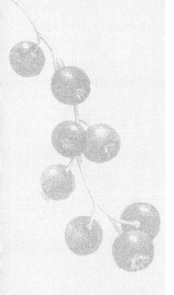

Black Currant

⅔ cup	apple juice	150 mL
½ cup	black currants	125 mL
1	ripe banana, peeled and chopped	1
⅓ cup	plain yogurt	75 mL
2 tbsp	liquid honey (or to taste)	25 mL

In blender, combine apple juice, black currants, banana, yogurt
and honey. Process as directed until smooth.

SERVES 2

Red, Black and Blue

½ cup	pineapple juice	125 mL
½ cup	black currants or blackberries	125 mL
½ cup	raspberries	125 mL
½ cup	blueberries	125 mL
1	ripe banana, peeled and chopped	1
2 tbsp	liquid honey (or to taste)	25 mL

In blender, combine pineapple juice, black currants, raspberries,
blueberries, banana and honey. Process as directed until smooth.

SERVES 2

Blueberry

⅔ cup	cranberry-raspberry juice	150 mL
1 cup	blueberries	250 mL
½ cup	red grapes	125 mL
¼ cup	silken tofu or plain yogurt	50 mL

In blender, combine cranberry-raspberry juice, blueberries, grapes
and tofu. Process as directed until smooth.

SERVES 2

Blue Cherry

1/2 cup	plain soy milk	125 mL
1 tbsp	lemon juice	15 mL
1 cup	blueberries	250 mL
1 cup	pitted cherries	250 mL
1/2 cup	seedless red grapes	125 mL
1/4 cup	silken tofu or fruit-flavored frozen yogurt	50 mL

In blender, combine soy milk, lemon juice, blueberries, cherries, grapes and tofu. Process as directed until smooth.

SERVES 3 OR 4

TIP
Try using
Fruit Yogurt Slush
(recipe, page 293)
for the frozen yogurt
in this smoothie.

Blue Water

3/4 cup	cranberry juice	175 mL
1/4 cup	crushed ice	50 mL
1 cup	chopped seeded peeled watermelon	250 mL
1/2 cup	blueberries	125 mL
1/4 cup	cranberry sauce	50 mL

In blender, combine cranberry juice, ice, watermelon, blueberries and cranberry sauce. Process as directed until smooth.

SERVES 3 OR 4

Pump It Up

3/4 cup	plain soy milk	175 mL
1/2 cup	pitted cherries	125 mL
1	ripe banana, peeled and chopped	1
1/4 cup	blueberries	50 mL
1 tbsp	protein powder	15 mL
2 tbsp	chopped almonds	25 mL

In blender, combine soy milk, cherries, banana, blueberries, protein powder and almonds. Process as directed until smooth.

SERVES 2

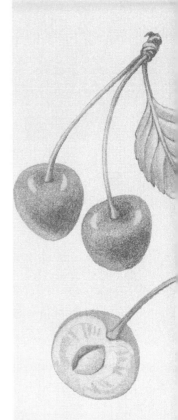

Fruit Smoothies

Cherry Berry

1	can (14 oz/398 mL) sweet cherries in juice	1
1/2 cup	raspberries or blueberries	125 mL
6	strawberries (hulled and halved if fresh)	6

In blender, combine cherries with juice, raspberries and strawberries. Process as directed until smooth.

SERVES 3

TIP
To substitute fresh cherries for canned in this recipe, use 1 cup (250 mL) chopped pitted cherries. Add 1/4 cup (50 mL) raspberry or orange juice.

Cherries Jubilee

1 cup	plain soy milk	250 mL
1 cup	pitted cherries	250 mL
2	wedges pineapple, peeled and chopped	2
1/2 cup	chopped peeled ripe banana	125 mL
1 tbsp	flax seeds	15 mL
1/8 tsp	almond extract	0.5 mL

In blender, combine soy milk, cherries, pineapple, banana, flax seeds and almond extract. Process as directed until smooth.

SERVES 3

Cherry Sunrise

1 cup	grapefruit juice	250 mL
1 cup	pitted cherries	250 mL
6	strawberries (hulled and halved if fresh)	6
1	apple, peeled, cored and chopped	1
1 tbsp	fresh chamomile flowers (optional)	15 mL

In blender, combine grapefruit juice, cherries, strawberries, apple, and chamomile flowers (if using). Process as directed until smooth.

SERVES 3 OR 4

Cran-Cherry

¾ cup	apple juice	175 mL
⅓ cup	dried cherries or cranberries	75 mL
¼ cup	frozen cherries	50 mL
¼ cup	cranberry sauce	50 mL

In blender, combine apple juice, dried cherries, frozen cherries and cranberry sauce. Process as directed until smooth.

SERVES 2 OR 3

General Directions
Always place the lid securely on the blender before processing. Blend on Low for 30 seconds. Gradually (if possible) increase speed to High and blend an additional 30 seconds or until smooth.

Eye Opener

⅓ cup	orange juice	75 mL
1 cup	pitted cherries	250 mL
12	strawberries (hulled and halved if fresh)	12
1	orange, peeled, seeded and chopped	1

In blender, combine orange juice, cherries, strawberries and orange. Process as directed until smooth.

SERVES 2

Citrus Cocktail

½ cup	orange juice	125 mL
¼ cup	grapefruit juice	50 mL
12	strawberries (hulled and halved if fresh)	12
1	piece (½ inch/1 cm) gingerroot, peeled and chopped	1
1 tbsp	wheat germ or chopped almonds	15 mL
¼ cup	plain or frozen yogurt	50 mL

In blender, combine orange juice, grapefruit juice, strawberries, gingerroot, wheat germ and yogurt. Process as directed until smooth.

SERVES 2 OR 3

TIP
The sweetness of this smoothie will increase significantly if you use sweetened frozen yogurt rather than plain yogurt. Try using Fruit Yogurt Slush (recipe, page 293) for the frozen yogurt in this recipe.

C-Blend

¼ cup	orange juice	50 mL
¼ cup	cranberry sauce	50 mL
	Juice of 1 lime	
2	oranges, peeled, seeded and chopped	2
Half	grapefruit, peeled, seeded and chopped	Half
1 tbsp	chopped fresh parsley*	15 mL
1 tbsp	liquid honey (optional)	15 mL

In blender, combine orange juice, cranberry sauce, lime juice, oranges, grapefruit, parsley, and honey (if using). Process as directed until smooth.

SERVES 2 OR 3

C-Blitz

¼ cup	orange juice	50 mL
	Juice of 1 lemon	
2	kiwis, peeled and chopped	2
1	orange, peeled, seeded and chopped	1
Half	grapefruit, peeled, seeded and chopped	Half
1 tbsp	chopped fresh parsley*	15 mL

In blender, combine orange juice, lemon juice, kiwis, orange, grapefruit and parsley. Process as directed until smooth.

SERVES 2 OR 3

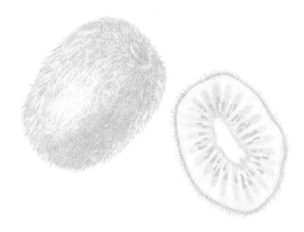

Fruit Smoothies

Mellow Mandarin

1	can (10 oz/284 mL) mandarin orange segments in juice	1
Quarter	honeydew melon, peeled, seeded and chopped	Quarter
6	frozen strawberries	6
1	piece (1/2 inch/1 cm) gingerroot, peeled and chopped	1

In blender, combine orange segments with juice, melon, strawberries and gingerroot. Process as directed until smooth.

SERVES 2

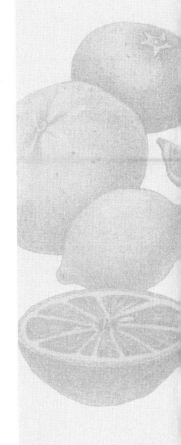

General Directions
Always place the lid securely on the blender before processing. Blend on Low for 30 seconds. Gradually (if possible) increase speed to High and blend an additional 30 seconds or until smooth.

Tangerine

1/2 cup	tangerine or orange juice	125 mL
2 tbsp	lemon juice	25 mL
2	tangerines, peeled, seeded and chopped	2
1 cup	seedless red grapes, halved	250 mL

In blender, combine tangerine juice, lemon juice, chopped tangerines and grapes. Process as directed until smooth.

SERVES 1 OR 2

Mellow Yellow

1/2 cup	white grape juice	125 mL
1	grapefruit, peeled, seeded and chopped	1
1	wedge pineapple, peeled and chopped	1
1	ripe banana, peeled and chopped	1

In blender, combine grape juice, grapefruit, pineapple and banana. Process as directed until smooth.

SERVES 2

Cranberry Pineapple

¾ cup	pineapple juice	175 mL
¼ cup	cranberries, chopped	50 mL
2	wedges pineapple, peeled and chopped	2
1	apple, peeled, cored and chopped	1

In blender, combine pineapple juice, cranberries, chopped pineapple and apple. Process as directed until smooth.

SERVES 2

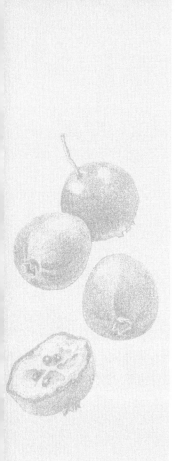

Cran-Apple

¾ cup	apple juice	175 mL
¼ cup	cranberry sauce	50 mL
1	apple, peeled, cored and chopped	1
1	orange, peeled, seeded and chopped	1
1 tbsp	flax seeds	15 mL

In blender, combine apple juice, cranberry sauce, apple, orange and flax seeds. Process as directed until smooth.

SERVES 2

Cran-Orange

¾ cup	orange juice	175 mL
¼ cup	silken tofu	50 mL
2 tbsp	dried cranberries	25 mL
1	orange, peeled, seeded and chopped	1
2 tsp	grated peeled gingerroot	10 mL

In blender, combine orange juice, tofu, cranberries, orange and gingerroot. Process as directed until smooth.

SERVES 1 OR 2

Fruit Explosion

¾ cup	apple juice	175 mL
¼ cup	dried cranberries	50 mL
Quarter	cantaloupe, peeled, seeded and chopped	Quarter
5	frozen strawberries	5

In blender, combine apple juice, cranberries, cantaloupe and strawberries. Process as directed until smooth.

SERVES 2

Fruit Splash

¾ cup	grapefruit juice	175 mL
¼ cup	cranberry sauce	50 mL
Quarter	cantaloupe, peeled, seeded and chopped	Quarter
¼ cup	frozen raspberries	50 mL

In blender, combine grapefruit juice, cranberry sauce, cantaloupe and raspberries. Process as directed until smooth.

SERVES 2

Almond Date

¾ cup	plain soy milk or Almond Milk (recipe, page 248)	175 mL
¼ cup	pitted dates, chopped	50 mL
2 tbsp	chopped almonds or pecans	25 mL
3 tbsp	cream cheese	45 mL
1	ripe banana, peeled and chopped	1
⅛ tsp	ground cinnamon	0.5 mL
Pinch	ground nutmeg	Pinch

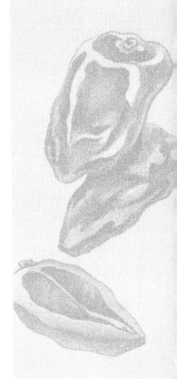

In blender, combine soy milk, dates, almonds, cream cheese, banana, cinnamon and nutmeg. Process as directed until smooth.

SERVES 2 OR 3

TIP
Using sweetened
cranberry sauce in
this smoothie will
produce a much
sweeter result than
fresh cranberries.

Date Time

3/4 cup	orange juice	175 mL
1/4 cup	pitted dates, chopped	50 mL
1/4 cup	chopped cranberries or cranberry sauce	50 mL
1	apple, peeled, cored and chopped	1

In blender, combine orange juice, dates, cranberries and apple.
Process as directed until smooth.

SERVES 2

Special Date

3/4 cup	orange juice	175 mL
2 tbsp	lemon juice	25 mL
1/4 cup	pitted dates, chopped	50 mL
1	orange, peeled, seeded and chopped	1

In blender, combine orange juice, lemon juice, dates and orange.
Process as directed until smooth.

SERVES 1 OR 2

Berry Bonanza

TIP
You can use fresh
and frozen fruit
interchangeably in
most smoothies,
although the results
will differ. Frozen
fruit not only chills
a smoothie, it also
makes it thicker.

1/2 cup	raspberry or cranberry-raspberry juice	125 mL
2 tbsp	lemon juice	25 mL
1/2 cup	fresh elderberries	125 mL
6	frozen strawberries	6
1/2 cup	frozen raspberries	125 mL

In blender, combine raspberry juice, lemon juice, elderberries,
strawberries and raspberries. Process as directed until smooth.

SERVES 2

Flu Fighter #1

½ cup	orange juice	125 mL
⅓ cup	lemon juice	75 mL
½ cup	elderberries	125 mL
¼ cup	cranberry sauce	50 mL
2 tbsp	black currant jelly or liquid honey	25 mL

In blender, combine orange juice, lemon juice, elderberries, cranberry sauce and black currant jelly. Process as directed until smooth.

SERVES 2

General Directions
Always place the lid securely on the blender before processing. Blend on Low for 30 seconds. Gradually (if possible) increase speed to High and blend an additional 30 seconds or until smooth.

Figgy Duff

½ cup	pineapple juice	125 mL
5	figs, chopped (peeled if fresh)	5
1 tbsp	flax seeds	15 mL
2 tsp	steel-cut or rolled oats	10 mL
1 tsp	extra-virgin olive oil or hemp oil	5 mL

In blender, combine pineapple juice, figs, flax seeds, oats and oil. Process as directed until smooth.

SERVES 1

Fruity Fig

½ cup	peach or apple juice	125 mL
	Juice of half a lemon	
¼ cup	chopped figs (peeled if fresh)	50 mL
¼ cup	chopped apricots	50 mL
½ cup	chopped pitted peeled peaches	125 mL
½ cup	chopped pitted peeled plums	125 mL

In blender, combine peach juice, lemon juice, figs, apricots, peaches and plums. Process as directed until smooth.

SERVES 2

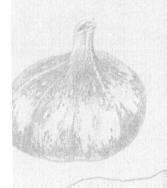

Gooseberry Fool

¼ cup	pineapple juice	50 mL
¼ cup	raspberry-flavored frozen yogurt	50 mL
1 cup	gooseberries	250 mL
1 tbsp	liquid honey (or to taste)	15 mL

In blender, combine pineapple juice, yogurt, gooseberries and honey. Process as directed until smooth.

SERVES 1

Loosey-Goosey

¼ cup	apple juice	50 mL
¼ cup	gooseberries	50 mL
1	apple, peeled, cored and chopped	1
3 tbsp	chopped pitted dates	45 mL
3 tbsp	chopped pitted prunes	45 mL
¼ tsp	ground licorice*, ginger or cinnamon	1 mL

In blender, combine apple juice, gooseberries, apple, dates, prunes and licorice. Process as directed until smooth.

SERVES 1

TIP

Be careful with this drink — it works as a laxative.

* Avoid licorice if you have high blood pressure. The prolonged use of licorice is not recommended under any circumstances.

Grape Glacé

½ cup	purple grape juice	125 mL
½ cup	ice cubes	125 mL
2 cups	seedless red grapes, halved	500 mL
1	plum, peeled, pitted and chopped	1

In blender, combine grape juice, ice cubes, grapes and plum. Process as directed until smooth.

SERVES 1

Grape Heart

1/2 cup	grape or grapefruit juice	125 mL
1 tbsp	chopped almonds	15 mL
2 cups	seedless red grapes, halved	500 mL
1/2 cup	blueberries	125 mL
Half	grapefruit, peeled, seeded and chopped	Half

In blender, combine grape juice, almonds, grapes, blueberries and grapefruit. Process as directed until smooth.

SERVES 2

Raisin Pie

1/2 cup	plain soy milk	125 mL
1 tbsp	lemon juice	15 mL
1 cup	seedless red grapes, halved	250 mL
1/4 cup	raisins	50 mL
1 tbsp	steel-cut or rolled oats	15 mL
1/4 tsp	ground cinnamon	1 mL

In blender, combine soy milk, lemon juice, grapes, raisins, oats and cinnamon. Process as directed until smooth.

SERVES 1

Sunrise Supreme

1/2 cup	white grape juice	125 mL
1 cup	seedless red grapes, halved	250 mL
12	strawberries (hulled and halved if fresh)	12
1/2 cup	raspberries	125 mL
1	orange, peeled, seeded and chopped	1

In blender, combine grape juice, grapes, strawberries, raspberries and orange. Process as directed until smooth.

SERVES 3 OR 4

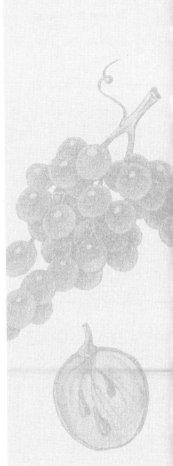

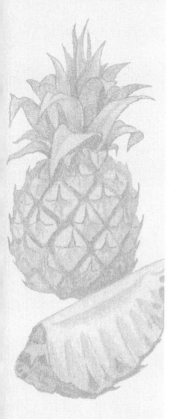

Pineapple Kiwi

1/2 cup	pineapple juice	125 mL
2	kiwis, peeled and chopped	2
2	apricots, peeled, pitted and chopped	2
1	mango, peeled, pitted and chopped	1
1/2 cup	plain yogurt	125 mL
1/4 tsp	ground ginger	1 mL

In blender, combine pineapple juice, kiwis, apricots, mango, yogurt and ginger. Process as directed until smooth.

SERVES 2

Ki-Lime

1/2 cup	white grape juice	125 mL
2 tbsp	lime juice	25 mL
2	kiwis, peeled and chopped	2
1 cup	chopped seeded peeled papaya	250 mL

In blender, combine grape juice, lime juice, kiwis and papaya. Process as directed until smooth.

SERVES 1

Sher-Lime

1/2 cup	orange juice	125 mL
3 tbsp	lime juice	45 mL
2	kiwis, peeled and chopped	2
1/4 cup	seedless green grapes	50 mL
1/4 cup	lime sherbet	50 mL

In blender, combine orange juice, lime juice, kiwis, grapes and sherbet. Process as directed until smooth.

SERVES 1 OR 2

Fruit Smoothies

Tropics

1/2 cup	coconut milk	125 mL
2	kiwis, peeled and chopped	2
Half	papaya, peeled, seeded and chopped	Half
1	ripe banana, peeled and chopped	1
1/2 cup	pineapple chunks	125 mL

In blender, combine coconut milk, kiwis, papaya, banana and pineapple. Process as directed until smooth.

SERVES 2

TIP
Use canned coconut milk or homemade Coconut Milk (recipe, page 250) in this smoothie.

Breakfast Cocktail

1/2 cup	carrot juice	125 mL
1	mango, peeled, pitted and chopped	1
1	papaya, peeled, seeded and chopped	1
1	apple, peeled, cored and chopped	1
1	piece (1/2 inch/1 cm long) gingerroot, peeled and chopped	1
1/4 cup	plain yogurt	50 mL

In blender, combine carrot juice, mango, papaya, apple, gingerroot and yogurt. Process as directed until smooth.

SERVES 3

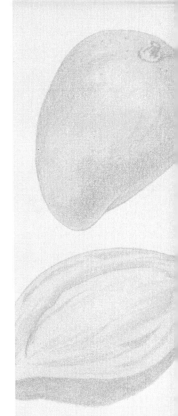

Mango Madness

1/2 cup	orange juice	125 mL
1	mango, peeled, pitted and chopped	1
1	ripe banana, peeled and chopped	1
1 cup	seedless green grapes, halved	250 mL
1	piece (1/4 inch/0.5 cm) gingerroot, peeled and chopped	1

In blender, combine orange juice, mango, banana, grapes and gingerroot. Process as directed until smooth.

SERVES 2 OR 3

Mango Mango

1/2 cup	mango or papaya nectar	125 mL
1	mango, peeled, pitted and chopped	1
1 cup	chopped seeded peeled watermelon	250 mL
1/2 cup	seedless red grapes	125 mL

In blender, combine mango nectar, chopped mango, watermelon and grapes. Process as directed until smooth.

SERVES 2

Mango Tango

1 cup	orange juice	250 mL
Half	mango, peeled, pitted and chopped	Half
1	wedge pineapple, peeled and chopped	1
1	slice (1 inch/2.5 cm thick) watermelon, peeled, seeded and chopped	1
1	slice (1/2 inch/1 cm thick) papaya, peeled, seeded and chopped	1
5	frozen strawberries	5

In blender, combine orange juice, mango, pineapple, watermelon, papaya and strawberries. Process as directed until smooth.

SERVES 3 OR 4

Fruit Smoothies

Tropi-Cocktail

1/4 cup	apricot nectar or orange juice	50 mL
1/2 cup	plain yogurt	125 mL
Quarter	cantaloupe or honeydew melon, peeled, seeded and chopped	Quarter
Half	mango, peeled, pitted and chopped	Half
1	slice (1/2 inch/1 cm thick) papaya, peeled, seeded and chopped	1
1	ripe banana, peeled and chopped	1

In blender, combine apricot nectar, yogurt, cantaloupe, mango, papaya and banana. Process as directed until smooth.

SERVES 2

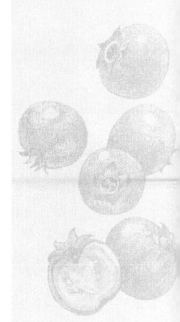

Berry Best

1/2 cup	raspberry juice	125 mL
1/2 cup	blueberries	125 mL
1/2 cup	pitted cherries	125 mL
1/2 cup	seedless grapes	125 mL
Quarter	cantaloupe, peeled, seeded and chopped	Quarter

In blender, combine raspberry juice, blueberries, cherries, grapes and cantaloupe. Process as directed until smooth.

SERVES 2

Beta Blast

1/2 cup	orange juice	125 mL
1/4 cup	carrot juice	50 mL
Half	cantaloupe, peeled, seeded and chopped	Half
1/4 cup	chopped apricots	50 mL
1/4 cup	silken tofu (optional)	50 mL

In blender, combine orange juice, carrot juice, cantaloupe, apricots, and tofu (if using). Process as directed until smooth.

SERVES 1 OR 2

Mega Melon Supreme

½ cup	orange juice or Apricot Milk (recipe, page 247)	125 mL
½ cup	chopped seeded peeled watermelon	125 mL
½ cup	chopped seeded peeled cantaloupe	125 mL
½ cup	chopped seeded peeled honeydew melon	125 mL
½ cup	vanilla-flavored frozen yogurt	125 mL

In blender, combine orange juice, watermelon, cantaloupe, honeydew and frozen yogurt. Process as directed until smooth.

SERVES 4

Melon Morning Cocktail

½ cup	orange juice	125 mL
1 cup	chopped seeded peeled watermelon	50 mL
Quarter	cantaloupe, peeled, seeded and chopped	Quarter
1	orange, peeled, seeded and chopped	1
1	wedge pineapple, peeled and chopped	1

In blender, combine orange juice, watermelon, cantaloupe, orange and pineapple. Process as directed until smooth.

SERVES 4

Green Goddess

TIP
You can substitute canteloupe for the musk melon in this recipe and the result will be a Goddess, just not a green one.

⅓ cup	kiwi or grapefruit juice	75 mL
	Juice of 1 lime	
Quarter	musk melon, peeled, seeded and chopped	Quarter
2	kiwis, peeled and chopped	2
½ cup	chopped peeled ripe banana	125 mL
1 tbsp	chopped fresh peppermint leaves	15 mL

In blender, combine kiwi juice, lime juice, melon, kiwis, banana and peppermint. Process as directed until smooth.

SERVES 4

Fruit Smoothies

Nectar of the Gods

1/2 cup	peach or apricot nectar or pineapple juice	125 mL
1 tbsp	lemon juice	15 mL
2	nectarines, peeled, pitted and chopped	2
2	peaches, peeled, pitted and chopped	2
1/2 cup	sparkling mineral water or soda water	125 mL

In blender, combine peach nectar, lemon juice, nectarines and peaches. Process as directed until smooth. Divide among glasses; divide mineral water evenly among glasses. Stir to combine.

SERVES 2 OR 3

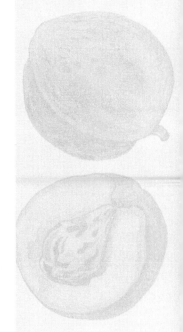

Nectarine on Ice

1/4 cup	frozen orange juice concentrate	50 mL
1/2 cup	water	125 mL
4	ice cubes	4
2	nectarines, peeled, pitted and chopped	2
2	apricots, peeled, pitted and chopped	2

In blender, combine orange juice concentrate, water, ice, nectarines and apricots. Process as directed until smooth.

SERVES 3

Nectarlicious

1 cup	orange juice	250 mL
2	nectarines, peeled, pitted and chopped	2
1/4 cup	blackberries	50 mL
1/4 cup	raspberries	50 mL

In blender, combine orange juice, nectarines, blackberries and raspberries. Process as directed until smooth.

SERVES 3

Orange Aid

3/4 cup	orange juice	175 mL
2 tsp	lemon juice	10 mL
2	nectarines, peeled, pitted and chopped	2
1	orange, peeled, seeded and chopped	1
1	wedge cantaloupe, peeled, seeded and chopped	1

In blender, combine orange juice, lemon juice, nectarines, orange and cantaloupe. Process as directed until smooth.

SERVES 3

Fruity Twist

3/4 cup	orange juice	175 mL
1	wedge pineapple, peeled and chopped	1
1	slice watermelon, peeled, seeded and chopped	1
Quarter	mango, peeled, pitted and chopped	Quarter
1/2 cup	chopped seeded peeled papaya	125 mL
1	ripe banana, peeled and chopped	1

In blender, combine orange juice, pineapple, watermelon, mango, papaya and banana. Process as directed until smooth.

SERVES 4

Papaya Passion

1/2 cup	orange juice	125 mL
1/4 cup	carrot juice	50 mL
1	wedge pineapple, peeled and chopped	1
1/2 cup	chopped seeded peeled papaya	125 mL

In blender, combine orange juice, carrot juice, pineapple and papaya. Process as directed until smooth.

SERVES 2

Hawaiian Silk

½ cup	coconut milk	125 mL
¼ cup	pineapple juice	50 mL
1 cup	chopped seeded peeled papaya	250 mL
1	wedge pineapple, peeled and chopped	1

In blender, combine coconut milk, pineapple juice, papaya and pineapple. Process as directed until smooth.

SERVES 2

TIP
Use canned coconut milk or homemade Coconut Milk (recipe, page 250) in this smoothie.

Taste of the Tropics

½ cup	orange juice	125 mL
	Juice of 1 lime	
Half	papaya, peeled, seeded and chopped	Half
1	wedge pineapple, peeled and chopped	1
1 tbsp	chopped fresh peppermint leaves	15 mL

In blender, combine orange juice, lime juice, papaya, pineapple and peppermint. Process as directed until smooth.

SERVES 4

Minty Peach

½ cup	peach or apricot nectar	125 mL
¼ cup	plain yogurt	50 mL
2 tbsp	lemon juice	25 mL
1 cup	frozen sliced peaches	250 mL
1	wedge honeydew melon, peeled, seeded and chopped	1
1 tbsp	chopped fresh peppermint leaves	15 mL

In blender, combine peach nectar, yogurt, lemon juice, peaches, melon and peppermint. Process as directed until smooth.

SERVES 2 OR 3

TIP
You can use fresh and frozen fruit interchangeably in most smoothies, although the results will differ. Frozen fruit not only chills a smoothie, it thickens it as well.

Peach Bliss

½ cup	grapefruit juice	125 mL
1 cup	frozen sliced peaches	250 mL
¼ cup	frozen raspberries	50 mL
¼ cup	chopped dried peaches or chopped mixed dried fruit	50 mL

In blender, combine grapefruit juice, sliced peaches, raspberries and dried peaches. Process as directed until smooth.

SERVES 2

Peach Cobbler

TIP
You can use fresh and frozen fruit interchangeably in most smoothies, although the results will differ. Frozen fruit not only chills a smoothie, it thickens it as well.

1	can (14 oz/398 mL) halved or sliced peaches in juice	1
4	ice cubes	4
½ cup	evaporated milk or Almond Milk (recipe, page 248)	125 mL
¼ cup	peach-flavored yogurt	50 mL
2	apricots, peeled, pitted and chopped	2
⅓ cup	peach sherbet	75 mL
Pinch	ground nutmeg	Pinch

In blender, combine peaches with juice, ice, evaporated milk, yogurt, apricots, sherbet and nutmeg. Process as directed until smooth.

SERVES 4

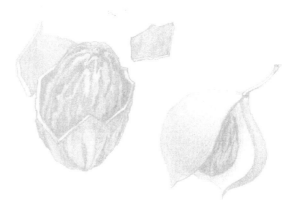

Peach Paradise

1/2 cup	evaporated milk	125 mL
1/4 cup	blueberries	50 mL
2	peaches, peeled, pitted and chopped	2
3 tbsp	plain or peach-flavored yogurt	45 mL
2 tbsp	chopped almonds	25 mL
1/4 tsp	ground cinnamon	1 mL

In blender, combine evaporated milk, blueberries, peaches, yogurt, almonds and cinnamon. Process as directed until smooth.

SERVES 3 OR 4

General Directions
Always place the lid securely on the blender before processing. Blend on Low for 30 seconds. Gradually (if possible) increase speed to High and blend an additional 30 seconds or until smooth.

Peaches and Cream

1	can (14 oz/398 mL) halved or sliced peaches, drained	1
1/2 cup	evaporated milk	125 mL
1/2 cup	frozen sliced peaches	125 mL
1/4 cup	silken tofu	50 mL
1/4 tsp	almond extract	1 mL

In blender, combine drained canned peaches, evaporated milk, frozen peaches, tofu and almond extract. Process as directed until smooth.

SERVES 3 OR 4

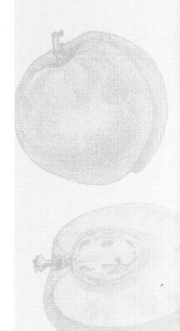

Peachy Melon

1/2 cup	peach nectar	125 mL
1/4 cup	orange juice or mango nectar	50 mL
2	peaches, peeled, pitted and chopped	2
2	apricots, peeled, pitted and chopped	2
1/2 cup	chopped pitted peeled mango	125 mL
Quarter	cantaloupe, peeled, seeded and chopped	Quarter

In blender, combine peach nectar, orange juice, peaches, apricots, mango and cantaloupe. Process as directed until smooth.

SERVES 3 OR 4

Apple Pear

1	can (14 oz/398 mL) pears in juice	1
1 tbsp	lemon juice	15 mL
1/4 cup	applesauce	50 mL
1	apple, peeled, cored and chopped	1
1/2 cup	seedless red or green grapes	125 mL

In blender, combine pears with juice, lemon juice, applesauce, apple and grapes. Process as directed until smooth.

SERVES 3 OR 4

Autumn Refresher

1/4 cup	orange juice	50 mL
3 tbsp	lime juice	45 mL
2	pears, peeled, cored and chopped	2
1	peach, peeled, pitted and chopped	1
1	apple, peeled, cored and chopped	1

In blender, combine orange juice, lime juice, pears, peach and apple. Process as directed until smooth.

SERVES 3

Pear Fennel

1/2 cup	pear nectar or apple juice	125 mL
1/4 cup	applesauce	50 mL
2	pears, peeled, cored and chopped	2
1	ripe banana, peeled and chopped	1
1/2 cup	chopped fresh fennel	125 mL
1/4 tsp	ground licorice* (optional)	1 mL

In blender, combine pear nectar, applesauce, pears, banana, fennel, and licorice (if using). Process as directed until smooth.

SERVES 3

Pear Pineapple

¼ cup	grapefruit juice	50 mL
	Juice of 1 lemon	
1	wedge pineapple, peeled and chopped	1
1	pear, peeled, cored and chopped	1
½ cup	seedless red or green grapes	125 mL

In blender, combine grapefruit juice, lemon juice, pineapple, pear and grapes. Process as directed until smooth.

SERVES 2 OR 3

Pear Raspberry

¼ cup	raspberry juice	50 mL
2 tbsp	lemon juice	25 mL
2	pears, peeled, cored and chopped	2
1 cup	raspberries	250 mL
¼ cup	vanilla-flavored frozen yogurt	50 mL

In blender, combine raspberry juice, lemon juice, pears, raspberries and frozen yogurt. Process as directed until smooth.

SERVES 3 OR 4

Liquid Gold

½ cup	orange juice	125 mL
3 tbsp	lemon juice	45 mL
2	apricots, peeled, pitted and chopped	2
2	peaches, peeled, pitted and chopped	2
1	wedge pineapple, peeled and chopped	1
Half	mango, peeled, pitted and chopped	Half
Half	ripe banana, peeled and chopped	Half

In blender, combine orange juice, lemon juice, apricots, peaches, pineapple, mango and banana. Process as directed until smooth.

SERVES 4

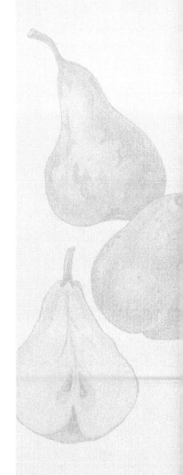

Fruit Smoothies

Pine-Berry

TIP
The sweetness
of this smoothie
will increase
significantly if you
use sweetened
frozen yogurt rather
than plain yogurt.

1	can (14 oz/398 mL) cherries in juice	1
1/4 cup	plain or frozen yogurt	50 mL
2	wedges pineapple, peeled and chopped	2
1 cup	blueberries	250 mL
1/2 cup	black currants	125 mL

In blender, combine cherries with juice, yogurt, pineapple, blueberries and black currants. Process as directed until smooth.

SERVES 4

Pineapple Citrus

1/4 cup	pineapple juice	50 mL
1/4 cup	orange juice	50 mL
	Juice of 1 lemon	
1	orange, peeled, seeded and chopped	1
1	wedge pineapple, peeled and chopped	1
1 tbsp	chopped fresh peppermint leaves	15 mL

In blender, combine pineapple juice, orange juice, lemon juice, orange, pineapple and peppermint. Process as directed until smooth.

SERVES 3

Pineapple Soy

TIP
Try using
homemade frozen
yogurt (see recipes,
pages 292 and 293)
in this smoothie.

1/4 cup	pineapple juice	50 mL
1/4 cup	plain soy milk	50 mL
1	ripe banana, peeled and chopped	1
2	wedges pineapple, peeled and chopped	2
1/2 cup	plain yogurt or fruit-flavored frozen yogurt	125 mL

In blender, combine pineapple juice, soy milk, banana, pineapple and yogurt. Process as directed until smooth.

SERVES 1 OR 2

Fruit Smoothies

B-Vitamin

1/2 cup	pineapple juice	125 mL
1/4 cup	plain soy milk	50 mL
1 cup	chopped peeled pineapple	250 mL
1/4 cup	chopped pitted peeled apricots	50 mL
1	ripe banana, peeled and chopped	1
1 tbsp	wheat germ	15 mL
2 tsp	flax seeds	10 mL
1 tsp	cod liver or hemp oil	5 mL

In blender, combine pineapple juice, soy milk, pineapple, apricots, banana, wheat germ, flax seeds and oil. Process as directed until smooth.

SERVES 4

General Directions
Always place the lid securely on the blender before processing. Blend on Low for 30 seconds. Gradually (if possible) increase speed to High and blend an additional 30 seconds or until smooth.

Plum Berry

3/4 cup	raspberry juice	175 mL
1/4 cup	black currant or raspberry jam	50 mL
2	plums, peeled, pitted and chopped	2
1 cup	raspberries	250 mL

In blender, combine raspberry juice, jam, plums and raspberries. Process as directed until smooth.

SERVES 3 OR 4

Plum Lico

* Avoid licorice if you have high blood pressure. The prolonged use of licorice is not recommended under any circumstances.

¼ cup	pineapple juice	50 mL
¼ cup	plain yogurt	50 mL
2	plums, peeled, pitted and chopped	2
1 cup	pitted cherries	250 mL
Half	grapefruit, peeled, seeded and chopped	Half
¼ tsp	ground licorice* (optional)	1 mL

In blender, combine pineapple juice, yogurt, plums, cherries, grapefruit, and licorice (if using). Process as directed until smooth.

SERVES 3 OR 4

Plums Up

¾ cup	orange juice	175 mL
2 tbsp	lemon juice	25 mL
2	plums, peeled, pitted and chopped	2
1	wedge pineapple, peeled and chopped	1
Quarter	cantaloupe, peeled, seeded and chopped	Quarter

In blender, combine orange juice, lemon juice, plums, pineapple and cantaloupe. Process as directed until smooth.

SERVES 3

Prune

1 cup	plain soy milk	250 mL
¼ cup	pitted prunes, chopped	50 mL
1	ripe banana, peeled and chopped	1

In blender, combine soy milk, prunes and banana. Process as directed until smooth.

SERVES 1 OR 2

TIP

Although many of these recipes call for plain soy milk, some flavored soy milks work equally well in fruit smoothies. Feel free to substitute your favorite flavor.

Berry Fine Cocktail

²/₃ cup	pineapple juice	150 mL
1 cup	raspberries	250 mL
12	strawberries (hulled and halved if fresh)	12
¼ cup	cranberries	50 mL
4	ice cubes	4

In blender, combine pineapple juice, raspberries, strawberries, cranberries and ice cubes. Process as directed until smooth.

SERVES 4

Raspberry

½ cup	orange juice	125 mL
1 cup	raspberries	250 mL
2	apricots, peeled, pitted and chopped	2
1	peach, peeled, pitted and chopped	1
¼ cup	plain yogurt	50 mL

In blender, combine orange juice, raspberries, apricots, peach and yogurt. Process as directed until smooth.

SERVES 4

Real Raspberry

½ cup	cranberry-raspberry juice	125 mL
1 cup	raspberries	250 mL
½ cup	pitted cherries	125 mL
½ cup	blueberries	125 mL
¼ cup	raspberry-flavored frozen yogurt	50 mL

In blender, combine cranberry-raspberry juice, raspberries, cherries, blueberries and frozen yogurt. Process as directed until smooth.

SERVES 2

TIP
Strawberries and raspberries vary in sweetness, depending upon the variety and/or growing conditions. Pineapple juice is a natural sweetener, but after blending taste for yourself and add honey, in 1-tsp (5 mL) increments, until this drink is sweet enough for you.

General Directions
Always place the lid securely on the blender before processing. Blend on Low for 30 seconds. Gradually (if possible) increase speed to High and blend an additional 30 seconds or until smooth.

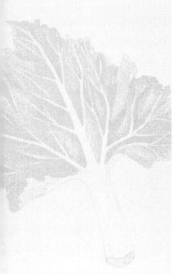

Razzy Orange

½ cup	orange juice	125 mL
½ cup	frozen raspberries	125 mL
1	orange, peeled, seeded and chopped	1
¼ cup	raspberry- or orange-flavored yogurt	50 mL

In blender, combine orange juice, raspberries, orange and yogurt. Process as directed until smooth.

SERVES 2 OR 3

Rhubarb Pineapple

½ cup	pineapple juice	125 mL
¼ cup	chopped fresh rhubarb	50 mL
1	wedge pineapple, peeled and chopped	1
1	peach, peeled, pitted and chopped	1

In blender, combine pineapple juice, rhubarb, pineapple and peach. Process as directed until smooth.

SERVES 3

Rhubarb Apple

TIP
See page 133
for how to
cook rhubarb.

¼ cup	apple juice	50 mL
½ cup	applesauce	125 mL
½ cup	canned or cooked rhubarb	125 mL
1	apple, peeled, cored and chopped	1

In blender, combine apple juice, applesauce, rhubarb and chopped apple. Process as directed until smooth.

SERVES 2

Best Berries

¾ cup	pineapple juice	175 mL
2 tbsp	lemon juice	25 mL
3 tbsp	plain or frozen yogurt	45 mL
12	strawberries (hulled and halved if fresh)	12
1	ripe banana, peeled and chopped	1

In blender, combine pineapple juice, lemon juice, yogurt, strawberries and banana. Process as directed until smooth.

SERVES 3

Pineapple-C

½ cup	orange or pineapple juice	125 mL
	Juice of 1 lime	
2 tbsp	lemon juice	25 mL
12	strawberries (hulled and halved if fresh)	12
1	wedge pineapple, peeled and chopped	1

In blender, combine orange juice, lime juice, lemon juice, strawberries and pineapple. Process as directed until smooth.

SERVES 3

Sea-Straw

½ cup	grapefruit juice	125 mL
6	strawberries (hulled and halved if fresh)	6
3 tbsp	chopped dried pitted dates	45 mL
1 tsp	crushed dried dulse	5 mL

In blender, combine grapefruit juice, strawberries, dates and dulse. Process as directed until smooth.

SERVES 2

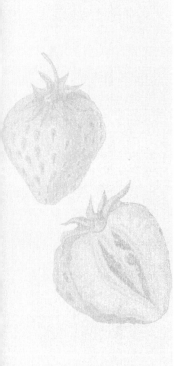

Strawberry Blush

1	can (14 oz/398 mL) diced beets	1
¼ cup	cranberry sauce	50 mL
½ cup	strawberries (hulled and halved if fresh)	125 mL
1 tbsp	chopped pitted dates	15 mL
6	ice cubes (see page 274)	6

In blender, combine beets with liquid, cranberry sauce, strawberries, dates and ice cubes. Process as directed until smooth.

SERVES 2

Strawberry Swirl

½ cup	cranberry-raspberry juice	125 mL
2 tbsp	lemon juice	25 mL
10	frozen strawberries	10
¼ cup	frozen raspberries	50 mL
2 tbsp	plain yogurt	25 mL

In blender, combine cranberry-raspberry juice, lemon juice, strawberries, raspberries and yogurt. Process as directed until smooth.

SERVES 3 OR 4

Perfect in Pink

¼ cup	cranberry juice	50 mL
1 tbsp	lemon juice	15 mL
1 cup	chopped seeded peeled watermelon	250 mL
½ cup	pitted cherries	125 mL
¼ cup	frozen raspberries	50 mL

In blender, combine cranberry juice, lemon juice, watermelon, cherries and raspberries. Process as directed until smooth.

SERVES 3

TIP
You can use fresh and frozen fruit interchangeably in most smoothies, although the results will differ. Frozen fruit not only chills a smoothie, it thickens it as well.

Fruit Smoothies

Watermelon

¼ cup	orange juice	50 mL
1 tbsp	lemon juice	15 mL
1 cup	chopped seeded peeled watermelon	250 mL
2	plums, peeled, pitted and chopped	2
⅓ cup	plain yogurt	75 mL

In blender, combine orange juice, lemon juice, watermelon, plums and yogurt. Process as directed until smooth.

SERVES 2 OR 3

Watermelon-Strawberry Splash

½ cup	raspberry or cranberry juice	125 mL
2 tbsp	lemon juice	25 mL
1 cup	chopped seeded peeled watermelon	250 mL
6	frozen strawberries	6

In blender, combine raspberry juice, lemon juice, watermelon and strawberries. Process as directed until smooth.

SERVES 2 OR 3

Watermelon Wave

¼ cup	orange juice	50 mL
1 tbsp	lime juice	15 mL
1 cup	chopped seeded peeled watermelon	250 mL
2	nectarines, peeled, pitted and chopped	2

In blender, combine orange juice, lime juice, watermelon and nectarines. Process as directed until smooth.

SERVES 1 OR 2

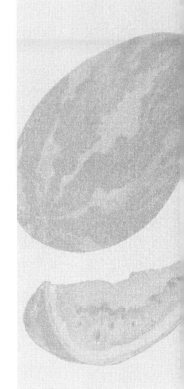

Fruit Smoothies

Vegetable Smoothies

WITH AN ALMOST OVERWHELMING VARIETY OF FRESH PRODUCE available in supermarkets year-round, adding vegetable smoothies to your diet — as a lunchtime beverage, a midafternoon pick-me-up or a predinner cocktail or appetizer — is one way of ensuring that you consume enough fresh vegetables to promote good health.

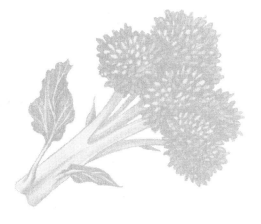

Fresh Organic Is Best

Fresh vegetables are packed with healthful vitamins, minerals and phytochemicals and, like fruits, are best eaten raw as soon after harvesting as possible. When you purchase organic fruits and vegetables, you support a sustainable system of soil regeneration that is important to our future food supply while reducing your exposure to toxins. To keep nutrient levels from diminishing, store fresh vegetables properly: they will stay fresh in the crisper drawer of your refrigerator for a few days to just over one week. Large quantities of fresh vegetables may be stored for longer in a root cellar.

THE RAW AND THE COOKED

Because cooking destroys some nutrients, try smoothies made with milder-tasting raw vegetables, such as celery, carrots, cucumbers, eggplants or zucchini first. Then try stronger-tasting raw vegetables, such as cauliflower, peas or broccoli. If you find their flavor too strong, you will know that you want to cook these vegetables before or after blending. Cooking softens both the taste and the texture of vegetables. Some vegetables, especially hard root vegetables — such as beets, potatoes and parsnips — must be cooked before you can use them in smoothies, because they cannot be liquefied in their raw state by ordinary blenders.

Cooking fresh vegetables: Broccoli, carrots, cauliflower, peas and beans may be parboiled (cooked for one to three minutes in boiling water) before adding to smoothies. Denser vegetables, such as beets, potatoes or parsnips, require a longer cooking time, five to seven minutes or until soft. Roasting vegetables before using them in smoothies adds a rich, sweet taste (see Roasted Eggplant, page 209). Alternatively, after blending, raw vegetable smoothies can be simmered on top of the stove for seven to 12 minutes or until the vegetables are tender. For convenience, save leftover cooked vegetables for use in smoothies.

Using Frozen Vegetables

Frozen vegetables are convenient for smoothies because, in addition to being consistently available, they save cooking time and are easy to measure. Add up to 1 cup (250 mL) cooked frozen vegetables to smoothie recipes.

To freeze fresh vegetables: Peel (if not organic), trim off stems and woody parts and cut into pieces or chunks. Drop vegetable pieces into a large pot of boiling water and return to a simmer (just under a full boil). Cook for one to two minutes or until the vegetables are tender-crisp. Remove from the water, transfer to a colander and rinse under cold running water until cool. Pat dry and arrange in a single layer on a baking sheet and freeze for one to two hours or until hard. Transfer to a resealable plastic freezer bag, then seal and label. Frozen vegetables will keep for up to six months in the freezer.

Canned Vegetables

When fresh vegetables are not in season, keep a variety of canned vegetables on hand for use in smoothies. Their nutrient value is comparable to that of cooked fresh vegetables. Unsalted water-packed organic vegetables, which are available in natural-food stores, are preferable.

Substituting canned and fresh vegetables: In all vegetable smoothie recipes, canned and fresh vegetables may be used interchangeably. Use one 14-oz (398 mL) can for each 1 cup (250 mL) of sliced or chopped fresh vegetables. Use the liquid in the can as well, and reduce the amount of liquid in the recipe by $1/4$ cup (50 mL). Alternatively, substitute 1 cup (250 mL) sliced or chopped cooked fresh vegetables for each 14-oz (398 mL) can of vegetables. Increase the liquid in the recipe by $1/4$ cup (50 mL).

Liquids for Vegetable Smoothies

- *Vegetable juices:* Tomato, carrot and beet are the most commonly used vegetable juices in smoothies. As with fruit juices, the best vegetable juices are made from fresh organic vegetables and should be consumed immediately. When it is not possible to make your own fresh vegetable juice, commercially made organic juice with no additives is the next best choice. Avoid monosodium glutamate (MSG), sugar and other unwanted additives in commercially prepared vegetable juices and cocktails.

- *Other liquids:* Homemade vegetable stock, meat broth and miso soup work well in smoothies, because no unwanted ingredients are added. Canned spaghetti sauce, clams, consommé or liquid soup bases may replace vegetable juices in vegetable smoothie recipes, but look for low-sodium products that contain no additives. Herbal teas (parsley, dandelion, burdock and others) may also be used in vegetable smoothies (see page 221 for how to use medicinal herbal teas in smoothies). Fruit and nut milks (see pages 247 to 250) give extra texture, flavor and/or sweetness to vegetable smoothies.

General Directions

Always place the lid securely on the blender before processing. Blend on Low for 30 seconds. Gradually (if possible) increase speed to High and blend an additional 30 seconds or until smooth.

Spring Celebration

1/2 cup	beet juice	125 mL
1 cup	cooked chopped asparagus	250 mL
1/2 cup	cooked diced beets	125 mL
1/2 cup	chopped fresh or frozen spinach	125 mL
2 tbsp	chopped figs (peeled if fresh) or pitted dates	25 mL
1 tsp	maple syrup or sap (optional)	5 mL

In blender, combine beet juice, asparagus, beets, spinach, dates, and maple syrup (if using). Process as directed until smooth.

SERVES 3

TIP

Substitute one 12-oz (375 mL) can asparagus tips or spears with liquid for the cooked chopped asparagus when fresh is not in season. Reduce beet juice to 1/4 cup (50 mL) if using canned asparagus.

Avocado Orange

1/2 cup	orange juice	125 mL
2 tbsp	lemon juice	25 mL
1	orange, peeled, seeded and chopped	1
4	figs (peeled if fresh), chopped	4
Half	avocado, peeled, pitted and chopped	Half
Half	frozen ripe banana, peeled and chopped	Half

In blender, combine orange juice, lemon juice, orange, figs, avocado and banana. Process as directed until smooth.

SERVES 2 OR 3

Avocado Pineapple

3/4 cup	raspberry juice	175 mL
1 cup	chopped peeled pineapple	250 mL
1	avocado, peeled, pitted and chopped	1

In blender, combine raspberry juice, pineapple and avocado. Process as directed until smooth.

SERVES 1

Creamy Chickpea

1 cup	chicken or vegetable broth	250 mL
½ cup	chopped or mashed cooked potato	125 mL
⅓ cup	cooked chickpeas	75 mL
1 tbsp	chopped onion	15 mL
Quarter	clove garlic, peeled	Quarter
1	sprig parsley*, chopped	1
¼ cup	half-and-half (10%) cream or milk	50 mL
¼ tsp	salt (or to taste)	1 mL

1. In a small saucepan over high heat, bring stock to a boil; pour half into blender. Reduce heat to low; keep remaining stock warm. Add potato, chickpeas, onion, garlic and parsley to blender. Cover with lid and blend on Low for 30 seconds.

2. With blender still running, add remaining hot stock through opening in center of lid. Replace center cover and increase speed to High; blend for another 30 seconds or until smooth. Add cream through opening in center of lid and blend just until combined. Season with salt. Serve hot or cold.

SERVES 4

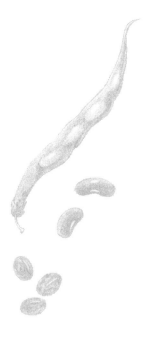

General Directions
Always place the lid securely on the blender before processing. Blend on Low for 30 seconds. Gradually (if possible) increase speed to High and blend an additional 30 seconds or until smooth.

Vegetable Smoothies

Lima Curry

1 cup	milk or table (18%) cream	250 mL
1	can (14 oz/398 mL) lima beans	1
1 tbsp	chopped onion	15 mL
1 tbsp	chopped fresh parsley*	15 mL
2 tsp	blackstrap molasses or maple syrup (optional)	10 mL
1/2 tsp	curry powder	2 mL
1/4 tsp	ground turmeric	1 mL
1/4 tsp	salt (or to taste)	1 mL

1. In a small saucepan over medium heat, bring milk just to a boil; reduce heat to low and keep warm. In blender, combine lima beans with liquid, onion, parsley, molasses (if using), curry powder and turmeric. Blend on Low for 1 minute.

2. With blender still running, add hot milk through opening in center of lid. Replace center cover and increase speed to High; blend for another 30 seconds or until smooth. Season with salt. Serve hot or cold.

SERVES 3 OR 4

TIP
Substitute 1 cup (250 mL) chopped cooked lima beans for the canned. Increase the milk by 1/4 cup (50 mL).

Peas Please

1	can (14 oz/398 mL) green peas or sliced green beans	1
1/2 cup	cooked chopped carrots	125 mL
1/4 cup	chopped fresh fennel	50 mL
1/4 cup	applesauce	50 mL

In blender, combine peas with liquid, carrots, fennel and applesauce. Process as directed until smooth.

SERVES 3 OR 4

TIP
You can substitute 1 cup (250 mL) cooked frozen or fresh green peas or sliced green beans for the canned. Add 1/2 cup (125 mL) chicken or vegetable broth to the recipe.

Pease Porridge

* If you are pregnant, limit your intake of parsley to ½ tsp (2 mL) dried or one sprig fresh per day. Do not take parsley if you are suffering from kidney inflammation.

1 cup	vegetable or chicken stock	250 mL
1 cup	fresh or frozen peas	250 mL
1	small potato, peeled and chopped	1
1	stalk celery, chopped	1
1	carrot, chopped	1
½ cup	chopped fresh or frozen spinach	125 mL
3 tbsp	steel-cut or rolled oats	45 mL
¼ cup	table (18%) cream or milk	50 mL
1 tbsp	chopped fresh parsley*	15 mL
¼ tsp	salt (or to taste)	1 mL

1. In a medium saucepan over medium heat, bring stock, peas, potato, celery and carrot just to a boil. Cover, reduce heat to low and simmer for 10 minutes. Stir in spinach and oats; simmer for another 4 to 7 minutes or until vegetables are tender. Pour into blender; blend on Low for 1 minute.

2. With blender still running, add cream and parsley through opening in center of lid. Replace center cover and increase speed to High; blend for another 10 seconds or until smooth. Season with salt. Serve hot or cold with a spoon.

SERVES 4

Apple Beet Pear

TIP
Substitute 1 cup (250 mL) cooked chopped beets for the canned. Increase apple juice by ¼ cup (50 mL).

1	can (14 oz/398 mL) diced beets	1
1 tbsp	lemon juice	15 mL
¼ cup	apple juice	50 mL
1	pear, peeled, cored and chopped	1
1	apple, peeled, cored and chopped	1
1 tsp	chopped fresh savory leaves	5 mL

In blender, combine beets with liquid, lemon juice, apple juice, pear, apple and savory. Process as directed until smooth.

SERVES 3 OR 4

Vegetable Smoothies

Beet

½ cup	beet or carrot juice	125 mL
¾ cup	cooked chopped beets	175 mL
½ cup	cooked chopped carrots	125 mL
½ cup	vegetable or chicken stock	125 mL
¼ tsp	salt (or to taste)	1 mL

In blender, combine beet juice, beets, carrots and stock. Process as directed until smooth. Season with salt.

SERVES 2 OR 3

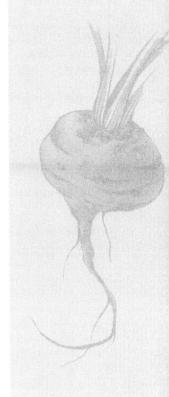

Blazing Beets

1	can (14 oz/398 mL) beets	1
½ cup	apple juice	125 mL
2	apples, peeled, cored and chopped	2
2	stalks celery, chopped	2
1	piece (½ inch/1 cm) gingerroot, peeled and chopped	1
Half	fresh chile pepper, chopped	Half
1	clove garlic, peeled and halved	1

In blender, combine beets with liquid, apple juice, apples, celery, gingerroot, chile pepper and garlic. Process as directed until smooth.

SERVES 3 OR 4

Clam Beet

1	can (10 oz/284 mL) clams (minced or whole)	1
1	can (14 oz/398 mL) diced beets	1
1	stalk celery, chopped	1
1 tbsp	chopped onion	15 mL
2 to 4	dashes hot pepper sauce (optional)	2 to 4

In blender, combine clams with juice, beets with liquid, celery and onion. Process as directed until smooth. Season with hot pepper sauce (if using).

SERVES 3 OR 4

TIP
Substitute 1 cup (250 mL) cooked chopped beets for the canned. Add ¼ cup (50 mL) vegetable or tomato juice.

Brocco-Carrot

½ cup	carrot juice	125 mL
1	can (14 oz/398 mL) spinach	1
½ cup	cooked chopped broccoli	125 mL
1	apple, peeled, cored and chopped	1
¼ tsp	salt (or to taste)	1 mL

In blender, combine carrot juice, spinach with liquid, broccoli and apple. Process as directed until smooth. Season with salt. Serve hot or cold with a spoon.

SERVES 1

TIP
Use 1 cup (250 mL) cooked or 2 cups (500 mL) well-washed uncooked fresh spinach in place of the canned. If desired, increase carrot juice until the desired consistency is achieved.

Cheesy Broccoli

1 cup	skim milk or plain soy milk	250 mL
Half	clove garlic, peeled and chopped	Half
1 cup	chopped cooked potato or cooked rice	250 mL
1 cup	cooked chopped broccoli	250 mL
⅓ cup	shredded Cheddar cheese	75 mL
¼ tsp	curry powder (optional)	1 mL
¼ tsp	ground turmeric	1 mL
¼ tsp	salt (or to taste)	1 mL

1. In a small saucepan over medium heat, bring milk just to a boil; pour half into blender. Keep remaining milk warm. Add garlic, potato, broccoli, cheese, curry powder (if using), and turmeric to blender. Cover with lid and blend on Low for 30 seconds.

2. With blender still running, add remaining hot milk through opening in center of lid. Replace center cover and increase speed to High; blend for another 30 seconds or until smooth. Season with salt. Serve hot or cold with a spoon.

SERVES 2

TIP
Taste and add up to double the amounts of curry and turmeric, if desired.

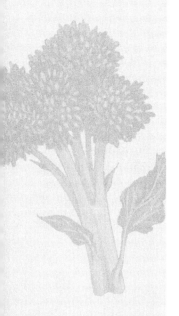

Cabbage Cocktail

1/2 cup	apple juice	125 mL
1/4 cup	carrot juice	50 mL
1 cup	shredded bok choy	250 mL
1	stalk celery, chopped	1
1	sprig parsley*, chopped	1
1 tsp	chopped fresh dill	5 mL
1/4 tsp	salt (or to taste)	1 mL

In blender, combine apple juice, carrot juice, bok choy, celery, parsley and dill. Process as directed until smooth. Season with salt.

SERVES 1 OR 2

General Directions
Always place the lid securely on the blender before processing. Blend on Low for 30 seconds. Gradually (if possible) increase speed to High and blend an additional 30 seconds or until smooth.

Minestrone

1 1/2 cups	vegetable or chicken stock, divided	375 mL
Half	clove garlic, peeled	Half
1	sprig parsley*, chopped	1
Half	onion, peeled and chopped	Half
2	stalks celery, chopped	2
1	carrot, chopped	1
2 tbsp	fresh oregano leaves	25 mL
1	tomato, cored and chopped	1
3/4 cup	sliced cabbage	175 mL
1/2 cup	cooked chickpeas (optional)	125 mL
1/4 tsp	salt (or to taste)	1 mL

* If you are pregnant, limit your intake of parsley to 1/2 tsp (2 mL) dried or one sprig fresh per day. Do not take parsley if you are suffering from kidney inflammation.

1. In blender, combine 1/2 cup (125 mL) stock, garlic, parsley, onion, celery and carrot. Cover with lid and blend on Low for 1 minute. Pour into saucepan; heat over medium heat until vegetables are soft.
2. Meanwhile, in blender, combine 1/2 cup (125 mL) vegetable stock, oregano, tomato and cabbage. Cover with lid and blend on Low for 1 minute. Remove lid and add chickpeas (if using); replace lid and blend on High (or Mix if your blender has that setting) for 1 to 2 minutes or until smooth. Add to saucepan. Bring to a boil; reduce heat to low and simmer for 2 to 3 minutes or until heated through.
3. Stir in enough of the remaining stock to make desired consistency. Season with salt. Serve hot or cold with a spoon.

SERVES 5 OR 6

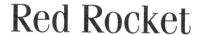

Red Rocket

¼ cup	apple juice	50 mL
¼ cup	cranberry juice	50 mL
1 tbsp	lemon juice	15 mL
½ cup	cooked chopped cabbage	125 mL
½ cup	cooked chopped beets	125 mL
1	stalk celery, chopped	1
1 tsp	chopped fresh thyme leaves	5 mL
1 tsp	rice vinegar	5 mL

In blender, combine apple juice, cranberry juice, lemon juice, cabbage, beets, celery, thyme and vinegar. Process as directed until smooth.

SERVES 1 OR 2

Carrot Raisin Cooler

¼ cup	orange juice	50 mL
½ cup	chopped carrots	125 mL
½ cup	plain yogurt	125 mL
¼ cup	raisins	50 mL
¼ tsp	ground nutmeg	1 mL
6	ice cubes (see page 274)	6

In blender, combine orange juice, carrots, yogurt, raisins, nutmeg and ice cubes. Process as directed until smooth.

SERVES 1 OR 2

Orange Zinger

½ cup	orange juice	125 mL
1 cup	cooked chopped carrots	250 mL
½ cup	seedless red grapes	125 mL
1	piece (½ inch/1 cm) gingerroot, peeled	1

In blender, combine orange juice, carrots, grapes and gingerroot. Process as directed until smooth.

SERVES 1

Vegetable Smoothies

Rustproofer #1

1/3 cup	carrot juice	75 mL
1 cup	cooked chopped carrots	250 mL
2	tomatoes, cored and chopped	2
1	sprig parsley*, chopped	1
1	apple, peeled, cored and chopped	1

In blender, combine carrot juice, carrots, tomatoes, parsley and apple. Process as directed until smooth.

SERVES 1 OR 2

Spiced Carrot

1/2 cup	apple juice	125 mL
1 cup	cooked chopped carrots	250 mL
1/4 cup	applesauce	50 mL
1	piece (1/2 inch/1 cm) gingerroot, peeled and chopped	1
1/4 tsp	ground cinnamon	1 mL
1/4 tsp	salt (or to taste)	1 mL
1/8 tsp	cayenne pepper (or to taste)	0.5 mL

In blender, combine apple juice, carrots, applesauce, gingerroot and cinnamon. Process as directed until smooth. Season with salt and cayenne.

SERVES 1

TIP
Substitute one 12-oz (375 mL) can diced carrots with liquid for the cooked fresh carrots and carrot juice.

* If you are pregnant, limit your intake of parsley to 1/2 tsp (2 mL) dried or one sprig fresh per day. Do not take parsley if you are suffering from kidney inflammation.

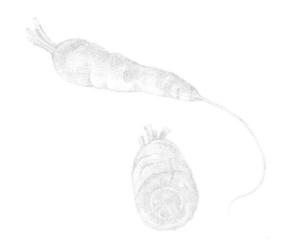

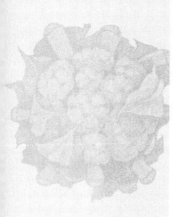

Cauliflower Cocktail

1 cup	carrot juice	250 mL
¼ cup	chopped parboiled cauliflower	50 mL
1	tomato, peeled, cored and chopped	1
½ cup	cooked chopped carrot	125 mL
1	stalk celery, chopped	1
1 tsp	flaked dried kelp	5 mL
¼ tsp	ground turmeric	1 mL

In blender, combine carrot juice, cauliflower, tomato, chopped carrot, celery, kelp and turmeric. Process as directed until smooth.

SERVES 2 OR 3

Herbed Cauliflower

1 cup	milk	250 mL
¾ cup	chopped cooked cauliflower	175 mL
Quarter	onion, peeled	Quarter
¼ cup	shredded Cheddar cheese	50 mL
2 tsp	chopped fresh oregano leaves	10 mL
1 tsp	chopped fresh thyme leaves	5 mL
¼ tsp	salt (or to taste)	1 mL

1. In a small saucepan over medium heat, bring milk just to a boil; pour ½ cup (125 mL) into blender. Reduce heat to low; keep remaining milk warm. Add cauliflower, onion, cheese, oregano and thyme to blender. Cover with lid and blend on Low for 30 seconds.
2. With blender still running, add remaining milk through opening in center of lid. Replace center cover and increase speed to High; blend for another 30 seconds or until smooth. Season with salt. Serve hot or cold.

SERVES 3 OR 4

Celery Cream

1/2 cup	plain soy milk	125 mL
1/4 cup	chopped celery	50 mL
1/4 cup	chopped fennel or celeriac (optional)	50 mL
1	tomato, peeled, cored and chopped	1
1/2 tsp	curry powder	2 mL
1/4 tsp	ground turmeric	1 mL
Pinch	ground cumin	Pinch

In blender, combine soy milk, celery, fennel, tomato, curry powder, turmeric and cumin. Process as directed until smooth.

SERVES 1

Cajun Cocktail

1/2 cup	tomato juice	125 mL
	Juice of 1 lime	
2	tomatoes, peeled, cored and chopped	2
1	small zucchini, peeled and chopped	1
1	clove garlic, peeled and halved	1
1	sprig parsley*, chopped	1
1	chile pepper, chopped	1
1/2 tsp	prepared horseradish	2 mL
1/4 tsp	dill seeds	1 mL

In blender, combine tomato juice, lime juice, tomatoes, zucchini, garlic, parsley, chile pepper, horseradish and dill seeds. Process as directed until smooth.

SERVES 1 OR 2

> ★ If you are pregnant, limit your intake of parsley to 1/2 tsp (2 mL) dried or one sprig fresh per day. Do not take parsley if you are suffering from kidney inflammation.

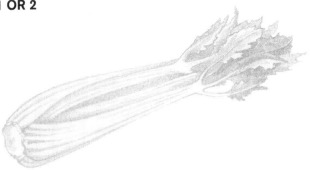

Corn Chowder

1 cup	chicken or vegetable stock	250 mL
1 cup	corn kernels	250 mL
1	small potato, peeled and chopped	1
2 tbsp	chopped onion	25 mL
1	sage leaf	1
1 tsp	fresh thyme leaves	5 mL
¼ cup	milk or table (18%) cream	50 mL
¼ tsp	salt (or to taste)	1 mL

1. In a medium saucepan over medium heat, bring stock, corn, potato, onion, sage and thyme just to a boil. Cover, reduce heat to low and simmer for 7 to 10 minutes or until vegetables are tender. Pour into blender and blend on Low for 30 seconds.

2. With blender still running, add milk through opening in center of lid. Replace center cover and increase speed to High; blend for another 30 seconds or until smooth. Season with salt. Serve hot or cold with a spoon.

SERVES 1 OR 2

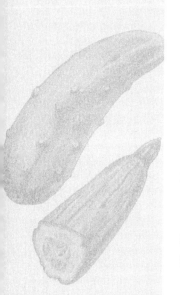

Flaming Antibiotic

½ cup	tomato juice	125 mL
2	tomatoes, peeled, cored and chopped	2
1	apple, peeled, cored and chopped	1
½ cup	cooked chopped carrots	125 mL
Half	cucumber, peeled and chopped	Half
Half	clove garlic, peeled	Half
1	chile pepper, chopped	1
2 tsp	fresh thyme leaves	10 mL

In blender, combine tomato juice, tomatoes, apple, carrots, cucumber, garlic, chile pepper and thyme. Process as directed until smooth.

SERVES 2 OR 3

Gazpacho

½ cup	tomato juice or spaghetti sauce	125 mL
2	tomatoes, peeled, cored and chopped	2
1	apple, peeled, cored and chopped	1
Half	cucumber, peeled and chopped	Half
1 tbsp	chopped onion	15 mL
Quarter	clove garlic, peeled	Quarter
2 tsp	chopped fresh cilantro	10 mL

In blender, combine tomato juice, tomatoes, apple, cucumber, onion, garlic and cilantro. Process as directed until smooth.

SERVES 2 OR 3

Roasted Eggplant

1	small eggplant, halved lengthwise	1
1	onion, peeled and quartered	1
2 tbsp	olive oil, divided	25 mL
1	clove garlic, peeled	1
2	peaches, peeled, pitted and halved	2
2	tomatoes, cored and halved	2
½ cup	spaghetti sauce	125 mL
¼ cup	apple juice	50 mL
1 tsp	chopped fresh oregano leaves	5 mL
½ tsp	salt (or to taste)	2 mL

TIPS
Italian plum, or paste, tomatoes stand up to broiling, so use that variety, if available, for this recipe.

Apples, plums, pears or nectarines may be substituted for the peaches.

1. On a lightly oiled baking sheet, arrange eggplant and onion, cut sides down, in a single layer. Drizzle with 1 tbsp (15 mL) olive oil. Broil for 12 minutes, rotating pan once to cook evenly.

2. Remove pan from oven. Turn eggplant and onions; arrange garlic, peaches and tomatoes, cut sides up, on pan. Drizzle with remaining olive oil. Broil, rotating pan once, for 7 to 10 minutes more or until vegetables are soft. Let cool enough to handle.

3. In blender, combine spaghetti sauce and apple juice. Scrape eggplant and tomato flesh into blender and discard skins. Add roasted garlic, peaches and onions and oregano. Cover with lid and blend on Low for 1 minute. Increase speed to High; blend for 1 minute more or until smooth. Season with salt. Serve warm or cold with a spoon.

SERVES 4 ● PREHEAT BROILER

TIP
Use canned coconut milk or homemade Coconut Milk (recipe, page 250) in this smoothie.

Creamy Fennel

1/2 cup	coconut milk	125 mL
1 cup	chopped fresh fennel	250 mL
1	apple, peeled, cored and chopped	1
1 tsp	fennel seeds	5 mL

In blender, combine coconut milk, chopped fennel, apple and fennel seeds. Process as directed until smooth.

SERVES 1 OR 2

Leafy Luxury

2/3 cup	orange or apple juice	150 mL
1 cup	chopped leafy greens (see page 140)	250 mL
1	apple, peeled, cored and chopped	1
1	pear, peeled, cored and chopped	1

In blender, combine orange juice, greens, apple and pear. Process as directed until smooth.

SERVES 1 OR 2

Garden Goodness

* If you are pregnant, limit your intake of parsley to 1/2 tsp (2 mL) dried or one sprig fresh per day. Do not take parsley if you are suffering from kidney inflammation.

3/4 cup	chopped cored fresh or canned tomatoes	175 mL
1 tbsp	lemon juice	15 mL
1/2 cup	chopped leafy greens (see page 140)	125 mL
1/4 cup	chopped carrots	50 mL
2 tbsp	chopped red or green bell pepper	25 mL
1	sprig parsley*, chopped	1
1 tbsp	raisins	15 mL
1 tsp	chopped onion	5 mL
1/4 tsp	celery seeds	1 mL
1 cup	ice cubes	250 mL

In blender, combine tomatoes, lemon juice, greens, carrots, pepper, parsley, raisins, onion, celery seeds and ice cubes. Process as directed until smooth.

SERVES 2

Vichyssoise

2 cups	vegetable stock	500 mL
1	potato, peeled and chopped	1
1	leek (white and light green parts only), chopped	1
2 tbsp	chopped onion	25 mL
1 tbsp	chopped fresh parsley*	15 mL
1/2 cup	milk, table (18%) cream or silken tofu	125 mL
	Salt and pepper to taste	

General Directions
Always place the lid securely on the blender before processing. Blend on Low for 30 seconds. Gradually (if possible) increase speed to High and blend an additional 30 seconds or until smooth.

1. In a small saucepan over high heat, bring stock to a boil. Add potato, leek and onion; reduce heat to low and simmer for 12 minutes or until vegetables are soft. Let cool.

2. Pour potato mixture into blender; add parsley. Cover with lid and blend on Low for 30 seconds.

3. With blender still running, add milk through opening in center of lid. Replace center cover and increase speed to High; blend for another 30 seconds to 1 minute or until smooth. Season with salt and pepper. Serve at room temperature or cold with a spoon.

SERVES 2 OR 3

Quick Vichyssoise

1/2 cup	vegetable stock	125 mL
1/2 cup	milk, table (18%) cream or silken tofu	125 mL
1	green onion, chopped	1
1/2 cup	cooked chopped potato	125 mL
1 tsp	chopped fresh parsley*	5 mL
	Salt and pepper to taste	

In blender, combine stock, milk, green onion, potato and parsley. Process as directed until smooth. Season with salt and pepper. Serve at room temperature or cold with a spoon.

SERVES 1

TIP
Vichyssoise is always served chilled, but this thick, smooth soup-drink is just as good right from the blender.

Creamed Onions

3/4 cup	milk	175 mL
2	onions, peeled and chopped	2
1	stalk celery, chopped	1
1	parsnip, chopped	1
1/4 cup	chopped fresh fennel	50 mL
1/4 tsp	ground star anise	1 mL
Pinch	ground nutmeg	Pinch

1. In a medium saucepan over medium heat, bring milk just to a boil. Add onions, celery, parsnip and fennel. Reduce heat to low and simmer for 12 minutes or until vegetables are soft.

2. Pour milk mixture into blender; add star anise and nutmeg. Process as directed until smooth. Thin with more milk, if desired. Serve hot or cold with a spoon.

SERVES 1 OR 2

Parsnip

2/3 cup	carrot or apple juice	150 mL
1 cup	cooked chopped parsnip	250 mL
1/2 cup	cooked chopped carrot	125 mL
Pinch	ground nutmeg	Pinch
1/4 tsp	salt (or to taste)	1 mL

In blender, combine carrot juice, parsnip, carrot and nutmeg. Process as directed until smooth. Season with salt.

SERVES 1 OR 2

Vegetable Smoothies

Peppery Tomato Cocktail

1/2 cup	tomato juice	125 mL
	Juice of half a lemon	
3	tomatoes, cored and chopped	3
Half	red or green bell pepper, chopped	Half
1/4 cup	chopped fresh fennel	50 mL
1	sprig watercress, chopped	1
Half	clove garlic, peeled	Half
1/4 tsp	cayenne pepper	1 mL

In blender, combine tomato juice, lemon juice, tomatoes, green pepper, fennel, watercress, garlic and cayenne. Process as directed until smooth.

SERVES 2 OR 3

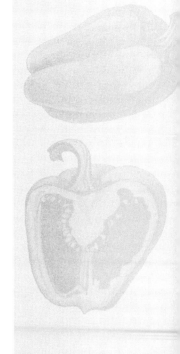

Peppered Potato

1 cup	vegetable or chicken stock	250 mL
1	potato, peeled and chopped	1
2 tbsp	chopped onion	25 mL
1/4 cup	chopped green or red bell pepper	50 mL
1 tbsp	chopped watercress or fresh parsley*	15 mL
1/2 tsp	chopped fresh thyme leaves	2 mL
Half to 1	chile pepper, chopped (optional)	Half to 1

1. In a medium saucepan over high heat, bring stock to a boil. Add potato and onion; reduce heat to low and simmer for 10 to 12 minutes or until vegetables are soft.
2. Pour stock mixture into blender. Add green pepper, watercress, thyme, and chile pepper (if using). Cover with lid and blend on Low for 1 minute. Increase speed to High; blend for 1 minute more or until smooth. Serve immediately with a spoon.

SERVES 1

> ∗ If you are pregnant, limit your intake of parsley to 1/2 tsp (2 mL) dried or one sprig fresh per day. Do not take parsley if you are suffering from kidney inflammation.

* If you are pregnant, limit your intake of parsley to $1/2$ tsp (2 mL) dried or one sprig fresh per day. Do not take parsley if you are suffering from kidney inflammation.

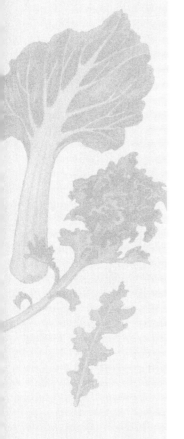

C-Green

3/4 cup	apple juice	175 mL
1 cup	chopped fresh or frozen spinach	250 mL
Half	avocado, peeled, pitted and chopped	Half
1 tbsp	chopped parsley*	15 mL
1 tbsp	chopped watercress	15 mL

In blender, combine apple juice, spinach, avocado, parsley and watercress. Process as directed until smooth.

SERVES 1

Green Gold

2/3 cup	carrot juice	150 mL
1/3 cup	apple juice	75 mL
1/2 cup	chopped fresh or frozen spinach	125 mL
Half	cucumber, peeled and chopped	Half
1	apple, peeled, cored and chopped	1
2 tsp	chopped fresh basil leaves	10 mL

In blender, combine carrot juice, apple juice, spinach, cucumber, apple and basil. Process as directed until smooth.

SERVES 1 OR 2

Rustproofer #2

1/2 cup	carrot juice	125 mL
1/2 cup	cooked yams, squash or pumpkin	125 mL
1/4 cup	cooked chopped broccoli	50 mL
4	apricots, peeled, pitted and chopped	4
1 tbsp	blackstrap molasses	15 mL
1 tbsp	chopped fresh peppermint leaves	15 mL

In blender, combine carrot juice, yams, broccoli, apricots, molasses and peppermint. Process as directed until smooth.

SERVES 1 OR 2

Vegetable Smoothies

Carrot Squash

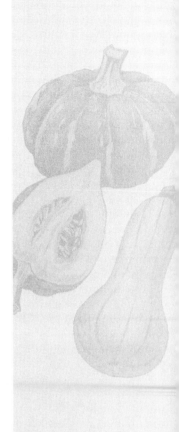

1 cup	vegetable or chicken stock	250 mL
1 cup	cooked squash	250 mL
1/2 cup	cooked chopped carrots	125 mL
1	apple, peeled, cored and chopped	1
Quarter	onion, peeled	Quarter
1/2 tsp	garam masala	2 mL
1/4 tsp	dry mustard	1 mL
Pinch	ground nutmeg	Pinch
1/2 cup	table (18%) cream or milk	125 mL
1/4 tsp	salt (or to taste)	1 mL

Garnish (optional):

1/4 cup	sour cream	50 mL
1/2 tsp	ground nutmeg	2 mL

1. In blender, combine stock, squash, carrots, apple, onion, garam masala, mustard and nutmeg. Cover with lid and blend on Low for 30 seconds.

2. With blender still running, add cream through opening in center of lid. Replace center cover and increase speed to High; blend for 1 minute or until smooth. Season with salt. Serve hot or cold with a spoon.

3. *Garnish:* Top with sour cream and nutmeg (if using).

SERVES 4

Squash Special

1/2 cup	apple juice	125 mL
1 cup	cooked squash or sweet potato	250 mL
1/4 cup	chopped pitted peeled apricots	50 mL
1/4 tsp	ground turmeric	1 mL
1/4 tsp	cayenne pepper	1 mL
Pinch	ground cumin	Pinch

In blender, combine apple juice, squash, apricots, turmeric, cayenne and cumin. Process as directed until smooth.

SERVES 2 OR 3

TIP
Subsitute an equal quantity of dried apricots in any smoothie recipe if fresh are not available.

Clam Tomato

TIP
This is a delicious nonalcoholic substitute for a Bloody Caesar, which is made with vodka.

1	can (10 oz/284 mL) clams (whole or minced)	1
4	tomatoes, cored and chopped	4
1/4 cup	spaghetti sauce	50 mL
	Juice of half a lemon	
1	stalk celery, chopped	1
1 tsp	chopped fresh thyme leaves	5 mL
1 or 2	dashes hot pepper sauce (optional)	1 or 2

In blender, combine clams with liquid, tomatoes, spaghetti sauce, lemon juice, celery, thyme, and hot pepper sauce (if using). Process as directed until smooth.

SERVES 3 OR 4

Pure Tomato

TIP
You can use 1/4 cup (50 mL) tomato juice and 3 ice cubes in place of the 4 tomatoes.

4	tomatoes, cored and halved	4
1/4 cup	spaghetti sauce	50 mL
	Juice of half a lemon	
1 tbsp	chopped fresh coriander	15 mL
	Salt and pepper to taste	

1. Working over a bowl to catch the juices, press tomatoes through a sieve to remove seeds and skins; discard seeds and skins.
2. Combine tomatoes, spaghetti sauce, lemon juice and coriander in blender. Process as directed until smooth. Season with salt and pepper.

SERVES 1

Tomato Juice Cocktail

1/4 cup	tomato juice	50 mL
1	can (14 oz/398 mL) diced beets	1
1	small zucchini, peeled and chopped	1
1 tbsp	chopped fresh basil leaves	15 mL
Half	clove garlic, peeled	Half
1/8 tsp	ground cumin	0.5 mL
1/8 tsp	cayenne pepper	0.5 mL
1/2 tsp	salt (or to taste)	2 mL

In blender, combine tomato juice, beets with liquid, zucchini, basil, garlic, cumin and cayenne. Process as directed until smooth. Season with salt.

SERVES 3 OR 4

General Directions
Always place the lid securely on the blender before processing. Blend on Low for 30 seconds. Gradually (if possible) increase speed to High and blend an additional 30 seconds or until smooth.

Zippy Tomato

1/4 cup	tomato juice	50 mL
2	tomatoes, cored and chopped	2
1	ripe pear, peeled, cored and chopped	1
Half	lemon, peeled, seeded and chopped	Half
1 tbsp	chopped parsley*	15 mL
1	piece (1/2 inch/1 cm) gingerroot, peeled and chopped	1
Half	chile pepper, chopped (or to taste)	Half
1/4 tsp	ground turmeric	1 mL
1/4 tsp	salt (or to taste)	1 mL

In blender, combine tomato juice, tomatoes, pear, lemon, parsley, gingerroot, chile pepper and turmeric. Process as directed until smooth. Season with salt.

SERVES 1 OR 2

* If you are pregnant, limit your intake of parsley to 1/2 tsp (2 mL) dried or one sprig fresh per day. Do not take parsley if you are suffering from kidney inflammation.

Vegetable Smoothies

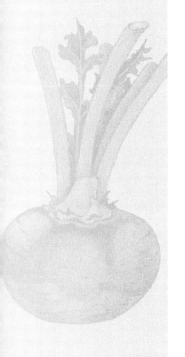

Turnip-Tomato Tango

1/2 cup	apple or carrot juice	125 mL
6	ice cubes (see page 274)	6
1	small turnip, peeled and chopped	1
1	cucumber, peeled and chopped	1
1	tomato, peeled, cored and chopped	1
1	stalk celery, chopped	1
1/4 cup	spaghetti sauce	50 mL
2 tbsp	lemon juice	25 mL

In blender, combine apple juice, ice, turnip, cucumber, tomato, celery, spaghetti sauce and lemon juice. Process as directed until smooth.

SERVES 2 OR 3

Turnip Parsnip Carrot

1 cup	vegetable or chicken stock	250 mL
1/2 cup	chopped peeled turnip	125 mL
1/2 cup	chopped parsnip	125 mL
1/2 cup	chopped carrot	125 mL
1/2 cup	milk	125 mL
1/4 tsp	ground cinnamon	1 mL
1/4 tsp	salt (or to taste)	1 mL

1. In a medium saucepan over high heat, bring stock just to a boil. Add turnip, parsnip and carrot; reduce heat to low and simmer for 7 to 10 minutes or until vegetables are tender.
2. Meanwhile, in a small saucepan, heat milk until small bubbles form around the outside of the pan. Pour stock mixture into blender; add cinnamon and milk. Process as directed or until smooth. Season with salt. Serve hot with a spoon.

SERVES 4

Watercress

1/2 cup	apple or carrot juice	125 mL
2 tbsp	lemon juice	25 mL
2	sprigs watercress, chopped	2
2	radishes, chopped	2
1	apple, peeled, cored and chopped	1
Half	cucumber, peeled and chopped	Half
1	stalk celery, chopped	1
1/4 tsp	salt (or to taste)	1 mL

In blender, combine apple juice, lemon juice, watercress, radishes, apple, cucumber and celery. Process as directed until smooth. Season with salt.

SERVES 1 OR 2

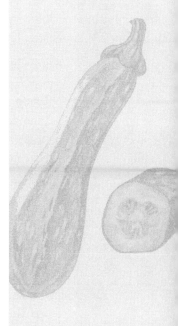

Zuke and Cuke

1/2 cup	apple or carrot juice	125 mL
2 tbsp	lemon juice	25 mL
1	small zucchini, peeled and chopped	1
Half	cucumber, peeled and chopped	Half
1	stalk celery, chopped	1
1/4 tsp	curry powder	1 mL
Pinch	celery salt	Pinch

In blender, combine apple juice, lemon juice, zucchini, cucumber, celery, curry powder and celery salt. Process as directed until smooth.

SERVES 2 OR 3

Herb Smoothies

HERBS ARE PLANTS THAT ARE OFTEN USED FOR MEDICINAL PURPOSES. Like fruits and vegetables, many herbs are high in antioxidants, which counteract the free radicals that can cause cellular damage, aging and susceptibility to cancers. Each medicinal herb has unique active components that offer specific health benefits to humans. In fact, modern drugs were derived from plants, and over half of the drugs prescribed today still have their origins in plants.

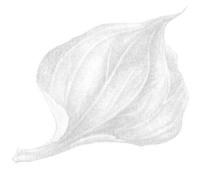

Fresh Organic Is Best

Like fruits and vegetables, fresh whole herbs — preferably organic — provide the maximum range of nutrients. Grow your own or look for fresh herbs in supermarkets and farmer's markets. Use dried herbs in smoothies when fresh are not available.

To substitute dried herbs for fresh in smoothies: Use one-half to one-third less dried herb than the quantity of fresh called for in a recipe. Crush or grind dried herbs to a powder, then add to smoothie ingredients before blending.

Herbal Teas (Infusions)

Medicinal teas made from herbs are called infusions and may be substituted for all or part of the liquid in any smoothie recipe. The issue is whether you like the taste. No one has ever said that all herbal infusions are delicious, but some, such as mint and chamomile, taste quite pleasant.

When making medicinal teas, most herbalists work with dried herbs because they are widely available and easy to store, transport and use. Purchase small quantities of dried organic herbs from a farm or health/alternative store (see Resources, page 303) and replace after eight to 10 months. Store dried herbs in a cool, dark, dry place.

To make an herbal tea (infusion): Bring 1 cup (250 mL) pure or filtered water to a boil. Remove the kettle from the heat. Measure 1 tsp (5 mL) — or the amount recommended under Infusion for a specific herb (see Herb Profiles, pages 90 to 124) — into a teapot. Pour the recommended amount of boiling water over top. Place lid on teapot and a cork in the spout to prevent steam from escaping. Steep for 10 to 15 minutes. Let cool before using in smoothies unless a hot drink is desired. Strain and discard bark, seeds or woody stems but blend leaves and flowers into smoothies along with other ingredients.

TIP

For convenience, make 1 to 2 cups (250 to 500 mL) herbal tea and store in a covered jar in the refrigerator for use throughout the day. Medicinal teas should be stored for no longer than one day. Keep them in a container that doesn't leave a large headspace above the liquid, because active ingredients will be lost through oxidization during storage.

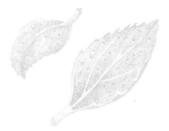

DECOCTIONS

When the woody parts (roots, bark and seeds) of herbs are simmered in water, the resulting solution is called a decoction.

To make a decoction: Measure the amount of the ground herb recommended under Decoction for a specific herb (see Herb Profiles, pages 90 to 124) into a small saucepan. Pour the recommended amount of filtered water into the pan and bring to a simmer. Simmer for the recommended amount of time. Use a saucepan made of a nonreactive material, such as glass, enamel or stainless steel and keep the lid on at all times, because some of the active ingredients will be lost if the steam is allowed to escape. Be sure to follow the instructions on the amount to use and the simmering time given for a particular herb.

Tinctures

A tincture is the solution made when herbs are steeped in alcohol and pure water. This technique extracts and preserves their active ingredients, and the resulting solution is so concentrated that only a few drops are required for each dose. Tinctures may be purchased at natural-food stores. To take a tincture, drop the amount recommended under Tincture for a specific herb (see Herb Profiles, pages 90 to 124) into water, juice or any fruit or vegetable smoothie and drink.

Spoonful of Medicine

Smoothies are a tasty way to add the medicinal benefits of herbs to your diet or to take conventional medicines. Gel capsules can easily be slit open and their contents blended with smoothie ingredients. Fresh or dried herbs, tinctures and herbal teas can also be added to blended drinks.

General Directions

Always place the lid securely on the blender before processing. Blend on Low for 30 seconds. Gradually (if possible) increase speed to High and blend an additional 30 seconds or until smooth.

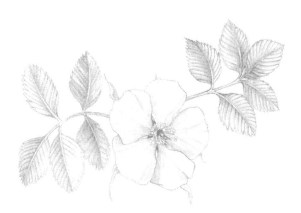

Good Health Elixir

¼ cup	orange juice	50 mL
¼ cup	alfalfa infusion (see page 90) or carrot juice	50 mL
Half	ripe banana, peeled and chopped	Half
4	frozen strawberries or raspberries	4

In blender, combine orange juice, alfalfa infusion, banana and strawberries. Process as directed until smooth.

SERVES 1

TIP
Alfalfa, humanity's oldest crop, feeds the cells and is safe to use every day.

Herb-eze

¼ cup	carrot juice	50 mL
¼ cup	astragalus decoction (see page 90)	50 mL
¼ cup	frozen blueberries	50 mL
¼ cup	chopped pitted peeled apricots	50 mL
Pinch	ground cloves	Pinch

In blender, combine carrot juice, astragalus decoction, blueberries, apricots and cloves. Process as directed until smooth.

SERVES 1

TIPS
Use an equal quantity of dried apricots in smoothie recipes if fresh are not available.

The Chinese call astragalus *huang qi* and add the roots to nourishing soups for the very young and the very old. It is safe to use every day.

Anti-Depression Tonic

¼ cup	carrot juice	50 mL
¼ cup	lemon balm infusion (see page 108)	50 mL
1 tbsp	lemon juice	15 mL
¼ cup	cooked chopped carrots	50 mL
Half	mango, peeled, pitted and chopped	Half
2	large fresh basil leaves, chopped	2

In blender, combine carrot juice, lemon balm infusion, lemon juice, carrots, mango and basil. Process as directed until smooth.

Pear Basil Raspberry

1/4 cup	raspberry juice	50 mL
1/4 cup	Apricot Milk (recipe, page 247)	50 mL
1 tsp	balsamic vinegar	5 mL
1 tbsp	chopped fresh basil leaves	15 mL
1/2 cup	frozen raspberries	125 mL
1/2 cup	frozen or fresh sliced peeled pears	125 mL

In blender, combine raspberry juice, apricot milk, balsamic vinegar, basil, raspberries and pears. Process as directed until smooth.

SERVES 1

Cramp Crusher

1/2 cup	orange juice	125 mL
2 tbsp	lemon juice	25 mL
1/2 cup	blueberries, blackberries or strawberries	125 mL
1/2 tsp	ground ginger	2 mL
8	drops black cohosh tincture	8

In blender, combine orange juice, lemon juice, blueberries, ginger and black cohosh tincture. Process as directed until smooth.

SERVES 1

TIP
**Borage, which was
believed to inspire
courage, was
traditionally made
into a drink for men
leaving to fight in
the Crusades.**

Courage

1/4 cup	borage infusion (see page 92)	50 mL
1/4 cup	orange juice	50 mL
1/2 cup	frozen sliced peaches	125 mL
1/4 cup	cooked diced beets or frozen raspberries	50 mL

In blender, combine borage infusion, orange juice, peaches and beets. Process as directed until smooth.

Herb Smoothies

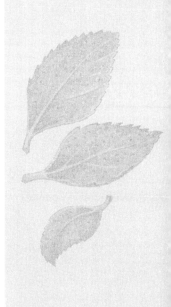

Healthy Bladder Blitz

¼ cup	buchu infusion (see page 92)	50 mL
¼ cup	cranberry juice	50 mL
¼ cup	frozen blueberries	50 mL
¼ cup	chopped celery	50 mL

In blender, combine buchu infusion, cranberry juice, blueberries and celery. Process as directed until smooth.

SERVES 1

Diuretic Tonic

¼ cup	burdock leaf infusion (see page 93)	50 mL
¼ cup	dandelion leaf infusion (see page 99)	50 mL
¼ cup	frozen blueberries	50 mL
½ cup	chopped seeded peeled cantaloupe	125 mL
1 tbsp	chopped parsley*	15 mL

In blender, combine burdock leaf infusion, dandelion leaf infusion, blueberries, cantaloupe and parsley. Process as directed until smooth.

SERVES 1

> ★ If you are pregnant, limit your intake of parsley to ½ tsp (2 mL) dried or one sprig fresh per day. Do not take parsley if you are suffering from kidney inflammation.

Gout Gone

¼ cup	burdock root decoction (see page 93)	50 mL
¼ cup	raspberry juice	50 mL
¼ cup	frozen strawberries	50 mL
1	ripe banana, peeled and chopped	1
1 tbsp	chopped parsley*	15 mL
1 tsp	crushed fennel seeds	5 mL

In blender, combine burdock root decoction, raspberry juice, strawberries, banana, parsley and fennel seeds. Process as directed until smooth.

SERVES 1

TIP
You can use fresh and frozen fruit interchangeably in most smoothies, although the results will differ. Frozen fruit not only chills a smoothie, it thickens it as well.

TIPS
This drink is a
cleansing tonic
that supports
hormone balance
and improves skin
problems, especially
during the
teenage years.

Use an equal
quantity of dried
apricots if fresh
are not available.

¼ cup	burdock seed infusion (see page 93)	50 mL
¼ cup	calendula infusion (see page 94) or carrot juice	50 mL
Half	mango, peeled, pitted and chopped	Half
¼ cup	chopped seeded peeled cantaloupe	50 mL
2	apricots, peeled, pitted and chopped	2
1 tsp	dandelion root tincture	5 mL

In blender, combine burdock seed infusion, calendula infusion, mango, cantaloupe, apricots and dandelion root tincture. Process as directed until smooth.

SERVES 1

Peptic Tonic

TIP
This healing tonic
is safe for an
everyday breakfast
drink if the slippery
elm bark powder
is eliminated.
See Peptic Ulcers,
page 76, for other
fruits, vegetables
and herbs to add
to this smoothie.

¼ cup	apple juice	50 mL
¼ cup	calendula infusion (see page 94)	50 mL
1	ripe banana, peeled and chopped	1
¼ cup	chopped pitted peeled mango	50 mL
¼ cup	chopped seeded peeled papaya	50 mL
1 tsp	slippery elm bark powder	5 mL

In blender, combine apple juice, calendula infusion, banana, mango, papaya and slippery elm bark powder. Process as directed until smooth.

SERVES 1

Herb Smoothies

Sleepytime Smoothie

¼ cup	catnip infusion (see page 95)	50 mL
¼ cup	chamomile infusion (see page 103)	50 mL
1	apple, peeled, cored and chopped	1
Half	ripe banana, peeled and chopped	Half
20 to 40	drops valerian* tincture	20 to 40

In blender, combine catnip infusion, chamomile infusion, apple, banana and valerian tincture. Process as directed until smooth.

SERVES 1

Digestive Drink

¼ tsp	crushed cardamom seeds	1 mL
¼ tsp	crushed cinnamon stick	1 mL
¼ tsp	crushed fennel seeds	1 mL
⅛ tsp	crushed cloves	0.5 mL
1	apple, peeled, cored and chopped	1
1	kiwi, peeled and chopped	1
¼ cup	seedless grapes	50 mL

1. In a teapot, pour ¼ cup (50 mL) boiling water over cardamom seeds, cinnamon, fennel seeds and cloves. Cover and steep for 10 minutes. Strain and discard spices. Let spice infusion cool.
2. In blender, combine spice infusion, apple, kiwi and grapes. Process as directed until smooth.

SERVES 1

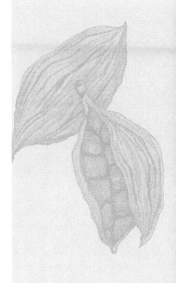

TIP
The range in the dosage of valerian reflects individual needs: some people need more than others. Try this first with 20 drops, then increase if required.

---

* Valerian has an adverse effect on some people.

General Directions
Always place the lid securely on the blender before processing. Blend on Low for 30 seconds. Gradually (if possible) increase speed to High and blend an additional 30 seconds or until smooth.

Pain Reliever

1/2 cup	tomato juice	125 mL
2 tbsp	lemon juice	25 mL
1/2 cup	shredded cabbage	125 mL
1/2 tsp	cayenne pepper (or to taste)	2 mL
8	drops black cohosh tincture	8

In blender, combine tomato juice, lemon juice, cabbage, cayenne and black cohosh tincture. Process as directed until smooth.

SERVES 1

TIP
Use raw or cooked cabbage in this smoothie. Although raw has more nutrients, cooked cabbage blends easily and the taste is not as strong.

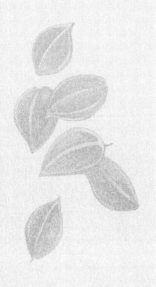

Muscle Relief

1/2 cup	beet juice	125 mL
1/4 cup	chopped celery	50 mL
1/4 cup	cooked chopped carrots or beets	50 mL
1 tsp	slippery elm bark powder	5 mL
1/4 tsp	crushed medicinal celery seeds	1 mL

In blender, combine beet juice, celery, carrots, slippery elm bark powder and celery seeds. Process as directed until smooth.

SERVES 1

TIP
Drink this smoothie one or two hours after eating. To minimize gas, never eat fruit at or immediately after mealtimes.

Gas Guzzler

1/2 cup	papaya nectar or apple juice	125 mL
1	apple, peeled, cored and chopped	1
1/2 cup	chopped seeded peeled papaya	125 mL
1/4 tsp	crushed cumin seeds	1 mL
1/4 tsp	crushed fennel seeds	1 mL
1/8 tsp	crushed mustard seeds	0.5 mL
1/8 tsp	ground cinnamon	0.5 mL

In blender, combine papaya nectar, apple, chopped papaya, cumin seeds, fennel seeds, mustard seeds and cinnamon. Process as directed until smooth.

SERVES 1

Popeye's Power

½ cup	beet or carrot juice	125 mL
1 cup	cooked diced beets	250 mL
½ cup	chopped fresh or frozen spinach	125 mL
½ cup	cooked chopped carrots	125 mL
1	piece (1 inch/2.5 cm) dandelion root, chopped	1
1 tbsp	blackstrap molasses (optional)	15 mL

In blender, combine beet juice, beets, spinach, carrots, dandelion root, and molasses (if using). Process as directed until smooth.

SERVES 1

TIP
Substitute 1 can (14 oz/398 mL) diced beets with liquid for the beet juice and cooked beets when fresh are not available.

Flu Fighter #2

¼ cup	pineapple juice	50 mL
¼ cup	echinacea decoction (see page 100)	50 mL
2 tbsp	lemon juice	25 mL
2 tbsp	cranberry sauce	25 mL
1	orange, peeled, seeded and chopped	1
¼ tsp	ground ginger	1 mL
⅛ tsp	ground cinnamon	0.5 mL
⅛ tsp	ground licorice*	0.5 mL

In blender, combine pineapple juice, echinacea decoction, lemon juice, cranberry sauce, orange, ginger, cinnamon and licorice. Process as directed until smooth.

SERVES 1

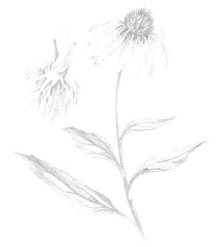

Take this drink at the first sign of cold or flu, before the virus can take hold.

* Avoid licorice if you have high blood pressure. The prolonged use of licorice is not recommended under any circumstances.

General Directions
Always place the lid securely on the blender before processing. Blend on Low for 30 seconds. Gradually (if possible) increase speed to High and blend an additional 30 seconds or until smooth.

Hot Flu Toddy

TIP
Take this drink
once a cold or flu
has taken hold.

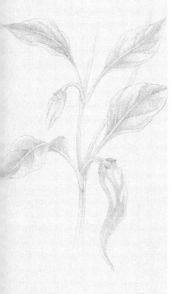

¼ cup	elderberry infusion (see page 100)	50 mL
¼ cup	cranberry juice	50 mL
2 tbsp	dried elderberries or blueberries (optional)	25 mL
¼ cup	chopped peeled pineapple	50 mL
4	frozen strawberries	4
¼ cup	frozen raspberries	50 mL
¼ tsp	ground ginger	1 mL
⅛ tsp	ground cinnamon	0.5 mL
⅛ tsp	cayenne pepper	0.5 mL

In blender, combine elderberry infusion, cranberry juice, dried elderberries (if using), pineapple, strawberries, raspberries, ginger, cinnamon and cayenne. Process as directed until smooth.

SERVES 1

Psoria-Smoothie

TIP
You can use fresh
and frozen fruit
interchangeably in
most smoothies,
although the results
will differ. Frozen
fruit not only chills
a smoothie, it
thickens it as well.

½ cup	apricot nectar or carrot juice	125 mL
¼ cup	blueberries	50 mL
¼ cup	chopped seeded peeled cantaloupe	50 mL
2	apricots, peeled, pitted and chopped	2
1 tsp	evening primrose oil	5 mL
½ tsp	crushed fennel seeds	2 mL
20	drops burdock root tincture	20

In blender, combine apricot nectar, blueberries, cantaloupe, apricots, evening primrose oil, fennel seeds and burdock root tincture. Process as directed until smooth.

SERVES 1

The Regular

1/2 cup	orange juice	125 mL
4	large strawberries (hulled and halved if fresh)	4
1	ripe banana, peeled and chopped	1
2 tbsp	wheat germ	25 mL
1 tsp	evening primrose oil	5 mL

In blender, combine orange juice, strawberries, banana, wheat germ and evening primrose oil. Process as directed until smooth.

SERVES 1

Migraine Tonic

1/4 cup	beet juice	50 mL
1/4 cup	carrot juice	50 mL
1/4 cup	chopped seeded peeled cantaloupe	50 mL
1	stalk celery, chopped	1
1 tbsp	chopped parsley*	1
1	slice (1/2 inch/1 cm) gingerroot, peeled and chopped	1
1 tsp	chopped fresh rosemary leaves	5 mL
1/4 tsp	cayenne pepper	1 mL
10	drops feverfew tincture	10

In blender, combine beet juice, carrot juice, cantaloupe, celery, parsley, gingerroot, rosemary, cayenne and feverfew tincture. Process as directed until smooth.

SERVES 1

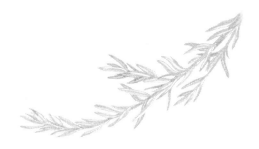

TIP
Evening primrose oil is sometimes available in small jars but is widely available in gel capsules. If the jars are not available, use a sharp knife to split open capsules, then pour into a measuring spoon and add to smoothies.

* If you are pregnant, limit your intake of parsley to 1/2 tsp (2 mL) dried or one sprig fresh per day. Do not take parsley if you are suffering from kidney inflammation.

General Directions
Always place the lid securely on the blender before processing. Blend on Low for 30 seconds. Gradually (if possible) increase speed to High and blend an additional 30 seconds or until smooth.

Allium Antioxidant

¾ cup	carrot juice	175 mL
1	stalk celery, chopped	1
Quarter	onion, peeled and chopped	Quarter
Half	clove garlic, peeled	Half
1	apple, peeled, cored and chopped	1

In blender, combine carrot juice, celery, onion, garlic and apple.
Process as directed until smooth.

SERVES 1 OR 2

In Europe,
chamomile is a
very popular herb.
In Germany, for
example, there
are 18 different
medicinal
preparations that
contain chamomile
on pharmacy shelves.

Calming Chamomile

½ cup	chamomile or chamomile-ginger tea	125 mL
1	apple, peeled, cored and chopped	1
Quarter	cantaloupe, peeled, seeded and chopped	Quarter
1 tbsp	fresh German chamomile flowers (or 1 tsp/5 mL dried)	15 mL
2 tbsp	plain yogurt	25 mL
1 tbsp	liquid honey (or to taste)	15 mL

In blender, combine chamomile tea, apple, cantaloupe, chamomile
flowers, yogurt and honey. Process as directed until smooth.

SERVES 1 OR 2

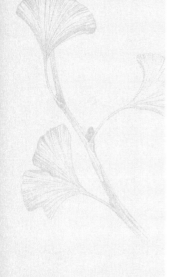

Green Energy

¾ cup	plain soy milk	175 mL
¼ cup	chopped dried apricots	50 mL
1 cup	fresh or frozen spinach, chopped	250 mL
2 tsp	chopped wheat or barley grass	10 mL
1 tbsp	pumpkin seeds	15 mL
1 tsp	dried ginkgo leaves	5 mL

In blender, combine soy milk, apricots, spinach, wheat grass, pumpkin
seeds and ginkgo leaves. Process as directed until smooth.

SERVES 1

Herb Smoothies

Day Starter

1/2 cup	orange juice	125 mL
3 tbsp	plain yogurt	45 mL
1/4 cup	frozen sliced peaches	50 mL
1/4 cup	raspberries or strawberries (hulled and halved if fresh)	50 mL
Half	ripe banana, peeled and chopped	Half
15	drops ginseng tincture	15

In blender, combine orange juice, yogurt, peaches, raspberries, banana and ginseng tincture. Process as directed until smooth.

SERVES 1

General Directions
Always place the lid securely on the blender before processing. Blend on Low for 30 seconds. Gradually (if possible) increase speed to High and blend an additional 30 seconds or until smooth.

Green Tea Smoothie

1/2 cup	green tea infusion (see page 106)	125 mL
1/4 cup	seedless grapes, halved	50 mL
1/4 cup	blueberries	50 mL
1	sprig parsley*, chopped	1

In blender, combine green tea infusion, grapes, blueberries and parsley. Process as directed until smooth.

SERVES 1

* If you are pregnant, limit your intake of parsley to 1/2 tsp (2 mL) dried or one sprig fresh per day. Do not take parsley if you are suffering from kidney inflammation.

** Avoid licorice if you have high blood pressure. The prolonged use of licorice is not recommended under any circumstances.

Bronchial Aid

1/4 cup	each hyssop and marshmallow infusion (see pages 107 and 110)	50 mL
1	pear, peeled, cored and chopped	1
2	apricots, peeled, pitted and chopped	2
1	sprig parsley*, chopped	1
1/4 tsp	ground licorice**	1 mL

In blender, combine hyssop and marshmallow infusions, pear, apricots, parsley and licorice. Process as directed until smooth.

SERVES 1

TIP
If fresh apricots are not available, use an equal quantity of dried in any smoothie.

TIP
If fresh apricots are not available, use an equal quantity of dried in any smoothie.

Lavender Smoothie

1 tsp	dried lemon balm flowers	5 mL
1/4 tsp	dried lavender flowers and leaves	1 mL
1	plum, peeled, pitted and chopped	1
2	apricots, peeled, pitted and chopped	2
1/4 cup	seedless grapes, halved	50 mL

1. In a teapot, pour 1/2 cup (125 mL) boiling water over lemon balm and lavender. Cover and steep for 10 minutes. Let infusion cool (no need to strain).

2. In blender, combine infusion, plum, apricots and grapes. Process as directed until smooth.

SERVES 1

Lemon Lemon

1 tsp	dried lemon balm	5 mL
1 tsp	dried lemon verbena	5 mL
1 tsp	dried linden leaves and flowers	5 mL
	Juice of 1 lemon	
1/4 cup	chopped peeled pineapple	50 mL
1/4 cup	frozen sliced peaches	50 mL
2	apricots, peeled, pitted and chopped	2

1. In a teapot, pour 1/2 cup (125 mL) boiling water over lemon balm, lemon verbena and linden. Cover and steep for 10 minutes. Let infusion cool (no need to strain).

2. In blender, combine infusion, lemon juice, pineapple, peaches and apricots. Process as directed until smooth.

SERVES 1

General Directions
Always place the lid securely on the blender before processing. Blend on Low for 30 seconds. Gradually (if possible) increase speed to High and blend an additional 30 seconds or until smooth.

The Cool Down

1/2 cup	carrot juice	125 mL
2	wedges pineapple, peeled and chopped	2
1	ripe banana, peeled and chopped	1
1 tbsp	chopped lemon balm	15 mL

In blender, combine carrot juice, pineapple, banana and lemon balm. Process as directed until smooth.

SERVES 1

Anise Anise

1/4 cup	licorice* decoction (see page 109)	50 mL
1/4 cup	apple juice	50 mL
1	apple, peeled, cored and chopped	1
3 tbsp	chopped fresh fennel	45 mL
1 tsp	crushed fennel seeds	5 mL

In blender, combine licorice decoction, apple juice, apple, fennel and fennel seeds. Process as directed until smooth.

SERVES 1

* Avoid licorice if you have high blood pressure. The prolonged use of licorice is not recommended under any circumstances.

Aspirin in a Glass

1/4 cup	meadowsweet infusion (see page 111)	50 mL
1/4 cup	cranberry juice	50 mL
1/4 cup	pitted cherries	50 mL
1/4 cup	chopped pitted peeled mango	50 mL
1 tbsp	chopped fresh alfalfa	15 mL
1/4 tsp	crushed fennel seeds	1 mL

In blender, combine meadowsweet infusion, cranberry juice, cherries, mango, alfalfa and fennel seeds. Process as directed until smooth.

SERVES 1

Anti-inflammatory salicylates were originally discovered in meadowsweet, then isolated and chemically duplicated for use in pill form, which was called Aspirin. The name "Aspirin" comes from the old botanical name for meadowsweet, *Spiraea ulmaria* (now known as *Filipendula ulmaria*).

Spa Special

¼ cup	milk thistle infusion (see page 111)	50 mL
¼ cup	silken tofu	50 mL
6	large strawberries (hulled and halved if fresh)	6
½ cup	blueberries	125 mL

In blender, combine milk thistle infusion, tofu, strawberries and blueberries. Process as directed until smooth.

SERVES 1

Woman's Smoothie

1 tsp	dried motherwort	5 mL
1 tsp	dried red clover	5 mL
1 tsp	grated peeled gingerroot	5 mL
¼ cup	orange juice	50 mL
¼ cup	frozen blueberries	50 mL
4	frozen strawberries	4

1. In a teapot, pour ¼ cup (50 mL) boiling water over motherwort, red clover and gingerroot. Cover and steep for 10 minutes. Let infusion cool (no need to strain).

2. In blender, combine infusion, orange juice, blueberries and strawberries. Process as directed until smooth.

SERVES 1

TIP
You can use fresh and frozen fruit interchangeably in most smoothies, although the results will differ. Frozen fruit not only chills a smoothie, it thickens it as well.

Morning After

½ cup	orange juice	125 mL
1	wedge pineapple, peeled and chopped	1
2 tbsp	chopped fresh parsley*	25 mL
2 tbsp	lemon juice	25 mL
1 tbsp	chopped peeled gingerroot	15 mL

In blender, combine orange juice, pineapple, parsley, lemon juice and gingerroot. Process as directed until smooth.

SERVES 1

Peppermint Aperitif

½ cup	peppermint infusion (see page 115)	125 mL
4	ice cubes	4
¼ cup	chopped fresh fennel	50 mL
1	kiwi, peeled and chopped	1
1	apple, peeled, cored and chopped	1

In blender, combine peppermint infusion, ice, fennel, kiwi and apple. Process as directed until smooth.

SERVES 1

This is a pleasing drink that cleanses the palate. When taking fruit drinks, wait a minimum of half an hour before eating a meal, as the fruit can cause gas if followed by other food. Allow one to two hours after meals before taking fruit drinks.

Raspberry Raspberry

¼ cup	red raspberry infusion (see page 116)	50 mL
¼ cup	raspberry juice	50 mL
2 tbsp	lemon juice	25 mL
¼ cup	frozen raspberries	50 mL
4	frozen strawberries	4

In blender, combine red raspberry infusion, raspberry juice, lemon juice, raspberries and strawberries. Process as directed until smooth.

SERVES 1

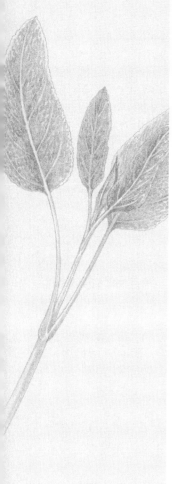

Rose Smoothie

¼ cup	fresh rose hip infusion (see page 117)	50 mL
¼ cup	apple juice	50 mL
2 tbsp	lemon juice	25 mL
¼ cup	seedless grapes, halved	50 mL
1	plum, peeled, pitted and chopped	1
4	frozen strawberries	4
1 tbsp	fresh rose petals	15 mL

In blender, combine rose hip infusion, apple juice, lemon juice, grapes, plum, strawberries and rose petals. Process as directed until smooth.

SERVES 1

Sage Relief

½ cup	beet juice	125 mL
1 tbsp	lemon juice	15 mL
¼ cup	cooked chopped beets	50 mL
1	apple, peeled, cored and chopped	1
½ tsp	chopped fresh sage leaves	2 mL

In blender, combine beet juice, lemon juice, beets, apple and sage. Process as directed until smooth.

SERVES 1

Prostate Power

½ cup	orange juice	125 mL
2 tbsp	lemon juice	25 mL
1	apple, peeled, cored and chopped	1
Half	ripe banana, peeled and chopped	Half
10 to 25	drops saw palmetto liquid extract	10 to 25

In blender, combine orange juice, lemon juice, apple, banana and saw palmetto extract. Process as directed until smooth.

SERVES 1

Smart Smoothie

½ cup	orange juice	125 mL
¼ cup	blueberries	50 mL
¼ cup	seedless red grapes, halved	50 mL
1 cup	fresh or frozen spinach, chopped	250 mL
1 tsp	dried or fresh ginkgo leaves (optional)	5 mL
1 tbsp	flax seeds	15 mL
1 tsp	dried skullcap	5 mL
1 tsp	lecithin	5 mL

In blender, combine orange juice, blueberries, grapes, spinach, ginkgo (if using), flax seeds, skullcap and lecithin. Process as directed until smooth.

SERVES 1

There is a large range in the amount of saw palmetto extract because people need more or less of it depending on their health, weight, age, the other herbs they are taking and the symptoms they have. Start with the smaller amount of saw palmetto and increase if necessary.

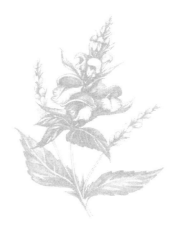

Hangover Remedy

½ cup	apple juice	125 mL
	Juice of 1 lemon	
2	apples, peeled, cored and chopped	2
1	ripe banana, peeled and chopped	1
1	piece (½ inch/1 cm) gingerroot, peeled and chopped	1
1 tsp	fresh chamomile flowers (or ½ tsp/2 mL dried)	5 mL
½ tsp	slippery elm bark powder	2 mL

In blender, combine apple juice, lemon juice, apples, banana, gingerroot, chamomile and slippery elm bark powder. Process as directed until smooth.

SERVES 1

Slippery Banana

¼ cup	chamomile infusion (see page 103)	50 mL
¼ cup	ginger infusion (see page 104)	50 mL
¼ cup	plain yogurt	50 mL
1	ripe banana, peeled and chopped	1
1 tsp	slippery elm bark powder	5 mL
¼ tsp	ground nutmeg	1 mL

In blender, combine chamomile and ginger infusions, yogurt, banana, slippery elm bark powder and nutmeg. Process as directed until smooth.

SERVES 1

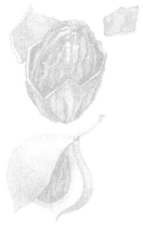

Mint Julep

1/2 cup	spearmint infusion (see page 120)	125 mL
1/4 cup	chopped seeeded peeled watermelon	50 mL
4	frozen strawberries or raspberries	4
1 tbsp	chopped fresh spearmint leaves	15 mL

In blender, combine spearmint infusion, watermelon, strawberries and chopped spearmint. Process as directed until smooth.

SERVES 1

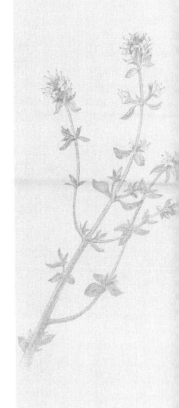

Thyme in a Glass

1/2 cup	beet juice	125 mL
1/4 cup	cooked chopped carrots	50 mL
1	apple, peeled, cored and chopped	1
1/4 tsp	dried thyme leaves	1 mL
1/8 tsp	dried rosemary leaves	0.5 mL

In blender, combine beet juice, carrots, apple, thyme and rosemary. Process as directed until smooth.

SERVES 1

Turmeric Cocktail

1/4 cup	carrot juice	50 mL
1/4 cup	tomato juice	50 mL
1	tomato, cored and chopped	1
1	stalk celery, chopped	1
2 tbsp	chopped fresh fennel (optional)	25 mL
1 tsp	ground turmeric	5 mL
1/8 tsp	celery seeds, crushed	0.5 mL
1/8 tsp	dill seeds, crushed	0.5 mL

In blender, combine carrot juice, tomato juice, chopped tomato, chopped celery, fennel (if using), turmeric, celery seeds and dill seeds. Process as directed until smooth.

SERVES 1 OR 2

Dairy and Dairy Alternative Smoothies

MAKING SMOOTHIES WITH MILK, YOGURT, TOFU OR FORTIFIED soy milk is a good way to add bone-building calcium and protein to your diet. Milk is also a good source of B vitamins, but many people cannot tolerate dairy products (see Milk Intolerance, below). Fortunately, a wide variety of nondairy liquids — such as soy milk, rice milk, fruit milks and nut milks, which are usually good sources of protein and calcium — may be used as substitutes for dairy products. As protein and calcium are essential for growth and maintenance of tissue, children, teenagers and many adults, especially postmenopausal women who are at risk of calcium depletion, will benefit from smoothies made with milk and yogurt, as well as tofu and fortified soy milk.

Dairy

Milk

Milk is a source of important nutrients, such as calcium, B vitamins, protein, minerals and vitamin D. This is true not only of whole milk but also of reduced-fat milks (2%, 1% and skim) and chocolate milk. All of the recipes for dairy smoothies may be made with whole or reduced-fat cow's milk, buttermilk, goat's milk, ewe's milk, or regular or low-fat evaporated milk. Milk is perishable, so always buy it and other dairy products that are well within the best-before date printed on the package and keep them refrigerated. Milk may be frozen in ice-cube trays, and the crushed cubes can be used in smoothies.

Milk Intolerance

A significant number of people have difficulty digesting the sugar in milk, which is called lactose. This condition is called lactose intolerance and is characterized by the appearance of painful symptoms, such as bloating, after milk or milk products are consumed. Eliminating milk and dairy products from the diet alleviates this condition. If you are lactose intolerant or allergic to milk, be aware that cream; butter; processed products, such as cereals and baking mixes; and baked goods that contain milk, milk solids, cheese, cheese flavoring, whey, curds or even margarine may trigger digestive problems.

Fruit and Nut Milks

Dairy Smoothies

Milk Shakes

Dairy Alternative Smoothies

Other Forms of Milk

- **Buttermilk** is a by-product of the butter-making process. A creamy, rich liquid with a natural bite, it contains no butter and imparts a characteristic flavor. Buttermilk is also available in powdered dried form (see Using Powdered Buttermilk, below). Use buttermilk in smoothies to add texture, with less fat than whole milk.

- **Powdered dried skim** or **whole milk solids** are pasteurized milk crystals made by air-drying milk to remove the water. They are a convenient and economical alternative to fresh milk (see Using Powdered Dried Milk, below).

- **Ewe's milk** has about 50% more calcium than cow's or goat's milk. It is high in essential vitamins and minerals and is easily digestible. Although it is used mainly in cheese making, it is sometimes available in specialty-food or natural-food stores.

- **Evaporated milk** is made by evaporating half of the water from fresh whole milk. The heat used to process and can it caramelizes the naturally occurring milk sugars, giving evaporated milk a slightly caramel-like flavor and light brown tint. Evaporated milk makes smoothies thicker and slightly sweeter than those made with regular milk. Do not confuse evaporated milk with sweetened condensed milk, which is very high in sugar. Low-fat evaporated milk is a good choice for smoothies. Cans of evaporated milk are easy to store but need to be refrigerated once they are opened.

- **Goat's milk** is available in most supermarkets and natural-food stores and can be comfortably consumed by many people with lactose intolerance.

USING POWDERED DRIED MILK

Keep powdered dried milk on the shelf and reconstitute just the amount required with water or add directly to smoothies for thicker, nutrient-enriched drinks. To make 1 cup (250 mL) of milk, whisk 2 to 4 tbsp (25 to 50 mL) with 1 cup (250 mL) water. You can add 2 or 3 tbsp (25 or 45 mL) powdered dried milk directly to a smoothie recipe, but be sure to increase the liquid by 1 or 2 tbsp (15 or 25 mL).

USING POWDERED BUTTERMILK

With a supply of powdered buttermilk in the cupboard, you will always be able to enjoy its rich, tart taste in smoothies. To make 1 cup (250 mL) buttermilk, whisk 3 tbsp (45 mL) powdered dried buttermilk with 1 cup (250 mL) water. You can add 1 or 2 tbsp (15 or 25 mL) powdered dried buttermilk directly to most smoothie recipes, but be sure to add 1 or 2 tbsp (15 or 25 mL) extra liquid or water as well.

Yogurt

Yogurt is a fermented milk product that contains a beneficial type of bacteria called lactobacillus, which restores and maintains normal microbial balance in the intestinal tract.

The nutritional value of yogurt is similar to that of milk but it is easier to digest. Check the label to ensure that yogurt contains active bacterial cultures and that it doesn't contain additives, preservatives or colorings.

For smoothies: Greek-style yogurt is popular for smoothies because it is thick, creamy and sweet. (Strain thin or watery yogurt through cheesecloth before adding to the blender.) Yogurt may be substituted for cream or milk to make thicker, creamier smoothies. Yogurt made from goat's milk is also readily available and may be used wherever regular yogurt is called for.

Alternative Sources of Calcium

Commercially produced cow's milk, which can be tainted with hormones and antibiotics fed to cattle, may be an overrated source of calcium. Legumes (dried beans and lentils) are an excellent alternative; for example, 1 cup (250 mL) of 2% milk has 121 g of calcium, but $1/2$ cup (125 mL) canned chickpeas with their canning liquid has 143 g of calcium. Other good sources of calcium are leafy greens, broccoli, nuts and sea herbs (see page 148). Raw sesame seeds contain more calcium than any other food (1 oz/30 g contains 162 g of calcium, compared with 1 oz/30 mL whole milk, which contains 18 g of calcium) and make an excellent addition to your diet.

Dairy Alternatives

Soy Milk

People seeking to reduce their saturated fat intake will find soy milk, which is made from soybeans, a versatile and tasty option. It may be substituted for regular milk in all smoothie recipes. Soy milk contains more protein and iron, less fat, fewer calories, no cholesterol and about one-fifth the calcium of cow's milk (for this reason, most soy milk is fortified with extra calcium). Soy milk can be frozen in ice-cube trays for use in smoothies.

Rice Milk

Rice milk, made from brown rice and filtered water, is slightly sweet and, when fortified, provides as much calcium and vitamins A and D as milk. Low in fat, it contains no lactose and is a tasty alternative for people who can not tolerate dairy products. Plain (unflavored) rice milk can be substituted for any milk in the recipes in this book.

Coconut Milk

Coconuts are the fruits of the coconut palm tree (*Cocos nucifera*) but are classified as nuts because they have an edible kernel inside a hard, brittle shell. Coconut meat can be eaten fresh or dried, and the thin, watery juice in fresh coconuts is used in cooking and drinks. (It should not be confused with coconut milk).

The dried meat may be shredded, flaked or compressed into hard cakes. These dried forms are often saturated with sucrose or fructose (sugar) solutions or corn syrup. To make your own Coconut Milk (recipe, page 250), use shredded fresh or unsweetened shredded dried coconut (available at natural-food stores).

Canned coconut milk is widely available but may contain sugar, water and other additives. Check the label and, if possible, purchase unsweetened coconut milk, which may be substituted for any dairy or nondairy milk or homemade coconut milk in smoothies.

Caution: Coconuts are high in saturated fat. One ounce (30 g) of sweetened shredded dried coconut contains 10.1 g of fat (8.9 g of which are saturated). One ounce (30 g) of pecans has 20 g of fat, but only 2 g are saturated, making pecans a healthier choice than coconut.

Nut Milks

When blended with water, nuts make a pleasant, thick liquid that can be used in smoothies. Nut milks (see recipes on pages 248 to 250) can be used to cut the sweetness of fruit smoothies. Nut milks make thicker shakes or smoothies than juice or soy milk and can be substituted for these liquids in most recipes.

Nuts contribute protein, vitamin E and fiber to the diet but should be eaten in small amounts because they are high in fat (although the fat in nuts is mostly unsaturated and contains healthful essential fatty acids). Because they are high in fat, nuts go rancid quickly. Purchase them in bulk-food or natural-food stores with high turnover and taste them before buying. You can store nuts in the freezer to keep them fresher longer.

To make nut milks: Use unsalted organic nuts with the skins intact or shell them yourself. You can also make milks using seeds. Raw sesame seeds are a good choice because they contain more calcium than any other food. Try making a milk using half nuts and half sesame seeds.

Fruit and Nut Milks

Apricot Milk

½ cup	chopped dried apricots	125 mL
1 tbsp	chopped vanilla bean	15 mL

1. In blender, combine 1 cup (250 mL) boiling water, apricots and vanilla bean. Cover with lid and blend on Low for 30 seconds. Gradually (if possible) increase speed to High and blend for 30 seconds more.

2. With blender still running, add another 1 cup (250 mL) boiling water through opening in center of lid. Replace center cover and blend for 30 seconds more or until smooth. Check consistency and add up to an additional ½ cup (125 mL) boiling water if desired, blending until smooth. Let cool. Cover and refrigerate for up to 1 week.

MAKES 2 TO 2½ CUPS (500 TO 625 ML)

TIP
This fruit milk has a unique sweet-tart taste. Use it in any of the fruit shakes or smoothies in this book in place of all or part of the liquid. Look for unsulphured organic dried apricots, to which sulphur dioxide has not been added in the drying process.

Date Milk

¼ cup	chopped pitted dates	50 mL
2 tsp	chopped vanilla bean	10 mL

In blender, combine ½ cup (125 mL) boiling water, dates and vanilla bean. Cover with lid and blend on Low for 30 seconds. Gradually (if possible) increase speed to High and blend for 30 seconds more. Let cool. Cover and refrigerate for up to 1 week.

MAKES ½ CUP (125 ML)

TIP
Date sugar is commonly used in commercial products as a sweetener. Using date milk is like using sugar (although it provides some fiber and a few nutrients), so use it sparingly.

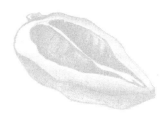

Fig Milk

¼ cup	chopped dried figs (or ⅓ cup/75 mL chopped peeled fresh figs)	50 mL
2 tsp	chopped vanilla bean	10 mL

In blender, combine ½ cup (125 mL) boiling water, figs and vanilla bean. Cover with lid and blend on Low for 30 seconds. Gradually (if possible) increase speed to High and blend for 30 seconds more. Let cool. Cover and refrigerate for up to 1 week.

MAKES ¾ CUP (175 ML)

TIP
Figs have antibacterial, cancer-fighting properties and make a sweet milk that can be used with yogurt or tofu in smoothies. Use fresh figs if available. Dried figs are difficult for machines to chop and should be coarsely chopped by hand before processing in the blender.

Almond Milk

1 cup	finely chopped almonds	250 mL
1 tbsp	finely chopped pitted dates	15 mL
1 tbsp	flax seeds	15 mL
1 tbsp	chopped vanilla bean	15 mL

1. In blender, combine 1 cup (250 mL) boiling water, almonds, dates, flax seeds and vanilla bean. Cover with lid and blend on Low for 30 seconds. Gradually (if possible) increase speed to High and blend for 30 seconds more.

2. With blender still running, add another 1 cup (250 mL) boiling water through opening in center of lid. Replace center cover and blend for 30 seconds more or until smooth. Let cool. Cover and refrigerate for up to 3 days.

MAKES 2 CUPS (500 ML)

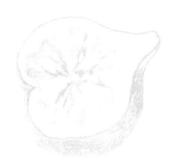

Walnut Milk

¾ cup	finely chopped walnuts	175 mL
1 tbsp	finely chopped pitted dates	15 mL
1 tbsp	flax seeds	15 mL
1 tbsp	chopped vanilla bean	15 mL

1. In blender, combine 1 cup (250 mL) boiling water, walnuts, dates, flax seeds and vanilla bean. Cover with lid and blend on Low for 30 seconds. Gradually (if possible) increase speed to High and blend for 30 seconds more.

2. With blender still running, add another 1 cup (250 mL) boiling water through opening in center of lid. Replace center cover and blend for 30 seconds more or until smooth. Let cool. Cover and refrigerate for up to 3 days.

MAKES 2 CUPS (500 ML)

Cashew Milk

¾ cup	finely chopped cashews	175 mL
1 tbsp	finely chopped dried dulse	15 mL
1 tbsp	finely chopped raisins	15 mL
1 tbsp	chopped vanilla bean	15 mL

1. In blender, combine 1 cup (250 mL) boiling water, cashews, dulse, raisins and vanilla bean. Cover with lid and blend on Low for 30 seconds. Gradually (if possible) increase speed to High and blend for 30 seconds more.

2. With blender still running, add another 1 cup (250 mL) boiling water through opening in center of lid. Replace center cover and blend for 30 seconds more or until smooth. Let cool. Cover and refrigerate for up to 3 days.

MAKES 2 CUPS (500 ML)

Pecan Milk

¾ cup	finely chopped pecans	175 mL
1 tbsp	finely chopped raisins	15 mL
1 tbsp	chopped vanilla bean	15 mL

1. In blender, combine 1 cup (250 mL) boiling water, pecans, raisins and vanilla bean. Cover with lid and blend on Low for 30 seconds. Gradually (if possible) increase speed to High and blend for 30 seconds more.

2. With blender still running, add another 1 cup (250 mL) boiling water through opening in center of lid. Replace center cover and blend for 30 seconds more or until smooth. Let cool. Cover and refrigerate for up to 3 days.

MAKES 2 CUPS (500 ML)

Coconut Milk

½ cup	shredded fresh coconut (or ⅓ cup /75 mL unsweetened shredded dried coconut)	125 mL
2 tsp	chopped vanilla bean	10 mL

In blender, combine ½ cup (125 mL) boiling water, coconut and vanilla bean. Process as directed until smooth. Let cool. Cover and refrigerate for up to 1 week.

MAKES ½ CUP (125 ML)

VARIATION: COCONUT CAROB MILK

Coconut is naturally sweet; when blended with carob, it is even sweeter. For this chocolaty version of coconut milk, add 1 tbsp (15 mL) carob powder to the blender along with the coconut.

TIP
To make this milk, use one fresh coconut and shred the flesh using a regular box grater (freeze any leftovers). If fresh coconut is unavailable, use unsweetened shredded dried coconut, which is available at some natural-food stores. Use coconut milk in frozen drinks, shakes, puddings and other desserts to replace both sugar and milk.

Dairy Smoothies

Always place the lid securely on the blender before processing.
Blend on Low for 30 seconds. Gradually (if possible) increase speed
to High and blend for an additional 30 seconds or until smooth.

Breakfast Blitz

1/2 cup	milk	125 mL
1/2 cup	frozen raspberries or strawberries	125 mL
1	ripe banana, peeled and chopped	1
2 tbsp	chopped almonds or sunflower seeds	25 mL
2 tbsp	wheat germ	25 mL
2 tsp	ground flax seeds	10 mL
1/4 cup	plain yogurt	50 mL
1 tsp	grated fresh ginseng root	5 mL

In blender, combine milk, raspberries, banana, almonds, wheat germ,
flax seeds, yogurt and ginseng. Process as directed until smooth.

SERVES 2

TIP
**This drink lends itself
to any combination of
fresh fruit. Add one
fresh peach, apple
or pear (peel, pit or
seed, and chop it
before adding to the
blender) or $1/4$ cup
(50 mL) chopped
seeded peeled melon,
orange or grapefruit.**

Buttermilk Blush

1/2 cup	buttermilk	125 mL
2	plums, peeled, pitted and chopped	2
1	peach, peeled, pitted and chopped	1
3	frozen strawberries	3

In blender, combine buttermilk, plums, peach and strawberries.
Process as directed until smooth.

SERVES 2

TIP
**You can use powdered
buttermilk in this
recipe. Substitute
$1/2$ cup (125 mL)
water and 1 tbsp
(15 mL) powdered
buttermilk for
the buttermilk.**

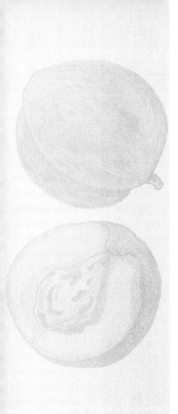

Fruity Splash

½ cup	milk	125 mL
2	nectarines, peeled, pitted and chopped	2
½ cup	pitted cherries	125 mL
½ cup	raspberries	125 mL

In blender, combine milk, nectarines, cherries and raspberries. Process as directed until smooth.

SERVES 2

Orange Juniper

Half	can (6 oz/175 mL can) frozen orange juice concentrate	Half
½ cup	water	125 mL
½ cup	evaporated milk	125 mL
¼ tsp	vanilla	1 mL
4	ice cubes	4

In blender, combine orange juice concentrate, water, milk, vanilla and ice. Process as directed until smooth.

SERVES 1 OR 2

Pink Lassi

½ cup	cranberry juice	125 mL
¼ cup	frozen raspberries	50 mL
6	frozen strawberries	6
¼ cup	plain yogurt	50 mL

In blender, combine cranberry juice, raspberries, strawberries and yogurt. Process as directed until smooth.

SERVES 1

Banan-o-rama

1/2 cup	orange juice	125 mL
1/2 cup	banana-flavored yogurt	125 mL
1	ripe banana, peeled and chopped	1

In blender, combine orange juice, yogurt and banana. Process as directed until smooth.

SERVES 1

General Directions
Always place the lid securely on the blender before processing. Blend on Low for 30 seconds. Gradually (if possible) increase speed to High and blend an additional 30 seconds or until smooth.

Blueberry Banana

2 cups	plain yogurt	500 mL
2 cups	blueberries	500 mL
1	ripe banana, peeled and chopped	1
2 tbsp	pure maple syrup (optional)	25 mL

In blender, combine yogurt, blueberries, banana, and maple syrup (if using). Process as directed until smooth.

SERVES 2

Very Cherry

1	can (12 oz /375 mL) pitted cherries in juice	1
1/2 cup	cherry-flavored or plain yogurt	125 mL
1/4 cup	frozen raspberries	50 mL
4	frozen yogurt or skim milk cubes (see page 273)	4

In blender, combine cherries with juice, yogurt, raspberries and yogurt cubes. Process as directed until smooth.

SERVES 1

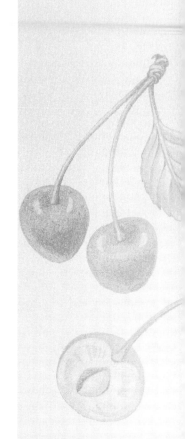

Apple Almond Feta

TIP
Dried apricots
may be substituted
for fresh in
any smoothie.

¼ cup	apple juice	50 mL
¼ cup	Almond Milk (recipe, page 248) or plain soy milk	50 mL
2	apples, peeled, cored and chopped	2
2	apricots, peeled, pitted and chopped	2
3 tbsp	crumbled feta cheese	45 mL

In blender, combine apple juice, almond milk, apples, apricots and cheese. Process as directed until smooth.

SERVES 1

Apricot Cantaloupe

½ cup	orange juice	125 mL
2 tbsp	lime juice	25 mL
3	apricots, peeled, pitted and chopped	3
Quarter	cantaloupe, peeled, seeded and chopped	Quarter
¼ cup	cottage cheese	50 mL

In blender, combine orange juice, lime juice, apricots, cantaloupe and cheese. Process as directed until smooth.

SERVES 2 OR 3

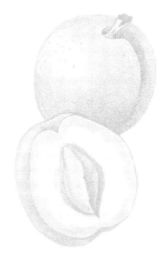

Blue Pear

1/2 cup	pear nectar or apple juice	125 mL
3	pears, peeled, cored and chopped	3
1/4 cup	crumbled blue cheese	50 mL
1/2 tsp	rice vinegar	2 mL
1 tsp	chopped fresh tarragon or basil leaves	5 mL

In blender, combine pear nectar, chopped pears, cheese, vinegar and tarragon. Process as directed until smooth.

SERVES 1

Cherry Cheesecake

1	can (12 oz/375 mL) pitted cherries in juice	1
1/2 cup	vanilla-flavored frozen yogurt	125 mL
3 tbsp	cream cheese	45 mL

In blender, combine cherries with juice, yogurt and cheese. Process as directed until smooth.

SERVES 2 OR 3

Coconut Cream Pie

1/2 cup	Coconut Milk (recipe, page 250)	125 mL
Half	frozen ripe banana, peeled and chopped	Half
1/4 cup	cream cheese	50 mL
2 tbsp	toasted fresh or dried shredded coconut	25 mL
1	container (3.5 oz/99 mL) prepared banana pudding	1

In blender, combine coconut milk, banana, cheese, shredded coconut and banana pudding. Process as directed until smooth.

SERVES 2 OR 3

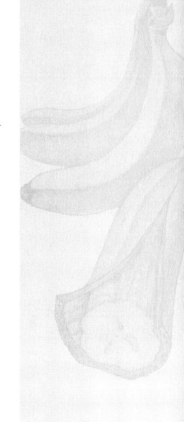

Milk Shakes

Blending Milk Shakes

In blender, combine ingredients (except ice cream). Cover with lid and blend on Low for 30 seconds. Gradually (if possible) increase speed to High and blend an additional 30 seconds or until smooth. Stop motor and add ice cream. Blend on Mix or Medium (or Low if using a two-speed blender) for 20 to 30 seconds or until ice cream is just mixed in. Add more liquid to thin or more ice cream to thicken, if desired.

Banana Chocolate Shake

1 cup	milk	250 mL
1 tbsp	unsweetened cocoa powder or carob powder	15 mL
1	frozen ripe banana, peeled and chopped	1
Pinch	ground nutmeg	Pinch
1 cup	chocolate or vanilla ice cream	250 mL

In blender, combine milk, cocoa powder, banana and nutmeg. Process as directed until smooth. Add ice cream and continue as directed until just mixed in.

SERVES 1

Black Cow

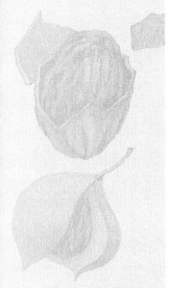

1 cup	chocolate milk	250 mL
1 tbsp	unsweetened cocoa powder or carob powder	15 mL
1	frozen ripe banana, peeled and chopped	1
1 cup	chocolate ice cream	250 mL

In blender, combine chocolate milk, cocoa powder and banana. Process as directed until smooth. Add ice cream and continue as directed until just mixed in.

SERVES 1

TIP
Try making your own blender ice cream using the recipes on pages 290 to 292.

Dairy and Dairy Alternative Smoothies

Blueberry Banana Shake

½ cup	milk	125 mL
½ cup	frozen blueberries	125 mL
1	ripe banana, peeled and chopped	1
1 tbsp	chopped pitted dates	15 mL
1 cup	vanilla-flavored frozen yogurt or ice cream	250 mL

In blender, combine milk, blueberries, banana and dates. Process as directed until smooth. Add frozen yogurt and continue as directed until just mixed in.

SERVES 1

Chocolate Malted

1 cup	milk	250 mL
2 tbsp	unsweetened cocoa powder or carob powder	25 mL
2 tbsp	malted milk powder (such as Ovaltine)	25 mL
1 cup	chocolate or coffee ice cream	250 mL

In blender, combine milk, cocoa powder and malted milk powder. Process as directed until smooth. Add ice cream and continue as directed until just mixed in.

SERVES 1

Chocolate Minted Shake

½ cup	milk	125 mL
1 tbsp	chopped fresh peppermint leaves	15 mL
2	small chocolate-covered peppermint patties	2
1 cup	chocolate ice cream	250 mL

In blender, combine milk, chopped peppermint and patties. Process as directed until smooth. Add ice cream and continue as directed until just mixed in.

SERVES 1

TIP
Try making your own **blender ice cream** (see recipes, **pages 290 to 292**) for **use in** these shakes.

Chocolate Peanut Butter Banana Slurry

¾ cup	milk or plain soy milk	175 mL
1	ripe banana, peeled and chopped	1
2 tbsp	peanut butter	25 mL
1 tbsp	carob powder or unsweetened cocoa powder	15 mL
2 cups	chocolate ice cream or frozen yogurt	500 mL

In blender, combine milk, banana, peanut butter and carob powder. Process as directed until smooth. Add ice cream and continue as directed until just mixed in.

SERVES 1

Gingered Cantaloupe Shake

½ cup	Coconut Milk (recipe, page 250)	125 mL
Half	cantaloupe, peeled, seeded and chopped	Half
1 tbsp	chopped candied ginger	15 mL
2 cups	vanilla ice cream or frozen yogurt	500 mL

In blender, combine coconut milk, cantaloupe and ginger. Process as directed until smooth. Add ice cream and continue as directed until just mixed in.

SERVES 1

Mocha Almond Shake

1/2 cup	Almond Milk (recipe, page 248)	125 mL
4	chocolate-covered coffee beans	4
1/8 tsp	almond extract	0.5 mL
2 cups	chocolate ice cream	500 mL

In blender, combine almond milk, coffee beans and almond extract. Process as directed until smooth. Add ice cream and continue as directed until just mixed in.

SERVES 1 OR 2

Peach Parfait

1/2 cup	peach nectar or orange juice	125 mL
1 cup	frozen sliced peaches	250 mL
1/2 cup	peach-flavored frozen yogurt or ice cream	125 mL

In blender, combine peach nectar and sliced peaches. Process as directed until smooth. Add frozen yogurt and continue as directed until just mixed in.

SERVES 1

Peanut Butter and Jelly Shake

1/2 cup	milk or plain soy milk	125 mL
1	container (6 oz/175 g) fruit-on-the-bottom yogurt	1
1	ripe banana, peeled and chopped	1
2 tbsp	peanut butter	25 mL
1/2 cup	vanilla ice cream	125 mL

In blender, combine milk, yogurt, banana and peanut butter. Process as directed until smooth. Add ice cream and continue as directed until just mixed in.

SERVES 1

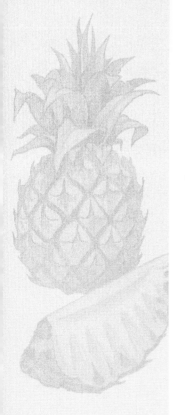

Pineapple Colada Shake

1/2 cup	Coconut Milk (recipe, page 250)	125 mL
1	can (8 oz/227 mL) crushed pineapple, drained	1
2 tbsp	toasted shredded fresh or dried coconut	25 mL
3 cups	vanilla ice cream	750 mL

In blender, combine coconut milk, pineapple and shredded coconut. Process as directed until smooth. Add ice cream and continue as directed until just mixed in.

SERVES 2

Pink Cow

1 cup	milk	250 mL
6	frozen strawberries	6
Half	frozen ripe banana, peeled and chopped	Half
1 cup	strawberry ice cream	250 mL

In blender, combine milk, strawberries and banana. Process as directed until smooth. Add ice cream and continue as directed until just mixed in.

SERVES 1

Razzy Chocolate Slush

1/2 cup	frozen raspberries	125 mL
1/4 cup	cranberry-raspberry juice	50 mL
4	frozen chocolate milk cubes (see page 273), crushed	4
1 cup	chocolate ice cream	250 mL

In blender, combine raspberries, cranberry-raspberry juice and chocolate milk cubes. Process as directed until smooth. Add ice cream and continue as directed until just mixed in.

SERVES 1

Dairy Alternative Smoothies

Always place the lid securely on the blender before processing. Blend on Low for 30 seconds. Gradually (if possible) increase speed to High and blend for an additional 30 seconds or until smooth.

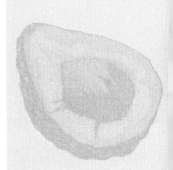

Avocado Shake

1 cup	plain soy milk	250 mL
	Juice of half a lemon	
1	avocado, peeled, pitted and chopped	1
1	grapefruit, peeled, seeded and chopped	1
1 tbsp	molasses	15 mL

In blender, combine soy milk, lemon juice, avocado, grapefruit and molasses. Process as directed until smooth.

SERVES 1

Breakfast in Brazil

¾ cup	plain soy milk or Coconut Milk (recipe, page 250)	175 mL
¾ cup	frozen strawberries	175 mL
1	ripe banana, peeled and chopped	1
2 tbsp	chopped Brazil nuts	25 mL
2 tbsp	wheat germ or steel-cut or rolled oats	25 mL
1 tsp	cod liver oil (optional)	5 mL
⅛ tsp	ground cinnamon	0.5 mL

In blender, combine soy milk, strawberries, banana, Brazil nuts, wheat germ, cod liver oil (if using), and cinnamon. Process as directed until smooth.

SERVES 2

Caribbean Crush

¾ cup	plain soy milk or Coconut Milk (recipe, page 250)	175 mL
	Juice of half a lime	
Half	mango, peeled, pitted and chopped	Half
1	kiwi, peeled and chopped	1

In blender, combine soy milk, lime juice, mango and kiwi. Process as directed until smooth.

SERVES 1

Orange Soy

½ cup	plain soy milk	125 mL
2	oranges, peeled, seeded and chopped	2
½ cup	frozen sliced peaches	125 mL
2	ice cubes	2

In blender, combine soy milk, oranges, peaches and ice. Process as directed until smooth.

SERVES 1 OR 2

Peach Coconut

1 cup	canned peaches with juice	250 mL
¼ cup	Coconut Milk (recipe, page 250)	50 mL
¼ cup	chopped peeled pineapple	50 mL
4	frozen plain soy milk cubes (see page 273)	4

In blender, combine peaches with juice, coconut milk, pineapple and soy milk cubes. Process as directed until smooth.

SERVES 2

Peach Pie

1/4 cup	pineapple juice	50 mL
1/4 cup	Coconut Milk (recipe, page 250)	50 mL
1 cup	sliced pitted peeled peaches	250 mL
1/4 cup	chopped peeled pineapple	50 mL
2 tbsp	plain or toasted unsweetened shredded dried coconut	25 mL
1/2 tsp	vanilla	2 mL

In blender, combine pineapple juice, coconut milk, peaches, chopped pineapple, shredded coconut and vanilla. Process as directed until smooth.

SERVES 2 OR 3

General Directions
Always place the lid securely on the blender before processing. Blend on Low for 30 seconds. Gradually (if possible) increase speed to High and blend an additional 30 seconds or until smooth.

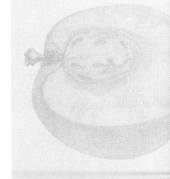

Strawberry Soy

1/2 cup	plain soy milk	125 mL
12	strawberries (hulled and halved if fresh)	12
1/2 cup	frozen sliced peaches	125 mL
2	ice cubes	2

In blender, combine soy milk, strawberries, peaches and ice. Process as directed until smooth.

SERVES 2

TIP
Using frozen fruit in smoothies thickens and chills the drink. Substitute the same quantity of fresh fruit, if desired.

Tropical Tonic

1/4 cup	plain soy milk	50 mL
1/4 cup	Coconut Milk (recipe, page 250)	50 mL
1/2 cup	chopped peeled pineapple	125 mL
1	ripe banana, peeled and chopped	1

In blender, combine soy milk, coconut milk, pineapple and banana. Process as directed until smooth.

SERVES 1

General Directions
Always place the lid securely on the blender before processing. Blend on Low for 30 seconds. Gradually (if possible) increase speed to High and blend an additional 30 seconds or until smooth.

TIP
You can substitute dried apricots for fresh in any smoothie.

Almond Cherry

½ cup	Almond Milk (recipe, page 248)	125 mL
½ cup	pitted cherries	125 mL
½ cup	frozen raspberries	125 mL
⅛ tsp	almond extract	0.5 mL

In blender, combine almond milk, cherries, raspberries and almond extract. Process as directed until smooth.

SERVES 1

Just Peachy Almond

¾ cup	Almond Milk (recipe, page 248)	175 mL
½ cup	frozen sliced peaches	125 mL
4	apricots, peeled, pitted and chopped	4
⅛ tsp	almond extract	0.5 mL

In blender, combine almond milk, peaches, apricots and almond extract. Process as directed until smooth.

SERVES 2

Almond Raspberry

¾ cup	Almond Milk (recipe, page 248)	175 mL
½ cup	frozen raspberries	125 mL
2	plums, peeled, pitted and chopped	2
⅛ tsp	almond extract	0.5 mL

In blender, combine almond milk, raspberries, plums and almond extract. Process as directed until smooth.

SERVES 1

Banana Frappé

1 cup	Almond Milk (recipe, page 248)	250 mL
1/2 cup	silken tofu	125 mL
1	frozen ripe banana, peeled and chopped	1
1 tbsp	carob powder or unsweetened cocoa powder	15 mL
1/8 tsp	almond extract (optional)	0.5 mL

In blender, combine almond milk, tofu, banana, carob powder, and almond extract (if using). Process as directed until smooth.

SERVES 1

Gingered Almond

3/4 cup	Almond Milk (recipe, page 248)	175 mL
1	piece (1 inch/2.5 cm long) candied ginger, chopped	1
1/4 cup	chopped peeled pineapple	50 mL
Half	frozen ripe banana, peeled and chopped	Half
1/8 tsp	almond extract	0.5 mL

In blender, combine almond milk, ginger, pineapple, banana and almond extract. Process as directed until smooth.

SERVES 1

TIP
Using frozen fruit in smoothies thickens and chills the drink. Substitute the same quantity of fresh fruit, if desired.

Chocolate Pecan

¾ cup	Pecan Milk (recipe, page 250)	175 mL
½ cup	frozen sliced peaches	125 mL
½ cup	chopped peeled pineapple	125 mL
1 tbsp	carob powder or unsweetened cocoa powder	15 mL
4	frozen juice (see page 273) or ice cubes	4

In blender, combine pecan milk, peaches, pineapple, carob powder and juice cubes. Process as directed until smooth.

SERVES 1

Baklava

¾ cup	Walnut Milk (recipe, page 249)	175 mL
1 tbsp	sesame seeds	15 mL
1 tbsp	liquid honey	15 mL
½ cup	frozen sliced peaches	125 mL

In blender, combine walnut milk, sesame seeds, honey and peaches. Process as directed until smooth.

SERVES 1

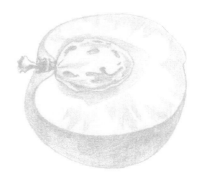

Coconut Carob Orange

¼ cup	Coconut Carob Milk (recipe, page 250)	50 mL
¼ cup	orange juice	50 mL
½ cup	plain yogurt	125 mL
1 tbsp	carob powder	15 mL
1 tsp	grated orange zest (optional)	5 mL
3	ice cubes	3

In blender, combine coconut carob milk, orange juice, yogurt, carob powder, orange zest (if using), and ice. Process as directed until smooth.

SERVES 2

Piña Colada

¾ cup	Coconut Milk (recipe, page 250)	175 mL
½ cup	chopped peeled pineapple	125 mL
1	kiwi, peeled and chopped	1
½ cup	frozen plain soy milk cubes (see page 273)	125 mL

In blender, combine coconut milk, pineapple, kiwi and soy milk cubes. Process as directed until smooth.

SERVES 1

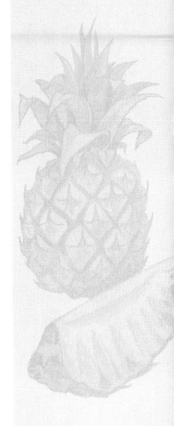

Date and Nut

TIP
Add 1 tbsp
(15 mL) chopped
pitted dates to
the ingredients if
you are using soy
milk instead of
Date Milk.

1 cup	Date Milk (recipe, page 247) or plain soy milk	250 mL
1/2 cup	silken tofu	125 mL
2	apples, peeled, cored and chopped	2
1 tbsp	chopped almonds	15 mL
Pinch	ground nutmeg	Pinch

In blender, combine date milk, tofu, apples, almonds and nutmeg.
Process as directed until smooth.

SERVES 1 OR 2

Beta Whiz

TIP
This drink is
thick and has the
refreshing taste of
cantaloupe. For a
thinner consistency,
increase the carrot
juice by 1/4 cup
(50 mL). Look for
buckwheat flakes in
natural-food stores.

1/2 cup	Fig Milk (recipe, page 248)	125 mL
1/4 cup	carrot or orange juice	50 mL
Quarter	cantaloupe, peeled, seeded and chopped	Quarter
1 tbsp	chopped almonds	15 mL
1 tbsp	buckwheat flakes	15 mL

In blender, combine fig milk, carrot juice, cantaloupe, almonds and
buckwheat flakes. Process as directed until smooth.

SERVES 1

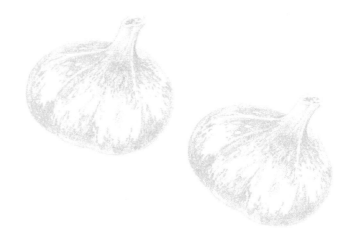

Peach Fuzz

½ cup	Fig Milk (recipe, page 248) or plain soy milk	125 mL
¼ cup	peach or apricot nectar or orange juice	50 mL
¾ cup	frozen sliced peaches	175 mL
2	apricots, peeled, pitted and chopped	2
4	ice cubes	4

In blender, combine fig milk, peach nectar, frozen peaches, apricots and ice. Process as directed until smooth.

SERVES 1 OR 2

TIP
You can use dried apricots instead of fresh in any smoothie.

Blueberry Frappé

1 cup	Apricot Milk (recipe, page 247) or apricot nectar	250 mL
½ cup	silken tofu	125 mL
½ cup	frozen blueberries	125 mL
4	ice cubes	4

In blender, combine apricot milk, tofu, blueberries and ice. Process as directed until smooth.

SERVES 1 OR 2

TIP
Any berries — blueberries, raspberries, strawberries, blackberries or even black currants — work well in this smoothie.

General Directions
Always place the lid securely on the blender before processing. Blend on Low for 30 seconds. Gradually (if possible) increase speed to High and blend an additional 30 seconds or until smooth.

Hot and Frozen Smoothies

SMOOTHIES ARE IDEAL AS ICY SUMMER COOLERS OR WARMING winter toddies because they are packed with potent nutrients — vitamins, minerals, phytochemicals and enzymes. Not only do they soothe or refresh (depending on their temperature), they promote health and supply energy at the same time. Made at home from nutritious ingredients, smoothies are far more healthful than hot powdered citrus drinks that may give temporary relief from the symptoms of a cold or flu, or chilled sugar-heavy beverages that provide an instant but short-lived energy boost.

Hot Smoothies

Comforting and soothing, warm toddies and mulled drinks hark back to earlier times, when thick, syrupy medicinal "robs" were stirred into hot teas and administered to relieve cold symptoms and bronchial problems.

The usual method for making hot smoothies is to add hot liquids (scalded milk, hot broth, herbal tea or boiling water) to the other ingredients before blending. Another technique is to cook the main ingredients before blending and add them to the remaining ingredients while they are still hot. Alternatively, ingredients may be blended while cold or at room temperature, then heated in a saucepan on the stovetop or in the microwave. Adding "hot" herbs, such as ginger, turmeric and cayenne (or other chile peppers), can add a unique warming touch to smoothies.

Blending Hot Liquids

Place half of any hot liquid in the blender jug with the solid ingredients and blend for 30 seconds. With the blender still running, add the remaining hot liquid gradually through the opening in the center of the lid. This prevents a surge of hot liquid from being forced upward, which might cause the lid to blow off.

Using boiling water: In recipes in which boiling water is required, bring a kettle of water to a boil, remove it from the heat and allow the bubbles to subside before measuring and adding to the ingredients in the blender.

Heating Milk

When milk or cream is heated for use in smoothies, it is scalded rather than boiled, which can result in scorching.

To scald milk or cream: Measure milk or cream into a small saucepan and heat over low heat, stirring occasionally, just until bubbles form around the edge of the pan. Remove from the heat and use immediately.

Frozen Smoothies

Thick, cold and refreshing, there is no better way to bring your body temperature down after a workout or during the intense heat of summer than with a frozen blended drink. Consuming nutrients along with water sends energy and food to muscles while rehydrating the system. You can easily turn ordinary fruit smoothies into slushy treats that require a spoon by adding ice, frozen fruit (see page 154 for how to freeze fresh fruit) and/or frozen unsweetened juice concentrates. Ice makes smoothies not only cold but also thicker.

Making Frozen Smoothies

In addition to ice (or other liquid that has been frozen into cubes), frozen fruit or frozen juice concentrates, some liquid (milk, yogurt, juice or nut or fruit milk) is required to make frozen smoothies. This liquid must be added to the jug before the frozen ingredients. Never add ice to the jug and try to process it unless there is some liquid in the bottom. The frozen smoothie recipes are very thick and require a spoon; add more liquid if a thinner drink is desired.

Using Ice in Frozen Smoothies

When adding ice to smoothies, you are actually adding liquid to the drink. If a large quantity of ice is used, the flavor of the smoothie will be diluted. To compensate, reduce the quantity of other liquids. Using undiluted frozen fruit juice concentrates instead of ice is one technique for maintaining flavor intensity while adding that frozen texture.

To facilitate the removal of frozen cubes, let ice-cube trays stand at room temperature for three to five minutes before using. This also makes it easier to chop the cubes.

LIQUID EQUIVALENTS FOR ICE

1 ice cube = approximately 1 1/2 tbsp (22 mL) liquid

6 ice cubes = approximately 1/2 cup (125 mL) liquid

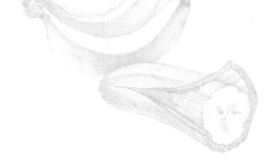

Add Flavor, Thicken and Chill

Flavored ice cubes

For a concentrated taste, substitute flavored ice cubes for regular ice cubes in smoothie recipes. Make flavored ice cubes by freezing juice, herbal teas, strong coffee, leftover smoothie mixtures, soy milk, nut or fruit milks, or yogurt in ice-cube trays.

Frozen yogurt cubes

Drain and discard liquid from a 16-oz (500 g) container of plain yogurt. Spoon into ice-cube trays and freeze. Use in smoothies where frozen yogurt is called for. Use six frozen yogurt cubes to replace one scoop or 1/2 cup (125 mL) frozen yogurt.

Frozen milk cubes

Plain or chocolate milk can be frozen in ice-cube trays to replace ice cream in milk-shake recipes. Use six frozen milk cubes to replace one scoop or 1/2 cup (125 mL) ice cream. To reduce the amount of fat in the drink, use low-fat or skim milk.

Frozen fruit juice concentrates

Frozen unsweetened fruit juice concentrates can be added straight from the can when making frozen smoothies. Run the container under hot water and soften just enough so that the contents can be squeezed directly into the blender jug. When only half a can is required, squeeze the remaining half into a resealable plastic freezer bag, label and refreeze immediately.

Blender Ice Cream, Frozen Yogurt and Sorbet

The recipes for blender ice cream, frozen yogurt and sorbet (see pages 290 to 293) may be used wherever similarly flavored ice cream, frozen yogurt or sorbet are called for in smoothie recipes. The blender ice creams and frozen yogurts are very soft and should really be called "ice milks" because most of them do not contain cream. Although cream may be used instead of milk, it is higher in fat. If a more-solid result is desired, freeze the blended mixture in a metal loaf pan for one to two hours. Due to their low sugar content, these frozen mixtures will freeze rock-solid if left in the freezer for longer, so plan to use them within two hours. With a stock of skim and chocolate milk cubes in the freezer, ice cream and frozen yogurt is quick and easy to make. In addition, these treats have the following benefits over their commercial equivalents:
- lower sugar content;
- all natural ingredients;
- no chemical additives or preservatives; and
- little (or very low) fat, without the gums and other additives used in commercial low-fat frozen desserts.

Adding a Large Number of Ice Cubes to Smoothies

With an Ice Crush setting:

If using more than five ice cubes in one recipe, add half of the ice cubes and all the other ingredients to the blender jug. Process on Ice Crush or Chop for 30 seconds, then add remaining ice cubes and process on Ice Crush or Chop for 30 seconds more or just until smooth.

Without an Ice Crush setting:

When making frozen drinks that require more than five ice cubes in a blender without an Ice Crush setting, the ice cubes must be crushed before you add them to the blender. Place cubes in a resealable plastic freezer bag, remove excess air, seal and place on a cutting board. Smash the cubes with a rolling pin or frying pan until the pieces are the size of quarters. Measure, add to the ingredients in the blender jug and blend for 10 seconds on Medium (or Low if you have a two-speed blender). Stop the motor, stir, replace the lid and blend for 10 seconds more. Repeat these steps until the ice is blended into the drink.

MAKING ICE CREAM, FROZEN YOGURT AND SORBET IN THE BLENDER

When making blender ice cream, frozen yogurt or sorbet, chill any liquid that you will be adding and keep frozen fruit or concentrates in the freezer until you are ready to use them. Allow ice or other frozen cubes to soften slightly at room temperature before adding to the blender. Add liquid ingredients to the blender jug first, then frozen ingredients and ice. Use the Ice Crush setting or crush first and use the blend/stop/stir/blend method described above.

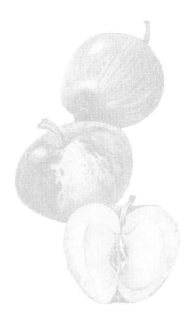

Hot Smoothies

General Directions

Place required amount of hot liquid in the blender with the other ingredients. Place the lid securely on the jug. Blend on Low for 30 seconds. With blender still running, add the remaining hot liquid gradually through the opening in the center of the lid. Replace center cover securely, increase speed to High and process for 30 seconds or until smooth.

Blazing Bullshot

2 cups	hot beef, chicken or vegetable stock, divided	500 mL
Half to 1	chile pepper, chopped	Half to 1
2	tomatoes, cored and chopped	2
1	stalk celery, chopped	1
1 tbsp	lemon juice	15 mL
1/2 tsp	Worcestershire sauce	2 mL
1/4 tsp	garam masala (optional)	1 mL

In blender, combine 1 cup (250 mL) stock, chile pepper, tomatoes, celery, lemon juice, Worcestershire sauce, and garam masala (if using). Process as directed above.

SERVES 2 OR 3

Café au Lait

1 cup	scalded skim milk (see page 271) or soy milk, divided	250 mL
1/4 tsp	vanilla	1 mL
1/8 tsp	ground cinnamon	0.5 mL
1 cup	hot strong brewed coffee	250 mL

In blender, combine 1/2 cup (125 mL) milk, vanilla and cinnamon. Process as directed above. To serve, combine milk mixture and coffee.

SERVES 2

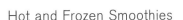

Citrus Toddy

TIP
This makes a thick drink. For a thinner result, use the juice of the orange and the juice of one whole grapefruit instead of the whole fruit.

1 cup	boiling water, divided	250 mL
2 tbsp	liquid honey (or to taste)	25 mL
	Juice of 1 lemon	
1	orange, peeled, seeded and chopped	1
Half	grapefruit, peeled, seeded and chopped	Half
1	piece ($\frac{1}{2}$ inch/1 cm) gingerroot, peeled and chopped	1
1 tsp	dried elderflowers (optional)	5 mL

In blender, combine $\frac{1}{2}$ cup (125 mL) boiling water, honey, lemon juice, orange, grapefruit, ginger, and elderflowers (if using). Process as directed at right.

SERVES 2 OR 3

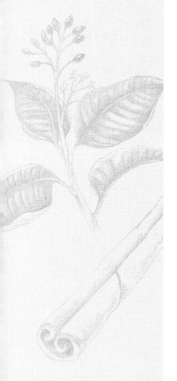

Hot Chai

2 cups	skim milk or soy milk	500 mL
1	green or black tea bag (or 2 tsp/10 mL loose tea)	1
1	piece ($\frac{1}{2}$ inch/1 cm) candied ginger, chopped	1
$\frac{1}{4}$ tsp	ground cinnamon	1 mL
3	black peppercorns	3
1	whole clove	1
$\frac{1}{8}$ tsp	ground cardamom (optional)	0.5 mL
2 tbsp	liquid honey (or to taste)	25 mL

1. In a medium saucepan over medium heat, bring milk, tea, ginger, cinnamon, peppercorns, clove, and cardamom (if using), just to a simmer. Remove from heat; strain and discard tea bags and herbs.
2. In blender, combine half of the milk mixture with the honey. Process as directed at right.

SERVES 2

Hot Chocolate

2 cups	scalded milk or table (18%) cream (see page 271), divided	500 mL
1 tbsp	unsweetened cocoa powder or carob powder	15 mL
1 tbsp	granulated sugar	15 mL
1 oz	bittersweet chocolate, chopped	30 g
¼ tsp	vanilla	1 mL

In blender, combine 1 cup (250 mL) scalded milk, cocoa powder, sugar, chopped chocolate and vanilla. Process as directed at right.

SERVES 2

General Directions
Place required amount of hot liquid in the blender with the other ingredients. Place the lid securely on the jug. Blend on Low for 30 seconds. With blender still running, add the remaining hot liquid gradually through the opening in the center of the lid. Replace center cover securely, increase speed to High and process for 30 seconds or until smooth.

Hot Gingered Apple Cider

1 cup	apple cider or apple juice	250 mL
2 tbsp	liquid honey (or to taste)	25 mL
1	piece (½ inch/1 cm) candied ginger, chopped	1
⅛ tsp	ground cinnamon	0.5 mL
⅛ tsp	ground cloves	0.5 mL
Pinch	ground nutmeg	Pinch
1	apple, peeled, cored and chopped	1
1 tsp	apple cider vinegar	5 mL

1. In a medium saucepan over medium heat, bring apple cider, honey, ginger, cinnamon, cloves and nutmeg just to a boil.
2. In blender, combine half of the cider mixture, the apple and cider vinegar. Process as directed at right.

SERVES 2

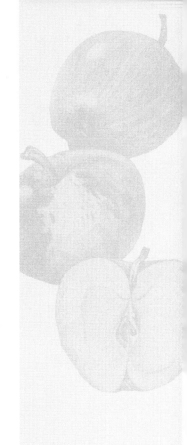

Hot Spiced Pear

³⁄₄ cup	pear nectar or apple cider	175 mL
1 tsp	balsamic vinegar	5 mL
¼ tsp	ground nutmeg	1 mL
Pinch	ground cloves	Pinch
3	pears, peeled, cored and chopped	3
2 tbsp	raisins	25 mL

1. In a medium saucepan over medium heat, bring pear nectar, vinegar, nutmeg and cloves just to a boil.

2. In blender, combine half of the pear nectar mixture, the pears and raisins. Process as directed at least.

SERVES 1

Mexican Hot Hot Chocolate

1 cup	scalded milk (see page 271), divided	250 mL
2 tbsp	liquid honey (or to taste)	25 mL
1 tbsp	chopped bittersweet chocolate	15 mL
1 tsp	chopped candied ginger	5 mL
¼ tsp	vanilla	1 mL
⅛ tsp	ground cinnamon	0.5 mL
⅛ tsp	hot pepper flakes or cayenne pepper	0.5 mL

In blender, combine ¹⁄₂ cup (125 mL) scalded milk, honey, chocolate, ginger, vanilla, cinnamon and hot pepper flakes. Process as directed at left.

SERVES 1

Wassail

4	apples	4
1/4 cup	raisins	50 mL
4 tsp	butter	20 mL
1/4 cup	liquid honey	50 mL
2 cups	apple cider or apple juice	500 mL
1/2 tsp	ground cinnamon, divided	2 mL
1/4 tsp	ground allspice, divided	1 mL
1/4 tsp	ground cloves, divided	1 mL
4	sticks (each 2 inches/5 cm long) cinnamon	4

1. Using a melon baller or teaspoon, core apples from tops, making a cavity but leaving bottoms intact. Place, hollow side up, on prepared baking sheet. Stuff each apple with one-quarter each of the raisins and butter. Drizzle each with one-quarter of the honey. Bake in preheated oven for 30 minutes or until tender. Let cool. Remove and discard skins.

2. Meanwhile, in a saucepan over medium-high heat, bring cider to a simmer. Reduce heat to low and keep cider warm.

3. In blender, combine 1 cup (250 mL) cider, 1/4 tsp (1 mL) cinnamon and 1/8 tsp (0.5 mL) each allspice and cloves. Blend on Low for 30 seconds. Stop blender and add 2 of the baked apples. Cover with lid and blend for 1 minute more. Gradually (if possible) increase speed to High and blend for 30 seconds more or until smooth. Pour into 2 warmed heatproof mugs and garnish each with 1 cinnamon stick. Repeat with remaining hot cider, cinnamon, allspice, cloves, baked apples and cinnamon sticks.

**SERVES 4 ● PREHEAT OVEN TO 375°F (190°C)
RIMMED BAKING SHEET, LIGHTLY GREASED**

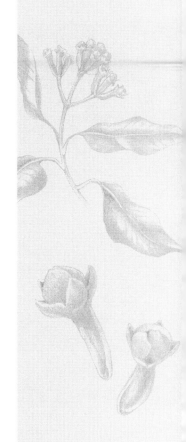

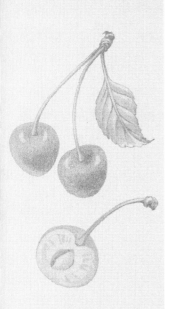

Frozen Smoothies

General Directions

Always place the lid securely on the blender before processing. If the recipe contains more than five ice cubes, follow the instructions on page 274, according to whether you have an Ice Crush setting. If the recipe does not contain more than five ice cubes, blend on Low for 30 seconds. Gradually (if possible) increase speed to High and blend for an additional 30 seconds or until smooth.

Chocolate Cherry Chiller

1 cup	chocolate milk	250 mL
1 cup	frozen pitted cherries	250 mL
1/2 cup	chocolate frozen yogurt (see recipe on page 292)	125 mL

In blender, combine chocolate milk, cherries and frozen yogurt. Process as directed until smooth.

SERVES 2

TIP
You can substitute 6 frozen chocolate milk cubes for the frozen yogurt in this smoothie.

Frozen Lemonade

1/4 cup	frozen lemonade concentrate	50 mL
2	lemons, peeled, seeded and chopped	2
6	ice cubes, divided and crushed, if necessary (see page 274)	6
3 tbsp	liquid honey (or to taste)	45 mL

In blender, combine lemonade concentrate, lemons, 3 ice cubes and honey. Process as directed on page 274 until smooth. Serve immediately with a spoon.

SERVES 1

TIP
Make frozen limeade by using frozen limeade concentrate and limes instead of lemons.

Frozen Mint Julep

½ cup	chilled brewed green or black tea	125 mL
½ cup	frozen pineapple juice concentrate	125 mL
1 tsp	grated lemon zest	5 mL
1 tbsp	lemon juice	15 mL
1 tsp	chopped candied ginger	5 mL
1 tbsp	granulated sugar (or to taste)	15 mL
1 tbsp	chopped fresh peppermint leaves	15 mL
6	ice cubes, divided and crushed if necessary (see page 274)	6

In blender, combine tea, pineapple juice concentrate, lemon zest and juice, ginger, sugar, peppermint and 3 ice cubes. Process as directed on page 274. Serve immediately with a spoon.

SERVES 2

Gingered Lemonade

¾ cup	lemon juice	175 mL
8	ice cubes, divided and crushed if necessary (see pages 274)	8
1 tbsp	chopped candied ginger	15 mL
2 tbsp	granulated sugar (or to taste)	25 mL
1 cup	sparkling mineral water or soda water	250 mL

In blender, combine lemon juice, 4 ice cubes, ginger and sugar. Process as directed on page 274 until smooth. Divide among glasses; divide mineral water evenly among glasses. Stir to combine.

SERVES 2 OR 3

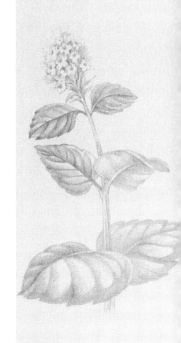

General Directions
Always place the lid securely on the blender before processing. If the recipe contains more then five ice cubes, follow the instructions on page 274, according to whether you have an Ice Crush setting. If the recipe does not contain more than five ice cubes, blend on Low for 30 seconds. Gradually (if possible) increase speed to High and blend for an additional 30 seconds or until smooth.

Golden Nectar Glacé

¾ cup	peach nectar	175 mL
¼ cup	frozen orange juice concentrate	50 mL
4	ice cubes	4
Quarter	cantaloupe, peeled, seeded and chopped	Quarter

In blender, combine peach nectar, orange juice concentrate, ice and cantaloupe. Process as directed until smooth. Serve immediately with a spoon.

SERVES 1 OR 2

Grapefruit Rosemary Granita

½ cup	grapefruit juice	125 mL
3	ice cubes	3
2 cups	lemon sorbet	500 mL
½ tsp	chopped fresh rosemary leaves	2 mL

In blender, combine grapefruit juice, ice, sorbet and rosemary. Process as directed until smooth. Serve immediately with a spoon.

SERVES 2

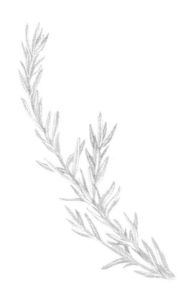

Iced Citrus Tea

1	lemon	1
1	orange	1
4 cups	boiling water	1 L
3	black or green tea bags	3
2	whole cloves	2
1	stick (2 inches/5 cm long) cinnamon	1
¼ cup	liquid honey (or to taste)	50 mL
16	ice cubes, divided and crushed, if necessary (see page 274)	16
6	slices orange or lemon	6

1. Peel lemon and orange; remove and discard bitter pith. Chop peel and set aside. Chop pulp and set aside separately.

2. In a large teapot, pour boiling water over chopped lemon and orange rinds, tea bags, cloves and cinnamon. Cover and steep for 5 minutes. Strain, discarding rind and spices. Chill tea.

3. In blender, combine half each of the tea, lemon and orange pulp, honey and ice. Process as directed on page 274 until smooth. Pour into 3 glasses; garnish each with 1 lemon or orange slice. Repeat with remaining tea, lemon and orange pulp, honey, ice, and lemon and orange slices.

SERVES 6

Green Tea on Ice

1 cup	boiling water	250 mL
1 tbsp	green or chai tea leaves	15 mL
2 tbsp	liquid honey (or to taste)	25 mL
¼ tsp	ground cinnamon or garam masala	1 mL
6	ice cubes, divided and crushed, if necessary (see page 274)	6

1. In a small teapot, pour boiling water over tea, honey and cinnamon. Cover and steep for 10 minutes. Strain, discarding leaves. Let cool. Chill in refrigerator if time allows.

2. In blender, combine cooled tea and 3 ice cubes. Process as directed on page 274 until smooth. Serve immediately with a spoon.

SERVES 1 OR 2

Hot and Frozen Smoothies

Iced Vanilla Custard

TIP
You can substitute
10 crushed frozen
skim milk cubes
(see page 273) for
the frozen yogurt.

1 cup	milk	250 mL
1	piece (2 inches /5 cm long) vanilla bean (or $1/2$ tsp/2 mL vanilla)	1
1 tbsp	granulated sugar	15 mL
2	egg yolks	2
1 cup	vanilla-flavored frozen yogurt or ice cream	250 mL

1. In a small saucepan over medium heat, heat milk, vanilla bean and sugar until small bubbles form around the edge of the pan. Meanwhile, in a medium bowl, beat egg yolks until pale and thickened.

2. Gradually whisk half of the hot milk mixture into egg yolks. Whisk egg mixture back into saucepan. Reduce heat to low and cook, stirring constantly, for 5 to 7 minutes or until custard is thick enough to coat the back of a spoon. Do not let custard boil. Strain into a small bowl. Place plastic wrap directly on surface and let cool. Chill in refrigerator if time allows.

3. In blender, combine cooled custard and frozen yogurt. Process as directed until smooth. Serve immediately with a spoon.

SERVES 1 OR 2

Lemon Mint Iced Tea

2 cups	chilled strong brewed tea	500 mL
6	ice cubes, divided and crushed, if necessary (see page 274)	6
$1/4$ cup	lemon juice	50 mL
3 tbsp	liquid honey (or to taste)	45 mL
1 tbsp	chopped fresh peppermint leaves	15 mL

In blender, combine tea, 3 ice cubes, lemon juice, honey and peppermint. Process as directed on page 274 until smooth. Serve immediately with a spoon.

SERVES 2

Lemon Peach Granita

1 cup	orange juice	250 mL
1 cup	frozen sliced peaches	250 mL
1 tbsp	chopped fresh lemon verbena leaves (optional)	15 mL
1 tbsp	liquid honey (or to taste)	15 mL
4	ice cubes	4

In blender, combine orange juice, peaches, lemon verbena (if using), honey and ice. Process as directed until smooth. Serve immediately with a spoon.

SERVES 1 OR 2

General Directions
Always place the lid securely on the blender before processing. If the recipe contains more then five ice cubes, follow the instructions on page 274, according to whether you have an Ice Crush setting. If the recipe does not contain more than five ice cubes, blend on Low for 30 seconds. Gradually (if possible) increase speed to High and blend for an additional 30 seconds or until smooth.

Mochaccino

1/2 cup	chilled espresso or strong coffee	125 mL
1/3 cup	half-and-half (10%) cream or evaporated milk	75 mL
3	chocolate-covered coffee beans	3
1 tbsp	unsweetened cocoa powder or carob powder	15 mL
1/8 tsp	ground cinnamon	0.5 mL
6	frozen skim milk cubes, divided and crushed, if necessary (see pages 273 and 274)	6

In blender, combine espresso, cream, coffee beans, cocoa powder, cinnamon and 3 skim milk cubes. Process as directed on page 274 until smooth. Serve immediately with a spoon.

SERVES 1

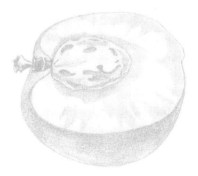

Mocha Mint

1/2 cup	chilled espresso or very strong coffee	125 mL
1/4 cup	evaporated partly skimmed milk	50 mL
1 tbsp	chopped fresh peppermint leaves	15 mL
1 tbsp	unsweetened cocoa powder or carob powder	15 mL
1 tbsp	liquid honey (or to taste)	15 mL
1/8 tsp	ground cinnamon	0.5 mL
6	frozen chocolate milk cubes, divided and crushed, if necessary (see pages 273 and 274)	6

In blender, combine espresso, evaporated milk, peppermint, cocoa powder, honey, cinnamon and 3 chocolate milk cubes. Process as directed on page 274 until smooth. Serve immediately with a spoon.

SERVES 1

Orange Lavender Ice

1/2 cup	frozen orange juice concentrate	125 mL
1	orange, peeled, seeded and chopped	1
1 tsp	chopped fresh lavender leaves and/or flowers	5 mL
1 tsp	balsamic vinegar	5 mL
6	ice cubes, divided and crushed, if necessary (see page 274)	6

In blender, combine orange juice concentrate, chopped orange, lavender, vinegar and 3 ice cubes. Process as directed on page 274 until smooth. Serve immediately with a spoon.

SERVES 1

Papaya Citrus Lassi

1/2 cup	orange juice	125 mL
3 tbsp	lemon juice	45 mL
2 cups	lemon sorbet	500 mL
Half	papaya, peeled, seeded and chopped	Half
6	frozen yogurt cubes, divided and crushed, if necessary (see pages 273 and 274)	6

In blender, combine orange juice, lemon juice, sorbet, papaya and 3 yogurt cubes. Process as directed on page 274 until smooth.

SERVES 2

Peach Granita

1 cup	cranberry juice	250 mL
4	ice cubes	4
1 cup	frozen sliced peaches	250 mL

In blender, combine cranberry juice, ice cubes and peaches. Process as directed until smooth. Serve immediately with a spoon.

SERVES 1

Pineapple Daiquiri

1/3 cup	frozen pineapple juice concentrate	75 mL
2	wedges pineapple, peeled and chopped	2
2 tbsp	lemon juice	25 mL
4	ice cubes	4

In blender, combine pineapple juice concentrate, chopped pineapple, lemon juice and ice cubes. Process as directed until smooth. Serve immediately with a spoon.

SERVES 1

TIP
Double the amount
of ice if you want
a thicker drink.

Pink Lemonade

½ cup	orange or cranberry juice	125 mL
½ cup	lemon juice	125 mL
6	ice cubes, divided and crushed, if necessary (see page 274)	6
2 cups	chopped seeded peeled watermelon, divided	500 mL
2 tsp	chopped candied ginger (optional)	10 mL
1 tbsp	liquid honey (or to taste)	15 mL

1. In blender, combine orange juice, lemon juice, 3 ice cubes, 1 cup (250 mL) watermelon, and ginger (if using). Cover with lid and blend on Low for 1 minute.

2. Stop blender. Add remaining watermelon and ice. Replace lid and process as directed until smooth. Sweeten with honey.

SERVES 4

Raspberry Flip

⅔ cup	raspberry juice	150 mL
2 tbsp	lemon juice	25 mL
1 cup	frozen raspberries	250 mL
2 tbsp	sugar (or to taste)	25 mL
6	ice cubes, divide and crushed, if necessary (see page 274)	6

In blender, combine raspberry juice, lemon juice, raspberries, sugar and 3 ice cubes. Process as directed on page 274 until smooth. Serve immediately with a spoon.

SERVES 1

Strawberry Daiquiri

1/3 cup	frozen lemonade or limeade concentrate	75 mL
6	strawberries (hulled and halved if fresh)	6
4	ice cubes	4

In blender, combine lemonade concentrate, strawberries and ice. Process as directed until smooth. Serve immediately with a spoon.

SERVES 1

Triple Chocolate Snowstorm

1 cup	chocolate milk	250 mL
1 tbsp	unsweetened cocoa powder or carob powder	15 mL
1 tbsp	liquid honey	15 mL
1 cup	chocolate frozen yogurt or ice cream (see recipes on pages 291 and 292)	250 mL

In blender, combine chocolate milk, cocoa powder, honey and frozen yogurt. Process as directed until smooth. Serve immediately with a spoon.

SERVES 1 OR 2

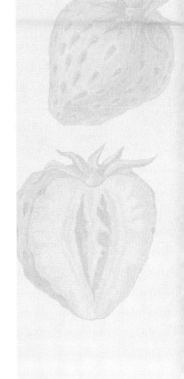

General Directions
Always place the lid securely on the blender before processing. If the recipe contains more then five ice cubes, follow the instructions on page 274, according to whether you have an Ice Crush setting. If the recipe does not contain more than five ice cubes, blend on Low for 30 seconds. Gradually (if possible) increase speed to High and blend for an additional 30 seconds or until smooth.

Blender Ice Cream, Frozen Yogurt and Sorbet

General Directions

Always place the lid securely on the blender before processing. If the recipe contains more than five ice cubes, follow the instructions on page 274, according to whether you have an Ice Crush setting. If the recipe does not contain more than five ice cubes, blend on Low for 30 seconds. Gradually (if possible) increase speed to High and blend for an additional 30 seconds or until smooth.

Almond Banana Ice Cream

$3/4$ cup	Almond Milk (recipe, page 248) or milk	175 mL
2 tbsp	granulated sugar	25 mL
1	frozen ripe banana, peeled and chopped	1
$1/2$ tsp	almond extract	2 mL
8 to 10	frozen skim milk cubes, divided and crushed, if necessary (see pages 273 and 274)	8 to 10

In blender, combine almond milk, sugar, banana, almond extract and skim milk cubes. Process as directed on page 274 until smooth. Use immediately or pour into a metal loaf pan and freeze for up to 2 hours.

SERVES 2

Chocolate Ice Cream

1/2 cup	Date Milk (recipe, page 247) or chocolate milk	125 mL
2 tbsp	granulated sugar	25 mL
2 tbsp	unsweetened cocoa powder or carob powder	25 mL
12	frozen skim milk cubes, divided and crushed, if necessary (see pages 273 and 274)	12

In blender, combine date milk, sugar, cocoa powder and 6 skim milk cubes. Process as directed on page 274 until smooth. Use immediately or pour into a metal loaf pan and freeze for up to 2 hours.

SERVES 1 OR 2

Coffee Ice Cream

1/2 cup	Coconut Carob Milk (recipe, page 250)	125 mL
2 tbsp	granulated sugar	25 mL
6	frozen espresso cubes, divided and crushed, if necessary (see pages 273 and 274)	6
3	frozen chocolate milk cubes (see page 273)	3

In blender, combine coconut carob milk, sugar, and espresso and chocolate milk cubes. Process as directed on page 274 until smooth. Use immediately or pour into a metal loaf pan and freeze for up to 2 hours.

SERVES 1

Strawberry Ice Cream

3/4 cup	Apricot Milk (recipe, page 247) or evaporated milk	175 mL
6	frozen strawberries	6
2 tbsp	sugar (or to taste)	25 mL
6	frozen milk cubes , divided and crushed, if necessary (see pages 273 and 274)	6

In blender, combine apricot milk, strawberries, sugar and 3 milk cubes. Process as directed on page 274 until smooth. Use immediately or pour into a metal loaf pan and freeze for up to 2 hours.

SERVES 2

Vanilla Ice Cream

¾ cup	evaporated partly skimmed milk	175 mL
3 tbsp	granulated sugar	45 mL
½ tsp	vanilla	2 mL
10	frozen skim milk cubes, divided and crushed, if necessary (see pages 273 and 274)	10

In blender, combine evaporated milk, sugar, vanilla and 6 skim milk cubes. Process as directed on page 274 until smooth. Use immediately or pour into a metal loaf pan and freeze for up to 2 hours.

SERVES 2

Chocolate Frozen Yogurt

½ cup	plain yogurt	125 mL
1 tbsp	unsweetened cocoa powder or carob powder	15 mL
2 tbsp	sugar (or to taste)	25 mL
12	frozen chocolate milk cubes, divided and crushed, if necessary (see pages 273 and 274)	12

In blender, combine yogurt, cocoa powder, sugar and 6 chocolate milk cubes. Process as directed on page 274 until smooth. Use immediately or pour into a metal loaf pan and freeze for up to 2 hours.

SERVES 1 OR 2

Fruit Yogurt Slush

¾ cup	plain yogurt	175 mL
¼ cup	evaporated partly skimmed milk	50 mL
12	frozen strawberries	12
2 tbsp	sugar (or to taste)	25 mL
6	frozen skim milk cubes, divided and crushed, if necessary (see pages 273 and 274)	6

In blender, combine yogurt, evaporated milk, strawberries, sugar and skim milk cubes. Process as directed on page 274 until smooth. Use immediately or pour into a metal loaf pan and freeze for up to 2 hours.

SERVES 2

TIP
Use frozen peaches, mangoes, apricots, cherries, raspberries, blueberries or other sweet berries instead of strawberries in this slush. For a change, try it without sugar — it's tart but tasty.

Citrus Sorbet

1	lemon	1
¼ cup	orange juice	50 mL
⅓ cup	sugar (or to taste)	75 mL
12	ice cubes, divided and crushed, if necessary (see page 274)	12

1. Grate 1 tsp (5 mL) zest from lemon. Peel and seed lemon; chop lemon pulp.
2. In blender, combine lemon zest and pulp, orange juice, sugar and 6 ice cubes. Process as directed on page 274 until smooth. Spoon into chilled glasses or cups.

SERVES 2

TIP
You can substitute a lime or an orange for the lemon. Or use the juice of one fruit in place of the whole fruit if desired.

Endnotes

Glossary

Adaptogen: A substance that builds resistance to stress by balancing the functions of the glands and immune response, thus strengthening the immune system, nervous system and glandular system. Adaptogens promote overall vitality. *Examples: Astragalus and ginseng.*

Allylic sulfides: See Organosulfides, page 300.

Alterative: A substance that gradually changes a condition by restoring health.

Amino acid: See Protein, page 300.

Analgesic: A substance that relieves pain by acting as a nervine, antiseptic or counterirritant. *Examples: German chamomile, meadowsweet and nutmeg.*

Anodyne: A substance that relieves pain. *Example: Clove.*

Anthocyanins: See Phenolic compounds, page 300.

Antibiotic: Meaning "against life," an antibiotic is a substance that kills infectious agents, including bacteria and fungi, without endangering health. *Examples: Garlic, green tea, lavender, sage and thyme.*

Anticatarrhal: A substance that reduces the production of mucus. *Examples: Garlic and marshmallow.*

Anti-inflammatory: A substance that controls or reduces swelling, redness, pain and heat, which are normal bodily reactions to injury or infection. *Examples: German chamomile and St. John's wort.*

Antimicrobial: A substance that destroys or inhibits the growth of disease-causing bacteria or other microorganisms.

Antioxidant: A compound that protects cells by preventing polyunsaturated fatty acids (PUFAs) in cell membranes from oxidizing, or breaking down. Antioxidants do this by neutralizing free radicals (see Free radical, page 299). Vitamins C and E and beta-carotene are antioxidant nutrients, and foods high in them have antioxidant properties. *Examples: Alfalfa, beet greens, dandelion leaf, parsley, garlic, thyme and watercress.*

Antipyretic: A substance that reduces fever. *Examples: German chamomile, sage and yarrow.*

Antiseptic: A substance used to prevent or reduce the growth of disease germs in order to prevent infection. *Examples: Cabbage, calendula, clove, garlic, German chamomile, honey, nutmeg, onions, parsley, peppermint, rosemary, salt, thyme, turmeric and vinegar.*

Antispasmodic: A substance that relieves muscle spasms or cramps, including colic. *Examples: German chamomile, ginger, licorice and peppermint.*

Astringent: A drying and contracting substance that reduces secretions from the skin. *Examples: Cinnamon, lemons, sage and thyme.*

Beta-carotene: The natural coloring agent (carotenoid) that gives fruits and vegetables (such as carrots) their deep orange color. It converts in the body to vitamin A. Eating foods high in beta-carotene helps prevent cancer, lowers your risk of heart disease, increases immunity, lowers your risk of cataracts and improves mental function. You can get beta-carotene in squash, carrots, yams, sweet potatoes, pumpkins and red peppers.

Betaine: A phytochemical that nourishes and strengthens the liver and gallbladder. It is found in high concentrations in beets.

Boron: A trace mineral that boosts the estrogen level in the blood, boron is also thought to help prevent calcium loss that leads to osteoporosis and to affect the brain's electrical activity. It is found in legumes, leafy greens and nuts.

Carbohydrates: An important group of plant foods that are composed of carbon, hydrogen and oxygen. A carbohydrate can be a single simple sugar or a combination of simple sugars. The chief sources of carbohydrates in a whole-food diet are grains, vegetables and fruits. Other sources include sugars, natural sweeteners and syrups.

Carminative: A substance that relaxes the stomach muscles and is taken to relieve gas and gripe. *Examples: Clove, dill, fennel, garlic, ginger, parsley, peppermint, sage and thyme.*

Carotenoid: See Beta-carotene, page 296.

Catechins: See Phenolic compounds, page 300.

Cathartic: A substance that has a laxative effect. See also Purgative, page 300. *Examples: Dandelion, licorice and parsley.*

Cellulose: See Fiber, page 298.

Chlorophyll: Found only in plants, chlorophyll has a unique structure that allows it to enhance the body's ability to produce hemoglobin, which, in turn, enhances the delivery of oxygen to cells.

Choline: A phytochemical that researchers believe improves mental function, and is therefore helpful for people with Alzheimer's disease. Good sources of lecithin (which contains choline) are dandelion, fenugreek, ginkgo, sage and stinging nettle.

Cruciferous vegetables: The name given to the *Brassica* genus of vegetables, which includes broccoli, brussels sprouts, cabbage, cauliflower, collard greens, kale, bok choy, rutabagas, turnips and mustard greens. The plants in this family were named *Cruciferae* because their flower petals grow in a cross shape.

Decoction: A solution made by boiling the woody parts of plants (roots, seeds and bark) in water for 10 to 20 minutes.

Demulcent: A soothing substance taken internally to protect damaged tissue. *Examples: Barley, cucumbers, figs, honey, marshmallow and fenugreek.*

Diaphoretic: A substance that induces sweating. *Examples: Cayenne, German chamomile, cinnamon and ginger.*

Digestive: A substance that aids digestion.

Diuretic: A substance that increases the flow of urine. These are meant to be used in the short term only. *Examples: Cucumbers, burdock (root and leaf), dandelion (leaf and root), fennel seeds, lemons, linden, parsley and pumpkin seeds.*

Dysmenorrhea: Menstruation accompanied by cramping pains that may be incapacitating in their intensity.

Elixir: A tonic that invigorates or strengthens the body by stimulating or restoring health.

Ellagic acid: A natural plant phenol (see Phenolic compounds, page 300) thought to have powerful anticancer and antiaging properties. It is found in cherries, grapes, strawberries, and other red, orange or yellow fruits; nuts; seeds; garlic; and onions.

Emetic: A substance taken in large doses to induce vomiting to expel poisons. Small quantities of some emetics, such as salt, nutmeg and mustard, are used often in cooking with no ill effects.

Emmenagogue: A substance that promotes healthy menstruation. *Examples: Calendula and German chamomile.*

Enzymes: The elements found in food that act as the catalysts for chemical reactions within the body, allowing efficient digestion and absorption of food and enabling the metabolic processes that support tissue growth, give you high energy levels and promote good health. Enzymes are destroyed by heat, but using fruits and vegetables raw in smoothies leaves enzymes intact and readily absorbable.

Essential fatty acids (EFAs): Fat is an essential part of a healthy diet — about 20 fatty acids are used by the human body to maintain normal function. Fats are necessary to maintain healthy skin and hair, transport the fat-soluble vitamins (A, D, E and K) and signal the feeling of fullness after meals. The three fatty acids considered the most important, or essential, are omega-6 linoleic, omega-3 linolenic and gamma linolenic acids. Evidence suggests that increasing the proportion of these fatty acids in the diet may increase immunity and reduce the risks of heart disease, high blood pressure and arthritis. The best vegetable source of omega-3 EFAs in the diet is flax seeds. Other sources of EFAs are hemp (seeds and nuts), nuts, seeds, olives, avocados and oily fish.

Expectorant: A substance that relieves mucus congestion caused by colds and flu. *Examples: Elder, garlic, ginger, hyssop and thyme.*

Fiber: An indigestible carbohydrate. Fiber protects against intestinal problems and bowel disorders. The best sources are raw fruits and vegetables, seeds and whole grains.

Types of fiber include *pectin*, which reduces the risk of heart disease (by lowering cholesterol) and helps eliminate toxins. It is found mainly in fruits, such as apples, berries and citrus fruits; vegetables; and dried legumes. *Cellulose* prevents varicose veins, constipation and colitis and plays a role in deflecting colon cancer. Because cellulose is found in the outermost layers of fruits and vegetables, it is important to buy only organic produce and leave the peels on. The *hemicellulose* in fruits, vegetables and grains aids in weight loss, prevents constipation, lowers the risk of colon cancer and helps remove cancer-forming toxins from the intestinal tract. *Lignin*, a fiber known to lower cholesterol, prevent gallstone formation and help people with diabetes, is found only in fruits, vegetables and Brazil nuts.

When raw fresh whole fruits or vegetables are used in smoothies, the pulp, or fiber, is still present in the drink and provides all the health benefits listed above.

Flatulence: Release of gas in the stomach and intestine caused by poor digestion. See also Carminative, page 297.

Flavonoids: These phytochemicals (e.g., genistein and quercetin) are antioxidants that have been shown to inhibit cholesterol production. They are found in cruciferous vegetables (see Cruciferous vegetables, page 297), onions and garlic.

Food combining: A disciplined method of eating foods in a specific order or combination (see page 306). It is used as a short-term aid to solve digestive problems and, in simple terms, requires eating fruit alone and never with meals. At mealtime, protein foods are combined with nonstarchy vegetables (leafy greens, asparagus, broccoli, cabbage, celery, cucumbers, onions, peppers, sea herbs, tomatoes and zucchini) only. Grains are also eaten separately and are combined with nonstarchy vegetables. Health conditions that may benefit from food combining are food allergies and intolerances, indigestion, irritable bowel syndrome, flatulence, fatigue and peptic ulcer.

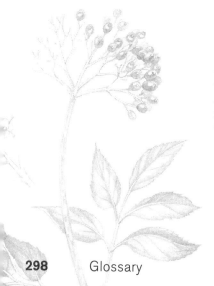

Free radical: A highly unstable compound that attacks cell membranes and causes cell breakdown, aging and a predisposition to some diseases. Free radicals come from the environment as a result of exposure to radiation, ultraviolet (UV) light, smoke, ozone and certain medications. Free radicals are also formed in the body by enzymes and during the conversion of food to energy. See also Antioxidant, page 296.

Glutamic acid: A naturally occurring substance that acts as a flavor enhancer. It is found in mushrooms and tomatoes.

Hemicellulose: See Fiber, page 298.

Hypotensive: A substance that lowers blood pressure. *Examples: Garlic, hawthorn, linden flower and yarrow.*

Indole: A phytochemical found in cruciferous vegetables (see Cruciferous vegetables, page 297) that may help prevent cancer by detoxifying carcinogens.

Isoflavone: A phytoestrogen, or the plant version of the human hormone estrogen, that is found in nuts, soybeans and legumes. Isoflavones help prevent several types of cancer — including pancreatic, colon, breast and prostate cancers — by preserving vitamin C in the body and acting as antioxidants.

Lactose intolerance: Deficiency of the enzyme lactase, which breaks down lactose, the sugar in both cow's and human milk. If you don't have sufficient lactase, milk sugar will ferment in the large intestine, causing bloating, diarrhea, abdominal pain and gas.

Laxative: A substance that stimulates bowel movements. Laxatives are meant to be used in the short term only. *Examples: Dandelion root, licorice root, prunes, rhubarb and yellow dock.*

Lignin: See Fiber, page 298.

Limonene: A type of limonoid (see Limonoid, below) thought to assist in detoxifying the liver and preventing cancer. It is found in lemons, limes, grapefruit and tangerines.

Limonoid: A subclass of terpenes (see Terpene, page 301) found in citrus fruit rinds.

Lutein: A carotenoid (see Carotenoid, page 297) found in beet greens; collard greens; mustard greens; and other red, orange and yellow vegetables.

Lycopene: An antioxidant carotenoid (see Beta-carotene, page 296) that's relatively rare in food. High levels are found, however, in tomatoes, pink grapefruit and watermelon. Lycopene is thought to reduce the effects of aging by maintaining physical and mental function and to reduce the risk of some forms of cancer.

Macrobiotic diet: Eating whole food that is seasonal and produced locally. Whole grains, vegetables, fruits (except tropical fruits), legumes, small amounts of fish or organic meat, sea herbs, nuts and seeds are appropriate foods for North Americans who eat macrobiotically.

Metabolism: The rate at which the body produces energy (or burns calories). It is measured by the amount of heat produced by the body, at rest or engaged in various activities, while maintaining its normal temperature.

Milk allergy: Many individuals, especially babies and young children, have allergic reactions to the protein in cow's milk, which causes wheezing, eczema, rashes, mucus buildup and asthma-like symptoms.

Mucilage: A thick, sticky, glue-like substance found in high concentrations in some herbs, which contains and helps spread the active ingredients of those herbs while soothing inflamed surfaces. *Examples: Marshmallow and slippery elm.*

Nervine: A substance that eases anxiety and stress and nourishes the nerves by strengthening nerve fibers. *Examples: German chamomile, lemon balm, oats, skullcap, St. John's wort, thyme and valerian.*

Nonreactive cooking utensils: The acids in foods can react with certain materials and promote the oxidation of some nutrients, as well as discolor the materials themselves. Nonreactive materials suitable for brewing teas are glass, enameled cast iron or enameled stainless steel. While cast-iron pans are recommended for cooking (a meal cooked in unglazed cast iron can provide 20% of the recommended daily intake of iron), and stainless steel is a nonreactive cooking material, neither is recommended for brewing or steeping teas.

Organosulfides: Compounds that have been shown to reduce blood pressure, lower cholesterol levels and reduce blood clotting. *Examples: Garlic and onions.*

Pectin: See Fiber, page 298.

Phenolic compounds: Found in red wine, phenolic compounds, including catechins, anthocyanins, ellagic acid and tannins, can prevent the oxidation of "bad" low-density lipoprotein (LDL) cholesterol, thus reducing the risk of heart disease.

Phytochemicals: Chemicals that come from plants. *Phyto*, from the Greek, means "to bring forth" and is used as a prefix to mean "from a plant."

Protein: The building block of body tissues. Protein is necessary for healthy growth, cell repair, reproduction and protection against infection. Protein consists of 22 parts called amino acids. Eight of the 22 amino acids in protein are especially important because they can not be manufactured by the body. Those eight are called essential amino acids.

A food that contains all eight essential amino acids is said to be a complete protein. Protein from animal products — meat, fish, poultry and dairy products — is complete. The only accepted plant sources of complete protein are soybeans and soy products, but research is establishing new theories that the protein content of legumes may be complete enough to replace animal protein.

A food that contains some, but not all, eight essential amino acids is called an incomplete protein. Nuts, seeds, legumes, cereals and grains are plant products that provide incomplete proteins. If your meals include foods from two complementary incomplete protein sources, your body will combine the incomplete proteins in the right proportions to make a complete protein. For example, many cultures have a tradition of using legumes and whole grains together in dishes. Scientifically, this combination provides a good amino-acid (complete protein) balance in the diet, because legumes are low in methionine but high in lysine, and whole grains are high in methionine but low in lysine. When eaten together, the body combines them to make complete proteins. Nuts and seeds must be paired with dairy or soy proteins in order to provide complete proteins.

Purgative: A substance that promotes bowel movements and increased intestinal peristalsis. *Example: Yellow dock.*

Quercetin: See Flavonoid, page 298.

Resveratrol: A fungicide that occurs naturally in grapes and has been linked to the prevention of clogged arteries by lowering blood cholesterol levels. Resveratrol is found in red wine and, to a lesser extent, in purple grape juice.

Rhizome: An underground stem that is usually thick and fleshy. *Examples: Ginger and turmeric.*

Rubefacient: A substance that, when applied to the skin, stimulates circulation in that area, bringing a good supply of blood to the skin and increasing heat in the tissue. *Examples: Cayenne; garlic; ginger; mustard seeds; and oils of rosemary, peppermint and thyme.*

Sedative: A substance that has a powerful quieting effect on the nervous system that relieves tension and induces sleep. *Examples: German chamomile, lettuce, linden, lavender and valerian.*

Stimulant: A substance that focuses the mind and increases activity. *Examples: Basil, cayenne, cinnamon, peppermint and rosemary.*

Tannin: A chemical constituent in herbs that causes astringency (see Astringent, page 296) and helps stanch internal bleeding. See also Phenolic compounds, page 300. *Examples: Coffee, tea and witch hazel.*

Terpene: A class of phytochemicals found in a wide variety of fruits, vegetables and herbs that are potent antioxidants. Ginkgo biloba is a good source of some terpenes. Limonoids (see Limonoid, page 299), which are found in citrus fruit rinds, are a subclass of terpenes.

Tincture: A liquid herbal extract made by soaking an herb in alcohol and pure water to extract the plant's active components. Some herbalists maintain that tinctures are the most effective way to take herbs, because they contain a wide range of the plant's chemical constituents and are easily absorbed.

Tisane: The "official" term used for a solution made by steeping fresh or dried herbs in boiling water. The term is interchangeable with the word *tea* when herbs are used.

Tonic: An infusion of herbs that tones or strengthens the system. Often tonics act as alteratives (see Alterative, page 296). Taken either hot or cold, tonics purify the blood and are nutritive. Tonic herbs support the body's systems in maintaining health. *Examples: Alfalfa, astragalus, dandelion (root and leaf) and ginseng.*

Vasodilator: A substance that relaxes blood vessels, increasing circulation to the arms, hands, legs, feet and brain. *Examples: Peppermint and sage.*

Volatile oil: Essential component found in the aerial parts of an herb. Often extracted to make essential oils, volatile oils are antiseptic and very effective at stimulating the body parts to which they are applied.

Wildcrafting: The practice of gathering herbs from the wild. Many plants today are endangered because of excessive wildcrafting. To avoid contributing to this problem, buy herbs that are organically cultivated.

Resources

Bibliography

Bartram, Thomas, *Bartram's Encyclopedia of Herbal Medicine* (Dorset, England: Grace Publishers, 1995), ISBN 0-9515984-1-4.

Brill, Steve, with Evelyn Dean, *Identifying and Harvesting Edible and Medicinal Plants* (New York: Hearst Books, 1994), ISBN 0-688-11425-3.

Carper, Jean, *Food: Your Miracle Medicine* (New York: HarperCollins Publishers, Inc., 1993), ISBN 0-06-018321-7.

Crocker, Pat, *The Healing Herbs Cookbook* (Toronto: Robert Rose, 1996), ISBN 0-7788-0004-0.

Crocker, Pat, and Susan Eagles, *The Juicing Bible* (Toronto: Robert Rose, 2000), ISBN 0-7788-0019-9.

Duke, James, Ph.D., *The Green Pharmacy* (Emmaus, PA: Rodale Press, 1997), ISBN 0-312-96648-2.

Foster, Stephen, and James A. Duke, *A Field Guide to Medicinal Plants* (New York: Houghton-Mifflin Company, 1990), ISBN 0-395-46722-5.

Gerras, Charles (editor), *Rodale's Basic Natural Foods Cookbook* (Emmaus, PA: Rodale Press, 1984), ISBN 0-87857-469-7.

Heatherley, Ana Nez, *Healing Plants: A Medicinal Guide to Native North American Plants and Herbs* (Toronto: HarperCollins Publishers, Inc., 1998), ISBN 0-00-638617-2.

Hoffman, David, *The New Holistic Herbal* (Rockport, MA: Element, Inc., 1992), ISBN 1-85230-193-7.

Lad, Vasant, *The Complete Book of Ayurvedic Home Remedies* (New York: Three Rivers Press, 1998), ISBN 0-609-80286-0.

McIntyre, Anne, *The Complete Woman's Herbal* (New York: Henry Holt and Company, 1995), ISBN 0-8050-3537-0.

Mortimer, Denise, *Nutritional Healing* (Boston: Element Books, Inc., 1998), ISBN 1-86204-176-8.

Murray, Michael, N.D., and Joseph Pizzorno, N.D., *Encyclopedia of Natural Medicine* (Rocklin, CA: Prima Publishing, 1991), ISBN 1-55958-091-7.

Pitchford, Paul, *Healing with Whole Foods: Oriental Traditions and Modern Nutrition* (Berkeley, CA: North Atlantic Books, 1993), ISBN 0-938190-64-4.

Turner, Lisa, *Meals that Heal* (Rochester, VT: Healing Arts Press, 1996), ISBN 0-89281-625-2.

Weed, Susun, *Healing Wise* (Woodstock, NY: Ash Tree Publishing, 1989), ISBN 0-9614620-2-7.

Werbach, Melvyn, M.D., *Nutritional Influences on Illness* (Tarzana, CA: Third Line Press, 1996), ISBN 0-9618550-5-3.

Herb and Organic Associations, Organizations and Agencies

Canadian Organic Growers (COG)
Box 6408, Station J
Ottawa, ON K2A 3Y6
Canada
Tel: (613) 231-9047
Web site: www.cog.ca
Canada's national information network for organic farmers, gardeners and consumers.

Herb Society of America (HSA)
9019 Chardon Road
Kirtland, OH 44094
USA
Tel: (440) 256-0514
Fax: (440) 256-0541
Web site: www.herbsociety.org
A well-organized group of herb enthusiasts, with many active local units.

International Herb Association (IHA)
910 Charles Street
Fredericksburg, VA 22401
USA
Tel: (540) 368-0590
Fax: (540) 370-0015
Web site: www.iherb.org
A professional organization of herb growers and business owners.

Organic Trade Association (OTA)
P.O. Box 547
Greenfield, MA 01302-0547
USA
Tel: (413) 774-7511
Fax: (413) 774-6432
Web site: www.ota.com
Promotes awareness and understanding of organic farming and provides a unified voice for the industry.

Herb Farms and Herb Mail-Order Sources

Frontier Natural Brands
3021 78th Street
P.O. Box 299
Norway, IA 52318 USA
Tel: (319) 227-7996
Fax: (319) 227-7966
Web site: www.frontiercoop.com
Supplier of bulk herbs.

Jekka's Herb Farm
Rose Cottage
Shellards Lane
Alveston, Bristol BS35 3SY
United Kingdom
Tel: (014) 54-418-878
Fax: (014) 54-411-988
Web site: www.jekkasherbfarm.com
Supplier of organic plants and seeds.

Laurel Farm Herbs
Main Road, Kelsale
Saxmundham, Suffolk
IP17 2RG
United Kingdom
Tel: (017) 28-668-223
Fax: (017) 28-668-468
Web site: www.theherbfarm.co.uk
Supplier who offers a wide range of herb plants for shipping.

Mountain Rose Herbs
85472 Dilley Lane
Eugene, OR 97405
USA
Tel: (800) 879-3337
Fax: (510) 217-4012
Web site: www.mountainroseherbs.com
Bulk organic herbs, oils, butters, clays and teas available for mail order.

Narnia Farms
R.R.# 2 S59C10
Smithers, BC V0J 2N0
Canada
Fax: (205) 847-3698
Web site: www.narniafarms.bc.ca
Organic seasonings, vinegars, mustard, honey, jellies and syrups.

Richters Herbs
357 Highway 47
Goodwood, ON L0C 1A0
Canada
Tel: (905) 640-6677
Fax: (905) 640-6641
Web site: www.richters.com
Herb specialist with over 800 varieties that has been selling herbs since 1969. Mail-order seeds, plants and books. Free color catalogue, seminars and herbal events.

Related Consumer Web Sites

www.OrganicConsumers.org
Activist organization with information and action strategies on organic foods, genetically modified foods, irradiation, mad cow disease and other issues.

www.ofrf.org
Organic Farming Research Foundation, which sponsors research related to organic-farming practices.

www.ewg.org
The United States–based Environmental Working Group, an activist organization around environmental issues.

www.ocia.org
Organic Crop Improvement Association, one of the international organic food certification bodies.

www.biodynamics.com
Information about biodynamic gardening and farming.

www.rodaleinstitute.org
In the mid-1900s, J.J. Rodale developed an emphasis on health and organic gardening through his publications and the Rodale Family Institute.

Appendix A

Food Allergies

CERTAIN FOODS CAN TRIGGER OR AGGRAVATE CONDITIONS SUCH AS asthma, chronic fatigue syndrome, depression, chronic digestive problems, eczema, headaches, hives, irritable bowel syndrome, migraines, rheumatoid arthritis and ulcerative colitis in adults, and ear infections and epilepsy in children.

Symptoms of food allergies and intolerances can include chronic infections or inflammations, diarrhea, fatigue, anxiety, depression, joint pain, skin rashes, dark circles or puffiness under the eyes, itchy nose or throat, water retention and swollen glands.

In the classic allergic reaction, a trigger (such as nuts) is mistakenly identified as an "enemy" by the immune system, which sets out to get rid of the offending toxin.

Food intolerances or sensitivities differ from "classic" allergies in that reactions do not happen immediately. As a result, allergy tests often cannot detect food intolerances. If you suspect that a food may be causing a chronic problem, the most effective method of identifying the culprit is to use an elimination diet.

Factors in food allergies include digestive system problems and lowered immune system function. While eliminating suspected foods from the diet, work to improve immunity (see Immune Deficiency, page 54) and digestion (see Indigestion, page 57). A key factor in digestion is liver function (see Liver Problems, page 65). Regular daily exercise and stress-reduction activities, such as meditation and yoga, improve immunity.

The most common foods that provoke chronic conditions are dairy products, wheat, corn, caffeine, yeast and citrus fruits. Other common food problems occur with processed and refined foods, artificial food additives and preservatives, eggs, strawberries, pork, tomatoes, peanuts and chocolate. In irritable bowel syndrome, potatoes and onions are also common triggers. Dairy products are the most common trigger for children's chronic ear infections.

Foods that are especially helpful in reducing allergic reactions are:
- antioxidant fruits and vegetables;
- yogurt with active bacterial cultures, which reestablish helpful digestive bacteria;
- flavonoids in the skins of fruits and vegetables;
- essential fatty acids in oily fish (herring, salmon, sardines, mackerel), fish oils, flax seeds and evening primrose oil, which are anti-inflammatory and reduce the severity of allergies; and
- foods that contain vitamin C (broccoli, lemon juice and rose-hip tea are sources that are unlikely to cause allergic reactions).

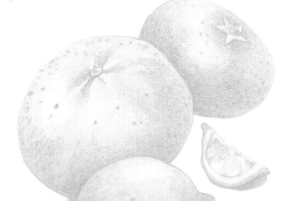

The Elimination Diet

Preparation

Before starting an elimination diet, consult with your health-care practitioner to eliminate the possibility of a serious disease causing your symptoms. If disease is not evident, ask for (and follow) your health-care practitioner's advice about trying the elimination diet.

Choosing Foods to Eliminate

Start by following the Guidelines to Good Health (see pages 10 and 11). This will eliminate refined and processed foods, which will improve immunity and digestion. Avoid artificial food additives and preservatives, which are common food allergens. If you regularly drink coffee or alcohol and are eliminating them, you may experience headaches. To avoid this side effect, cut down on them gradually.

You can choose to eliminate one food at a time or multiple foods. It is important that you consume a wide variety of different types of food in your diet. Choose to eliminate the most-common food allergens from the list on page 304. Do not add foods to which you have known allergies.

Steps in the Elimination Diet

1. Start a daily diet diary, noting all the foods you eat each day and the symptoms you experience.
2. Eliminate one food item from your diet for a period of one week. Start with a food that most commonly causes symptoms, especially one that you eat regularly. The food must be completely eliminated. If you are eliminating eggs, avoid cakes, salad dressings and any other foods that may contain eggs. If you are eliminating dairy products, check the ingredient lists of all foods for lactose, lactic acid and whey, which are all dairy. Margarine commonly contains these ingredients.
3. If you have fewer symptoms while eliminating the chosen food or foods, proceed to Step 4 to check each food you have eliminated. If there is no improvement in your symptoms, go back to the Guidelines to Good Health diet while you choose another food to eliminate.
4. Add the suspected food item back to your diet by eating two servings a day for the next three days. If you experience any symptoms, stop eating the food immediately and avoid it for six months while you work on improving your immunity, digestion and liver function.

Reintroducing Foods that Cause Adverse Reactions

After eliminating the food from your diet for six months, it often can be slowly reintroduced to the diet without adverse effects.

Appendix B

Food Combining

FOOD COMBINING IS A DISCIPLINED METHOD OF EATING FOODS IN A specific order or combination. It is used as a short-term aid to digestive problems and, in simple terms, requires eating protein foods, carbohydrate foods and fruits at different times, thus allowing for complete and efficient digestion of each food.

Protein foods — meat, poultry, fish, eggs, nuts, seeds, dairy products, soy products — require the most time and energy for the body to digest.

Carbohydrates are the starches and sugars found in foods that furnish most of the energy needed for the body's activities. Squash, legumes, grains (wheat, oats, rice, rye, etc.), pasta, beets, parsnips, carrots, sweet potatoes and pumpkin are starchy carbohydrate foods that break down faster than protein foods but not as quickly as fruits. Fruits are high-sugar carbohydrate foods that are digested very quickly and are thus considered separately in food combining.

Fruits require the least time and energy for the body to digest and should be eaten before a meal or at least two hours after a meal. When taken this way, fruit acts as a digestive cleanser, promoting digestive function. Fruit taken with a meal causes digestive problems. Melons and bananas should be eaten separately from other fruits.

The best food-combining meals are given below.

- Fruits alone — this is best taken as a variety of fruits at breakfast.
- Proteins with non-starchy vegetables (leafy greens, asparagus, broccoli, cabbage, celery, cucumber, onion, sweet peppers, sea herbs, tomatoes, zucchini).
- Grains with non-starchy vegetables.

Health conditions that may improve with food combining are food allergies and intolerances, indigestion, inflammatory bowel, flatulence, fatigue and peptic ulcer.

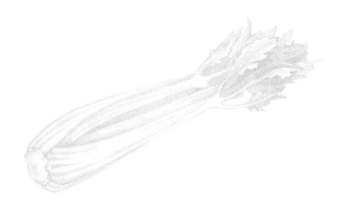

Eating Protein and Carbohydrate Foods in the Same Meal

PROTEIN FOODS NEED TO BE IN THE STOMACH FOR THREE TO FOUR HOURS. Protein requires an acid medium in which to be digested. Pepsin, the enzyme that begins the digestion of protein, is active only in an acid medium.

Starches (elements that break down into sugars) and sugars (honey, sugar and sugar products) pass through the stomach in 20 to 45 minutes and are digested in the small intestine. Starch requires an alkaline medium in which to be digested. The enzyme ptyalin (salivary amylase), which initiates starch breakdown, is active in an alkaline medium only and is destroyed by the hydrochloric acid that the stomach secretes.

When starches and proteins are eaten together, acidic gastric juices destroy the ptyalin and the salivary digestion of starch. Starches cannot pass through the stomach to the small intestine and are left to rot and ferment, causing gas and abdominal pain. The undigested starch in the stomach interferes with the breakdown and absorption of protein, leading to undigested protein in the stool and protein deficiency in the body.

The hydrochloric acid normally produced by a healthy system can neutralize the putrefactive process if it is present in significant amounts. For many people, especially those over age 35 and those with weak secretions, hydrochloric acid is not produced in sufficient amounts.

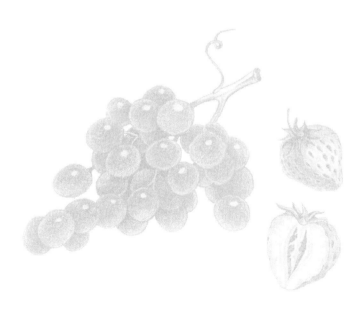

Appendix C

AVOID MEDICINAL DOSES OF ALL HERBS WHILE PREGNANT UNLESS YOU have full knowledge of the actions of the herb or recipe-specific advice from a midwife. Following are some of the most common herbs to avoid during pregnancy.

- Alder buckthorn *Rhamnus frangula*
- Aloe *Aloe vera* (use externally only)
- Angelica *Angelica archangelica*
- Arborvitae *Thuja occidentalis*
- Autumn crocus *Colchicum autumnale*
- Barberry *Berberis vulgaris*
- Bethroot *Trillium* (all species)
- Black cohosh *Cimicifuga racemosa* (except as advised by midwife)
- Blood root *Sanguinaria canadensis*
- Blue cohosh *Caulophyllum thalacthroides* (except as advised by midwife)
- Bogbean *Menyanthes trifoliata*
- Broom *Sarothamnus scoparius*
- Bryony *Bryonia dioica*
- Buchu *Barosma betulina*
- Calamus *Acorus calamus*
- Cascara sagrada *Rhamnus purshiana*
- Cayenne *Capsicum frutescens* (use sparingly)
- Celandine *Chelidonium majus*
- Coffee *Coffea arabia*
- Coltsfoot *Tussilago farfara*
- Comfrey *Symphytum officinale*
- Cotton root *Gossypium herbaceum*
- Dong quai *Angelica sinensis*
- Elecampane *Inula helenium*
- Essential oils (except floral oils, use sparingly)
- Fenugreek *Trigonella foenum-graecum*
- Feverfew *Tanacetum parthenium*
- Gentian *Gentiana lutea*
- Ginger *Zingiber officinale* (use sparingly)
- Ginkgo *Ginkgo biloba*
- Ginseng *Panax ginseng, Panax quinquefolius, Eleutherococcus senticosus*
- Goldenseal *Hydrastis canadensis*
- Hops *Humulus lupulus*
- Horehound *Marrubium vulgare*
- Horseradish *Amoracia lapathifolia*
- Hyssop *Hyssopus officinalis*
- Jamaican dogwood *Piscidia erythrina*
- Jimsonweed *Datura stramonium*
- Juniper *Juniperus communis*
- Licorice *Glycyrrhiza glabra*
- Lobelia *Lobelia inflata*
- Lomatium *Lomatium dissectum*
- Ma huang (Ephedra) *Ephedra sinensis*
- Male fern *Dryopteris felix-mas*
- Mandrake *Podophyllum peltatum*
- Mistletoe *Viscum album*
- Mugwort *Artemesia vulgare*
- Nutmeg *Myristica fragrans* (use sparingly)
- Oregon/Mountain grape *Mahonia aquifolium*
- Osha root *Ligusticum porterii*
- Parsley *Petroselinum crispum* (use sparingly)
- Pennyroyal *Mentha pulegium*
- Peruvian bark *Cinchona* (all species)
- Pleurisy root *Aesclepius tuberosa*
- Poke root *Phytolacca decandra*
- Poppy *Papaver somniferum*
- Purging buckthorn *Rhamnus cathartica*
- Rue *Ruta graveolens*
- Sage *Salvia officinalis*
- Saw palmetto *Seranoa serrulata*
- Senna *Cassia senna*
- Snake root *Polygala senega*
- Southernwood *Artemesia arboratum*
- Tansy *Tanacetum vulgare*
- Thuja *Thuja occidentalis*
- Thyme *Thymus vulgaris*
- Turkey rhubarb root *Rheum palmatum*
- Vervain *Verbena officinalis*
- Wild indigo *Baptisia tinctoria*
- Wormwood *Artemesia absinthum*
- Yarrow *Achillea millefolium*
- Yellow jasmine *Gelsemium sempervirens*
- Yellow dock *Rumex crispus*

National Library of Canada Cataloguing in Publication

Crocker, Pat
    The smoothies bible / Pat Crocker.

Includes index.
ISBN 0-7788-0063-6

1. Smoothies (Beverages) 2. Blenders (Cookery) I. Title.

TX840.B5C76 2003   641.8'75   C2002-905891-0

Index